Bedlam in the New World

Bedlam in the New World
A Mexican Madhouse in the Age of Enlightenment

Christina Ramos

The University of North Carolina Press CHAPEL HILL

© 2022 The University of North Carolina Press
All rights reserved
Set in Merope Basic by Westchester Publishing Services
Manufactured in the United States of America

The University of North Carolina Press has been a member of the Green Press Initiative since 2003.

Library of Congress Cataloging-in-Publication Data
Names: Ramos, Christina (Historian), author.
Title: Bedlam in the New World : a Mexican madhouse in the Age of Enlightenment / Christina Ramos.
Description: Chapel Hill : University of North Carolina Press, [2022] | Includes bibliographical references and index.
Identifiers: LCCN 2021041592 | ISBN 9781469666563 (cloth) | ISBN 9781469666570 (paperback) | ISBN 9781469666587 (ebook)
Subjects: LCSH: Hospital de San Hipólito (Mexico City, Mexico)—History. | Psychiatric hospitals—Mexico—Mexico City—History. | Psychiatry—Mexico—History. | Enlightenment—Mexico.
Classification: LCC RC451.M62 M697 2022 | DDC 362.2/1097253—dc23
LC record available at https://lccn.loc.gov/2021041592

Cover illustration: Detail of drawing by José "Tebanillo" Ventura Gonzalez, a patient at San Hipólito, ca. 1789. Courtesy Archivo General de la Nación, Mexico City, Mexico.

For my parents,
Antonio and Ruth Ramos,
and for
Skye Marie Garcia

Contents

Acknowledgments xi

Introduction 1
Casting Light from the Margins

CHAPTER ONE
Bedlam in the New World 23

CHAPTER TWO
An Enlightened Madhouse 48

CHAPTER THREE
It Is Easy to Mistake a Heretic for a Madman 80

CHAPTER FOUR
Medicalization and Its Discontents 114

CHAPTER FIVE
Crime and Punishment 143

Conclusion 175
A Defense of Bedlam

Appendix 183
Notes 193
Bibliography 219
Index 239

Figures and Tables

FIGURES

1.1 Bernardino Alvarez, founder of the Hospital de San Hipólito, 1762 26

1.2 Potential ground design of the Hospital de San Hipólito, ca. 1690s 41

2.1 Remodeled ground design of the Hospital de San Hipólito, ca. 1777 66

2.2 Nineteenth-century lithograph of Church and Hospital de San Hipólito 67

2.3 Representative patient register, 1752 71

3.1 Salacious sketch by José "Tebanillo" Ventura Gonzalez, ca. 1789 100

3.2 Salacious sketch by José "Tebanillo" Ventura Gonzalez, ca. 1789 101

3.3 Salacious sketch by José "Tebanillo" Ventura Gonzalez, ca. 1789 102

3.4 Salacious sketch by José "Tebanillo" Ventura Gonzalez, ca. 1789 103

3.5 Salacious sketch by José "Tebanillo" Ventura Gonzalez, ca. 1789 104

3.6 Salacious sketch by José "Tebanillo" Ventura Gonzalez, ca. 1789 105

5.1 Assault weapons used by María Getrudis Torres, 1806 160

TABLES

1.1 Patient population, Hospital de San Hipólito, 1697–1706 39

2.1 Records of admissions, discharges, and deaths, 1751–1785 72

2.2 Overview of San Hipólito's patients, 1751–1786 77

A.1 Monthly tally of the Indigenous patients at San Hipólito 183

A.2 San Hipólito's criminal inmates 185

Acknowledgments

This book began in the summer of 2009, when I first visited the archives in Mexico City to conduct research on hospitals in New Spain. I was inspired by Josefina Muriel's *Hospitales de la Nueva España* and saw in her two-volume compendium of hospital development a research agenda for my career. My focus quickly turned to the case of San Hipólito because I wanted to write a hospital history that was peopled with patients. As this book documents, San Hipólito's patients (some, at least) were not quiet; their social world, their pain and suffering, and particularly their encounters with the law were documented and preserved—albeit not without ample mediation—in the archives of the Inquisition and secular criminal courts. The ability to place San Hipólito into dialogue with other colonial institutions and the social and emotional lives of its patients set the foundations for my research. I later discovered the scholarship of María Cristina Sacristán, who has excavated Inquisition and criminal records for cases involving madness to reconstruct a multiplicity of colonial worldviews. I want to acknowledge at the outset that *Bedlam in the New World* would not exist in quite the same way as it does without the research, labor, and insights of these pioneering historians.

A number of institutions have extended generous resources that have made research and writing possible. I am endlessly grateful to the Ford Foundation for predoctoral and postdoctoral fellowships that supported me during critical phases of my career and for its powerful mission to enhance diversity in academia. At Washington University in St. Louis, the Center for the Humanities secured a semester of revising while providing intellectual camaraderie; the History Department also cheered me on while providing generous funding for indexing and the editing services of Peter Hohn, whom I warmly thank. Research for this book would not have been possible without a Mellon Fellowship, which facilitated a boot camp in Spanish paleography; I hold fond memories of that summer in Austin and the friendships that were forged. At Harvard University, I benefited from a Frederick Sheldon Traveling Fellowship; numerous grants and fellowships from the David Rockefeller Center for Latin American Studies; and an Erwin N. Hiebert Fellowship from the History of Science Department. Finally, a José Amor y

Vázquez Fellowship enabled research at the John Carter Brown Library and introduced me to a lovely cohort of early Americanists.

Deborah Harkness kindled my love of history and helped me visualize a career as a historian and professor—I cannot thank her enough. Deb always praised my abilities as a writer, so I will simply state that I am at a total loss for words in expressing my profound gratitude and admiration. At Harvard University, I feel deeply fortunate to have worked with Katharine Park. I thank Katy for her generous mentorship, rigor, and warmth; for her unwavering support during especially difficult times; and for her beautiful, commanding scholarship, which consistently sets the bar high—too high, it seems, at times.

My debts extend to the numerous friends and colleagues who have nurtured and sustained me throughout this journey. Martha Few offered early guidance for my research and continues to shine as an inspiration. Pete Sigal deserves much praise for guiding this project through its earliest iterations. At UC Davis, Margaret W. Ferguson, along with Deb, nurtured my early development as a scholar. At Duke, I learned important lessons in social history from Cynthia Herrup and Judith Bennet. At Harvard, Charles E. Rosenberg and David S. Jones endured early drafts and provided encouragement and incisive, thoughtful feedback, while the History of Science Department fostered stimulating intellectual community. I forged many friendships during my years living in the Cambridge-Boston area and continue to rely on the kindness and support of Raquel Kennon, Leandra Swanner, and Mariel Wolfson. At UC Merced, Susan Amussen and David Torres-Rouff helped me transition from graduate student to teacher. I also thank Whitney Pirtle for inviting me back to present my research at the Humanities Center and for introducing me to like-minded colleagues. It has been a true pleasure to see my home, the Central Valley, become a site of intellectual thriving. I owe a major debt to Elizabeth Mellyn for our overlapping interests and for providing a model for how to study madness when I desperately needed one; to Paola Bertucci and Mariselle Meléndez for their careful reading of drafts of this book's introduction; and to the two anonymous readers secured by UNC Press for their generous feedback, which has only made this book more robust. I also thank my editor, Elaine Maisner, and her wonderful production team for bringing this book to life.

At Washington University in St. Louis, the History Department has served as my academic home for the last five years, and I extend a heartfelt thanks to each of my colleagues. This book bears the imprint of Corinna Treitel's compassionate mentorship, and I cannot thank her enough for slugging through numerous drafts and for supporting me during especially challenging phases of writing. Peter Kastor offered invaluable advice at various stages in my early career and has served as a wonderful chair and mentor. Daniel Bornstein, Christine Johnson, and Alexandre Dubé shared their love of all things early modern and welcomed me into their intellectual cohort. I am indebted to Christine Johnson for reading through an early and unpolished draft of the manuscript, and to Kenneth Ludmerer for his helpful comments and encouragement on a tidier version. I have benefited tremendously from the collegiality of Nancy Reynolds, Anika Walke, Monique Bedasse, Douglas Flowe, Sowande' Muskateem, Andrea Friedman, Shefali Chandra, Diana J. Montaño, Lori Watt, and Sonia Lee, among many others. Across the university, I have found a vibrant intellectual community. I am grateful to Billy Acree, Stephanie Kirk, Ignacio Sánchez Prado, Mabel Moraña, Miguel Valerio, Ignacio Infante, Rene Esparza, Bahia Munem, Trevor Sangrey, Rebecca Wanzo, Rebecca Messbarger, Tilli Boon Cuillé, Luis Salas, Jean Allman, and Adrienne Davis. Rebecca Messbarger has been an enthusiastic supporter of this project, and her love for the eighteenth century is infectious. I thank her and Tilli for welcoming me to the Eighteenth-Century Salon and for helping me think through the Enlightenment. I also thank the members of the Early Modern Reading Group, the Eighteenth-Century Salon, and the Medical Humanities Reading Group for their intellectual community and sustenance.

I have shared many meals, drinks, and laughs with Miguel Valerio, AJ Neff, Bahia Munem, and Diana J. Montaño, and I thank them effusively for sustaining me through the final stages of writing. My academic *hermano*, Miguel Valerio, has been a wonderful friend and interlocutor. Many of these pages were nurtured by our daily walks during a frightening global pandemic in which we discussed topics ranging from politics to race to our shared love of colonial Mexico. May our friendship and competitive book hoarding continue, *amigo*. I am overwhelmed with gratitude for Diana Montaño, my treasured colleague and friend, who instantaneously treated me like family and provided Mexican cooking away from home. I thank the forces of the universe for placing us in the same department; life as junior faculty would not be the same without our daily doses of *chisme*, mutual respect, and admiration. Obadiah J. Miles arrived in my life as I was completing this book, provided the greatest of company, indulged my chattiness, and lovingly nudged me to the finish line.

I am overjoyed to acknowledge my family, both in Mexico and the United States, for their unsurpassed love and patience. My family in Mexico—most of them authentic *chilangos*—was enormously supportive during the research phase of this project, and I offer this book as a small token of repayment. In these pages, I hope they find the history they wanted to see written. While I never met tía Carmen, in relating this story, I hope to honor her memory and suffering, which haunts these pages. The physical distance separating me from my loved ones in California hurts sometimes, but I thank them for their unwavering support as I pursued my dreams and for selflessly rejoicing in my successes, large and small. I especially want to thank my aunt, Sandra Garcia, who has cared for me like a daughter, and honor my uncle, Henry Garcia, who lamentably did not live to witness me finish.

It is with a humble heart that I dedicate this book to my selfless parents, Ruth and Antonio Ramos. I hope this labor of love does small justice to the countless sacrifices they have made. My father's difficult journey from Mexico to the United States has imbued my intellectual enterprises with meaning; my mom has been my rock through everything and my most cherished friend. Finally, I dedicate this book to Skye as a gesture of appreciation for blessing me with her presence.

Bedlam in the New World

Introduction
Casting Light from the Margins

> We were seven days out at sea, and during that time, my head was brimming with a thousand delirious visions of my viceroyalty. Decrees, embroidered uniforms, Your Excellencies, gifts, submissiveness, banquets, fine china, parades, coaches, lackeys, liveries, and palaces were the puppets dancing without a rest in my mad brain and entertaining my foolish imagination. . . . That's how the new Quixote went off in his chivalrous madness, which increased so much from day to day and moment to moment that if God had not allowed the winds to shift, by now I would be taking office in a cage in San Hipólito.
> —JOSÉ JOAQUÍN FERNÁNDEZ DE LIZARDI,
>   *El periquillo sarniento*, 1816

In 1877, Dr. Sebastián Labastida, newly appointed director of Mexico City's oldest public institution for the insane, the Hospital de San Hipólito, meditated at length on the hospital's rich colonial heritage. At a moment when the institution had deteriorated into a national embarrassment—resembling, in Labastida's own words, little more than a "prison for violent madmen"—he looked nostalgically to the colonial era as a time when Mexico had pioneered the way in providing rational and humane treatment to those afflicted with mental illness.[1]

Founded by a penitent conquistador centuries earlier in 1567, San Hipólito holds a bold if unappreciated claim to being the first hospital for the mad in the Western Hemisphere. Its modest but precocious beginnings, Labastida argued, had set Mexico, then a colony of Spain, apart from many "civilized countries" in Europe, which not only lacked comparable facilities but were mired in backward notions of madness as having divine or demonic origins. While in New Spain colonial charity fueled an institution that nourished, clothed, and medically treated an unfortunate body of individuals who were unable to care for themselves, in many parts of the world the mad were treated with the utmost callousness and ignorance, "subjected to exorcisms and torture, burnt alive, oppressed by chains, [and] encaged like ferocious

1

beasts." At best, these poor and miserable creatures were "relegated to the darkest, dankest, and most insalubrious dungeons of convents and prisons" or, just as unfortunate, were abandoned and left to roam helplessly through the streets, "the objects of terror, contempt, and ridicule."[2]

Labastida's lecture continued. It was not until the eighteenth century, he opined, that conditions in Europe improved dramatically, guided in no small part by the currents of Enlightenment thinking. In England, London's St. Luke's Hospital and the York Retreat represented formidable efforts to provide institutional and medical care to the mentally ill. Meanwhile, in France, as the revolution raged and the Old Regime collapsed, the "sage Pinel" enjoyed the "glory of devising the most useful and humane measures of treatment." While these achievements were undeniably commendable, Labastida reiterated that in Mexico, similar practices, ideas, and institutions regarding madness and its management had existed for centuries.[3]

Recent historians, widely disinclined to take golden age narratives at face value, will take issue with Labastida's account of Mexican psychiatry's colonial origins. This skepticism is not unwarranted. Although he alerted his audience to Mexico's stunningly early participation in the provisioning of institutional care to the mentally disturbed, Labastida's message disclosed more about the late nineteenth century than its colonial precursor. At the time he was writing, Mexico's incipient psychiatric profession and the hospital itself were at a critical crossroads. The decades of civil strife and foreign invasions that followed the Mexican War of Independence had taken their toll on the capital's once vibrant welfare institutions. Meanwhile, Porfirio Díaz, who had only a year earlier usurped the presidency, was about to inaugurate, under the dictum of "order and progress," a period of unprecedented stability and industrial growth.[4] In the decades that followed, Mexico would embark on a concerted campaign to shed itself of its colonial past in the dogged pursuit of modernization. In the realm of psychiatry, a small but budding profession had already begun to adopt the latest trends emanating from Europe in a bid for scientific legitimacy and expertise.[5] State recognition of the profession's growing authority would culminate in the establishment of the nation's first psychiatric facility, La Castañeda, an institution that would ultimately eclipse San Hipólito, a remnant of a bygone era when Spanish colonialism and Christian charity combined to propel a tradition in which the mentally disturbed and impoverished were offered free shelter and medical care. Thus, evidently worried that a new generation of psychiatrists, in their fixation with European models and theories, would ignore Mexico's distinctive national character and traditions, Labastida reminded his contemporaries that in matters pertaining to the institutional care of the mad, Mexico had not always lagged behind.[6]

Labastida had erred on numerous fronts. The New World's first mental hospital was not a beacon of a glorious era in mental health care, to employ modern terminology; its history cannot be reduced to facile claims of premodern mental hospitals and their practices as being either humane or barbaric. While it certainly was the first of its kind to appear in the Americas—no minor accomplishment—it drew inspiration from hospitals in Iberia and coexisted with similar institutions located throughout Europe. Like mental hospitals in both the Old World and the New, San Hipólito reflected growing acknowledgment that madness was a social problem—intimately connected to the perils of poverty, or the threat of violent harm—as well as a physical condition, and that charitable institutions could offer limited relief. Yet its centuries of operation in what was once the viceregal capital of New Spain, as colonial Mexico was then called, coupled with its long-standing neglect in an otherwise vast and robust scholarship on madness and its institutions, merits deeper scrutiny.[7] And here Labastida was onto something: in insisting that San Hipólito presaged developments across the Atlantic, he inadvertently articulated what would ultimately become the origin story of psychiatry and Mexico's erasure from that narrative.

This book interrogates psychiatry's overlooked colonial legacy to provide the first in-depth account of the Hospital de San Hipólito and the patients who occupied its wards. It argues that attention to the Spanish colonial experience calls into question enduring assumptions about medicalization, confinement and its uses, and the role of colonialism and the Enlightenment in these processes and practices. While San Hipólito enjoyed remarkable longevity—its life span encompassing 1567 to 1910—the pages that follow draw attention to the late eighteenth century as a pivotal moment in which the hospital gained prominence among secular and ecclesiastical authorities as an institutional strategy for managing disordered mental states. This book uncouples confinement from the mechanisms of state centralization and social control that have traditionally informed how madness gets narrated. Instead, it proposes that the hospital offers a window into a contested, uneven, and imperfect history of medicalization that not only entangled a wide array of actors but featured religious personnel, including inquisitors, at the pioneering forefront. Treating the hospital as both a microcosm and a laboratory of the world beyond its walls, *Bedlam in the New World* positions the Spanish colonial experiment as integral to histories of madness, medicine, the Enlightenment, and modernity.

Lamenting the miserable state of nineteenth-century Mexican psychiatry, Labastida nearly foretold the extent to which colonial Mexico's contribution would go ignored. The history of psychiatry's birth has often been told as geographically seated in Europe—France and England especially—with the Enlightenment as a critical turning point. Indeed, the oft-repeated and potentially dubious account of Philippe Pinel's unchaining of the mad at the Bicêtre and Salpêtrière hospitals in Paris has taken on almost mythical status, symbolizing a heroic gesture of liberation that ushered in an era of rational psychiatry—or its polar opposite: the moment at which society began to exert if no longer physical force than medical and moral control over those deemed marginal and deviant.[8] In England and the continental United States, accounts of the rise of the asylum system often begin with reformers like the Tukes, who, along with Pinel, introduced the so-called moral treatment within institutions of confinement; here, too, such events have often been interpreted in light of positivist or declensionist polemics.[9]

Of course origin stories, by their very nature, are problematic, often overlooking meaningful continuities shaping the transition to modernity as well as unexpected actors. But even histories of early modern mental hospitals, which are few and far between, are haunted by the specter of "Bedlam," the corrupted name for London's Bethlem hospital, whose reputation as one of the earliest madhouses was immortalized by the notable likes of Shakespeare and Hogarth. While the history of Bedlam has been richly documented, its caricature as a site where marginality and mayhem commingled—the world gone topsy-turvy—remains more widely accepted, fueling distortions of the institutions that confined the mad before the dawning of psychiatry and the age of the asylum.[10] As one scholar succinctly put it, "Historians of psychiatry actually do not want to know about Bethlem as a historical fact because Bethlem as a reach-me-down historical cliché is far more useful."[11] To date, they have likewise not wanted to know about San Hipólito, the first mental hospital of the New World, quite possibly because traditional narratives of psychiatry's history have made its mere existence unfathomable.

But the archive and historical precedent alike reveal that San Hipólito's sixteenth-century appearance in the capital of New Spain was fathomable indeed. One need only reference Cervantes's *Don Quixote* or Lope de Vega's *Los locos de Valencia* to know that early modern Spaniards were keenly interested in states of unreason, or what they called *locura*. While such texts circulated among elite audiences or were performed on stage, hospitals for the mad sheltered and cared for the most extreme cases: mad paupers (*pobres dementes*), who lacked family and livelihood, and the raving insane (*locos furio-*

sos), whose violent outbreaks posed a danger to themselves and society. Such institutions designed exclusively for the care and custody of the mentally incapacitated first appeared in the Spanish kingdoms in the fourteenth century, owing in part to the influence of Islamic precedents in that multiethnic region, and multiplied in the centuries that followed. When the Spanish colonized the New World, unlike the Dutch or Portuguese they sought to re-create in their colonies a society that mirrored their own, modeled on Iberian ideas, practices, and institutions. Just as they erected churches and convents, so too they built hospitals as part of a larger campaign to reproduce Iberian culture, spread Catholicism, and secure hegemony. Of course, the world they ultimately resurrected only partially resembled that of Spain, as wholesale social and cultural transplantation was never possible. This was true even for the viceroyalty of New Spain, crown jewel of the Spanish Empire, and Mexico City, its cosmopolitan and administrative center. New Spain's environment; its multiracial inhabitants; and the social, political, and material conditions of coloniality, among other factors, produced an intricate world that fundamentally differed from its Iberian counterpart. Life in the New World was Spanish inspired but not wholly Spanish.

San Hipólito was both an outcome and a microcosm of this process. Established a half century after the fall of Tenochtitlán adjacent to the Church of San Hipólito, which commemorated Spanish triumph over the Mexica (Aztecs), it appeared alongside a diverse range of hospitals founded to address the material, medical, and spiritual needs of the colony's multiracial inhabitants. While it originally opened its doors as a convalescent hospital, from its inception it expressed a unique commitment to sheltering *pobres dementes*, and it gradually came to concentrate on this marginal and vulnerable group exclusively. As such, it participated in and upheld a nascent colonial health-care system rooted in the Christian ideal of charity (*caridad*) by taking in a class of chronic patients who could neither be housed nor treated in general hospitals. In so doing, it not only functioned to keep mad paupers off the streets of the capital and neighboring areas but helped to legitimize the colonial enterprise that cast the king as the bountiful and benevolent distributor of charity, medical services included. At least initially it appears to have received both men and women, but by the seventeenth century, the institution solely confined a male population. While patients of all races and ethnicities occupied its facilities, the largest constituency were American-born criollos, or Creoles, thus indicating the hospital's role in buttressing a colonial socio-racial order that favored citizens of Spanish ancestry as most "deserving" of charitable assistance. It came to operate, moreover, alongside a handful of smaller establishments with a similar dedication to managing states of *locura* concentrated in the central valley of what is now modern-day Mexico: San Roque in the city of Puebla de los Ángeles, and both the Hospital de San Pedro, which exclusively admitted retired priests suffering from age-related dementia, and the Hospital del Divino Salvador, founded in the late seventeenth century for poor mad women (*pobres mujeres dementes*), in Mexico City. San Hipólito was thus no historical aberration. Its history is intimately connected to an overlooked Iberian tradition of providing charitable succor to the mad and its subsequent transfer to the Americas as an integral part of Spanish colonization.

While all colonial hospitals preserved core features of their Spanish antecedents, they assimilated aspects of their surrounding context and embarked on distinct historical trajectories. In New Spain, for instance, long marked by a dearth of university-trained practitioners, the role of the regular clergy in hospital care was accentuated. This was especially the case for madness, a condition that had long posed challenges to curability and whose symptoms were just as receptive to spiritual counseling as medical intervention. *Bedlam in the New World* examines how medicalization unfolded within a Spanish American colonial setting, documenting the centrality of religious authorities, institutions, and personnel to this process. I argue that it was in the late eighteenth century, a time of imperial realignment and pretenses to modernization, when madness became understood in increasingly medical terms, with San Hipólito serving as a site of care, confinement, and knowledge production that, taken together, shed light on overlooked aspects of the Hispanic Enlightenment, particularly its religious incarnations. What follows is a history of madness that not only decenters Europe but decenters physicians, who were but peripheral protagonists in generating new notions about how madness was to be understood, institutionally managed, and potentially cured.

The history that unfolds in the following pages may have parallels to developments in Europe—particularly southern Europe, where the regular clergy constituted a forceful presence in hospital care. To date, however, these patterns have remained largely invisible to historians, partly because prevailing historiographies have pitted religion against the Enlightenment, privileged the writings and activities of doctors, or focused on dismantling Foucault's misleading if enduring "great confinement" narrative.[12] An emerging scholarship on medicine in colonial Latin America has remained largely impervious to these trends.[13] Unencumbered by historiographies that have thwarted meaningful conversations about the social histories of the institutions that confined and cared for the mad—their daily functioning rather than hyperbolic representation—colonial Mexico provides an ideal setting to explore alternative histories of madness and medicine in the Age of Enlightenment.

A Mexican Madhouse in the Age of Enlightenment

Between 1793 and 1794, while recovering from an undisclosed illness, Francisco de Goya painted a scene of an enclosed courtyard in a madhouse, which he linked to a spectacle he witnessed at the Zaragoza hospital.[14] One of two paintings in which the Spanish artist dealt explicitly with the subject of mental hospitals and their theatrics, *Yard with Lunatics* depicts two naked madmen engaged in a physical struggle while their warden, visibly bewildered, attempts in vain to subdue the violence by beating them with a limp switch. A haunting cast of characters—the hospital's other inmates, some clothed in sacks, others seminude—surround the scene's central image, their visages and bodily gestures eerily conveying madness's delusional, all-consuming grip. It is more than likely that the impressionable scene reflected Goya's own conjuring rather than an authentic illustration of events at Zaragoza, an institution that Pinel himself effusively praised for its innovative therapeutic techniques.[15] Perhaps the mayhem of the madhouse was intended to mirror the social and political upheaval of revolutionary Spain and its collapsing empire, or the artist's own inner afflictions and physical distress. Perhaps, as Foucault insisted, Goya was trying to convey that unreason and its confinement represented the dark underbelly of the Age of Enlightenment.

As evocative now as it was then, Goya's painting is yet one more example of how the late eighteenth century represented madness—an incurable affliction that left a person not much more than an imbecile or a brute. The exasperated expression of the warden telegraphs the futility of his efforts, while the dark, thick walls of the courtyard signify the need for removal. Yet like the caricatures of Bedlam, Goya's sensationalized image did not reflect historical reality, certainly not within the walls of San Hipólito. Although it housed a marginal population in what was ostensibly a marginal part of the world, San Hipólito was embedded—materially, socially, intellectually—in larger historical processes and developments that have often been considered in isolation from one another. Its brick-and-mortar edifice weathered the tide of different colonial regimes and their shifting policies, from the paternalistic ethos of the Habsburgs to the reformist, centralizing agenda of the Bourbon monarchy and its agents. Its coffers, often in straits, speak to a broader history of medical charity in New Spain, of its promises and pitfalls, waxes and wanes. Its nurses, members of the Order of San Hipólito, recall a long tradition, however imperfect, in which the regular clergy assumed primary responsibility for the institutional care of the mad and penniless, delivering both spiritual and secular medicine. The Inquisition and secular criminal courts haunted the hospital's corridors, shipping allegedly mad criminals to its premises for medical treatment and custodial surveillance. Cases from their archives capture the experiences of some of the hospital's most troubled and troublesome patients and the unique set of circumstances under which they fell afoul of colonial authorities, were judged to be mad, and involuntarily confined. They too offer a window into the inner machinations of colonial power when confronted with crime and marginality, and point to wider medical and legal changes unfolding during the late colonial period.

Bedlam in the New World argues that San Hipólito served as both a microcosm and a colonial laboratory of the Hispanic Enlightenment.[16] From its inception, the hospital performed a prominent if limited role in Spanish efforts to secure legitimacy and hegemony in the Americas, reproducing the colonial world in which it was firmly entrenched. However, it was in the late eighteenth century that the Enlightenment ideals of order, utility, rationalism, and the public good fueled renewed attention to states of unreason in the Spanish colonies and came to impinge on the institutional management of *locura*. These changes expressed themselves in a variety of ways—most conspicuously in the hospital's modernized and amplified facilities, most provocatively in its swelling and diversifying patient population, which at the time included a growing body of suspects from the Inquisition and the secular criminal courts charged with an array of crimes, ranging from murder to blasphemy.

This book asks what such changes reveal about colonial Mexico's *Ilustración* (Enlightenment), resurrecting, rather intentionally, the ghost of Foucault. It does so, however, less for Foucault's controversial and flawed claim for a state-driven "great confinement" of the mad, idle, and deviant than for his more stimulating premise that "reason" and "unreason" exist in a dialectical relationship, and that institutions of madness offer an unconventional, indeed uncomfortable, window into the so-called age of reason.[17] Here, too, I follow Chris Philo's provocation, building on Foucault's insights, that scholars engage "the *geographies* of reason, unreason, and their encounter as key components of the Enlightenment." Like Philo, I treat the Enlightenment "as a 'process' permitted of different geographies: some obvious, illuminated, and celebrated; others hidden, shadowy, and unannounced, but all in different ways integral to what this thing called Enlightenment entailed then and has since come to represent."[18]

In framing the hospital's history in this manner, this book builds on recent studies that have positioned the Hispanic world at the center, rather than on the margins, of the Enlightenment, thereby forcing us to rethink the geography of modernity and its overlooked actors and agents.[19] As recent scholarship has emphasized, attention to the Spanish American colonial experience challenges parochial conceptions of the Enlightenment as a predominately intellectual affair promulgated by *philosophes* and directly opposed to the institutions of the church and inherited monarchy.[20] In the Spanish Empire, as is increasingly shown to be the case elsewhere, Enlightenment ideas were consistently funneled through traditional venues of authority, employed in efforts to augment state power and craft and endorse empire-wide reforms and imperialist projects.[21] So too were they championed by church reformers who embraced varying degrees of secularization; regalism, or the subordination of church to state; and a moderated, antibaroque brand of Catholicism they appropriately termed *la piedad ilustrada* (enlightened piety).[22] While on the ground local rebels may have harbored illicit copies of "Wolter" (Voltaire) and whispered rumors of the coming of revolution, colonial authorities and the educated elite alike advocated for an empire built on the enlightened principles of social improvement, *felicidad pública* (public happiness), *salud pública* (public health), *policía* (rational order), utilitarian knowledge, and the rule of reason over superstition.

As a laboratory of empire during this period, Mexico City's *casa de locos* (madhouse) put these ideas and processes to the test, variously exposing the Enlightenment's promises, paradoxes, failures, and unexpected twists. In particular, this book contends that the hospital became a site that at once enacted and refracted a process of medicalization, unfolding both within and outside its walls. In his classic interpretation of the Enlightenment, Peter Gay identified advancements in medicine as the "most tangible" and "visceral" contributor to what he called the "recovery of the nerve"; by this he referred to mankind's unshackling from the constraints of religion and growing optimism in individual agency and critical inquiry.[23] Enlightenment thinkers ranging from Descartes to Locke praised medicine not just for its ability to cure disease and preserve a healthy body and mind capable of abstract, lofty reasoning but also for its potential to reveal higher philosophical and empirical truths. "It was in medicine," Gay asserts, "that the philosophes tested their philosophy by experience; medicine was at once the model of the new philosophy and proof of its efficacy."[24] But if laboratories confirm hypotheses, so too do they produce unexpected surprises. This book accepts Gay's premise that the embrace of medical knowledge was fundamental to the Enlightenment project, especially in the colonies where public health campaigns were inextricably tied to concerns over population management and Spain's imperial might on the global stage.[25] However, building on the insights of scholars who have reconstructed a plurality of Enlightenments enacted and experienced by a wide range of actors, I contend that in the case of *locura*, the key agents of medicalization were not philosophers or even physicians; they were the clergy, in particular the brothers of San Hipólito, and, more surprisingly still, inquisitors—in short, men of religion, not science.[26]

This is a complicated story to tell. The medicalization of mental disorder— that is, the transformation of human behavior considered irrational into a medical condition with an underlying physiological basis—unfolded in a manner that was contested, uneven, and at times haphazard, and with doctors as secondary rather than primary agents.[27] Up until Mexico's independence from Spain in 1821, San Hipólito remained firmly under the grip of the religious, who provided not only custodial services but medical ones as well, and even boasted about their ability to cure madness. While the hospital modernized and medicalized to some extent from within, it did so while never fully discarding its religious persona and charitable commitment to *pobres dementes*. Meanwhile, university-trained physicians were peripheral to the hospital, but they began to penetrate the courts as experts in diagnosing *locura*. Inquisition and secular criminal trials involving allegedly mad suspects chart the rise of the insanity defense, a development that went hand in hand with the growing recognition on the part of colonial magistrates that madness was a physical impairment that warranted medical treatment and judicial lenience rather than punishment. By the eighteenth century, they increasingly marshaled medical evidence and turned to San Hipólito or its counterpart for women, the Divino Salvador, as a means of managing the problem of criminals who were judged or suspected to be mad. Occasionally, they even transformed San Hipólito's confines into a site of knowledge production, a veritable laboratory where experts eagerly scrutinized and debated rationalist models of madness. Ironically, it was the Inquisition that frequently used the hospital for such purposes. A tribunal obsessed with inward states of reasoning and conscience, the Holy Office by the eighteenth century had not only honed its age-old techniques for probing the intricacies of the mind and will but increasingly tethered itself to medical standards of proof in cases involving suspicions of madness, becoming in the process a powerful, if at times unwitting and reluctant, tool of medicalization.

If this history seems deeply counterintuitive, there is ample explanation for it. In spite of recent works on the "Catholic Enlightenment," the notion that religion was vehemently opposed to the forces of science and secular rational thought widely persists.[28] Within this line of reasoning, the Holy Office of the Inquisition, especially its Iberian variant, has served as an emblem of modernity's antithesis—in Irene Silverblatt's words, "an implacable, premodern institution, manned by greedy fanatics who gleefully and brutally defended Spain's religious purity."[29] While this caricature, central to Spain's black legend, has origins dating to the Reformation, when it was weaponized by Protestant reformers, it was reinvigorated in the eighteenth century as intellectuals across the confessional and political spectrum advocating for greater religious tolerance pitched their arguments against the backdrop of a generic Inquisition that became shorthand for the inhumanity of religious persecution. From Voltaire's satiric portrayal of an auto-da-fé in Lisbon in *Candide* to Beccaria's systematic assault on Inquisition procedure in arguing for the reform of criminal law, various Enlightenment thinkers furthered an intellectual agenda, with the Inquisition as their chief foil. By the nineteenth century, these characterizations had become fully universalized, immortalized in the art of Goya, in the histories of martyred scientific heroes like Galileo, and elsewhere.[30] They remain, to date, ingrained in the popular imaginary, even in the face of histories that document far more nuanced historical realities.

In all fairness, the Inquisition's very own activities made it vulnerable to its overblown portrayal as both anti-modern and anti-Enlightenment. By the late eighteenth century, Spanish royal officials debated how to rein in "the most fanatical state body," while elite clerics, sensitive to accusations of superstition and intellectual backwardness, sought to reform the institution from within to bring its activities and prerogatives tightly in line with those of the absolutist state.[31] In keeping with the intellectual tenor of the Hispanic Enlightenment, Spanish *ilustrados* (men of enlightened thinking) desired tempered reform rather than wholesale change, even when it came to one of the empire's most maligned institutions. Since the Inquisition had always served as a tentacle of the state, conflating heresy with treason, it naturally opposed and censored Enlightenment works and ideas that questioned the king's divine and absolute authority, in addition to its routine enforcement of Catholic orthodoxy. However, it was following the outbreak of the French

Revolution that its policing of revolutionary activity and thought intensified, aligned with the agenda of an increasingly reactionary and fearful state.[32] In doing so, it found itself directly if ineffectually opposed to a strain of Enlightenment thought that would become canonical and celebrated for ushering in the modern world.

Perhaps unsurprisingly, many of the personalities that populate this book's pages fell afoul of the Inquisition and made their way to San Hipólito precisely for spewing ideas that reflected the Enlightenment's poignant critique of traditional authority. From a Basque Freemason in possession of a Protestant text to a melancholic military lieutenant lauding the French Revolution, San Hipólito's criminal patients engaged in the gamut of offenses that reflected the Inquisition's varied late eighteenth-century concerns and activities. In reconstructing their experiences, this book documents the ways in which the Inquisition's age-old procedures—developed in the fifteenth century for the purposes of eradicating crypto-Judaism and other heresies, then transported and readapted to the New World's diverse population—accommodated and even promoted the shifting view of madness as a physical disorder that could be medically diagnosed and potentially even cured. From the vantage point of San Hipólito, the Holy Office looked quite different from what Edward Peters called "*The Inquisition* of modern folklore," outdated, perhaps, yet also strikingly humane when it came to dealing with individuals judged to lack their full senses and deeply invested in empirical proof when issuing its verdicts.[33]

In characterizing San Hipólito as a "laboratory" of the Hispanic Enlightenment, I do so metaphorically rather than literally. The hospital was not, in other words, a controlled arena manned by experts—in Warwick Anderson's words, a "delibidinized" space marked by "somatic control and closure, organized around avoidance of contamination."[34] As rampant instances of patient flight indicate, the hospital's walls were exceedingly porous, and fears over feigned madness (often imagined, sometimes not) illustrate the degree to which colonial subjects destabilized authority. Moreover, while medicalization unfolded, it did so all the while confinement remained an ad hoc arrangement—a "custodial experiment" that could be put to both traditional and novel uses.[35] If doctors occasionally penetrated the hospital's spaces, they exerted only modest sway, their expertise consistently mediated by the imperatives of the representatives of religious and secular law—one concerned with religious orthodoxy and the salvation of the soul, the other with the maintenance of law and order.

Furthermore, if the hospital's spaces refract a complex history of medicalization and its unexpected agents, so too did they reproduce in microcosm the vulnerabilities and limitations of the colonial state during its touted era of enlightened administration. As studies of enlightened absolutism and the Bourbon reforms demonstrate, the Spanish monarchy's varied reform projects were ambitious in vision, conceptualized and orchestrated in a vast effort to fortify state power, extract greater revenue, and rein in the colonies. In practice, however, its policies often unmasked the state's impotence, exposed fissures between different factions of government, and cast into bold relief its inconsistencies and incoherence, especially on matters of social reform.[36] Thus, at no point in its history was San Hipólito a brick-and-mortar embodiment of a hegemonic colonial state; at no point was confinement tightly tethered to the mechanisms of state centralization in a universal scheme to discipline, criminalize, and control.

In the last decade, scholars of colonialism have come to conceptualize the colonies as "laboratories of modernity"—that is, experimental settings where social engineering projects were tentatively implemented and new knowledge produced.[37] Thinking of the colonies in this manner not only expands modernity's cartography but underscores the ways in which Europe and its others were mutually coproduced.[38] In a crucial sense, San Hipólito was a laboratory within a laboratory, its enclosed if porous spaces and the madness of its patients unearthing deeper truths about the larger processes and transformations reverberating throughout the empire. As Richard Butterwick has written regarding the centrality of the periphery to global engagements with the Enlightenment: "A flash of light can be disorienting, even blinding at its source. Projected, refracted and altered, light can be clearer, and its effects more easily analyzed, at a distance from the peripheries of illuminated space."[39] It is in the spirit of casting light from the margins that this book is written.

Writing the History of Madness in Colonial Spaces

In search of the mythic Amazonian city of El Dorado, the sixteenth-century soldier Lope de Aguirre earned the nickname El Loco (The Madman) for his feverish, unbridled displays of treachery and cruelty. Indeed, contemporary chronicles portray the earliest conquistadores as crazed and obsessed in their relentless appetite for glory, power, and riches (especially the latter), explicitly linking New World exploits with states of irrationality. For the Spanish official Baltasar Dorantes de Carranza, who participated in a failed expedition to Florida, the Indies were nothing short of "a reservoir of lies and deceit" that brought "confusion" to the "wise and discrete" and inflicted "madness" on the "sane."[40] In a different register, medical and scientific texts warned Spaniards of the physical dangers of the hot and unfamiliar American climate, which not only sapped energy and weakened the body but could potentially even dull the intellect.[41] Meanwhile, across the Atlantic, within the lecture halls of Spanish universities, intellectuals and theologians debated the mental capabilities of the New World's Indigenous inhabitants, characterizing them as brutes ruled by passions until finally conceding that they were natural-born children whose capacities for abstract reasoning remained weak and developmentally stunted.[42]

As this discussion suggests, Spanish colonization, from its violent onset, shaped how madness was expressed, understood, and experienced. Since San Hipólito was not just the first mental hospital of the Americas but the first colonial institution of its kind, it inherently raises questions about the intersection of madness, medicine, and colonialism. I am not, of course, the first person to wrestle with these connections. While practicing psychiatry in colonial Algeria, Frantz Fanon came to the conclusion that the subjectivity of the colonized was akin to a kind of madness.[43] More recently, historians focused mostly on North and sub-Saharan Africa and India have examined the workings of psychiatry and the modern asylum within colonial frameworks.[44] This scholarship has left me with an understanding of the ways in which institutions and expertise are embedded in systems of power and knowledge, and of the limits of European hegemony within colonial settings. I am aware, however, that the emphasis on expert discourse informing much of this work ("discourse" here understood in the Foucauldian sense) does not shed light on an institution like San Hipólito, which preceded the rise of psychiatry and systems of "biopower." *Bedlam in the New World* therefore departs from the approach often taken by historians of colonial psychiatry and focuses more intently on the social history of the hospital itself.[45] In so doing, it unveils the act of confinement to be the product of complex—albeit uneven—local exchanges among a variety of participants: hospital nurses, priests and friars, inquisitors, physicians and surgeons, legal experts, prison guards, laypeople, and the patients themselves.

In drawing attention to the ways in which confinement was an ad hoc arrangement and a negotiated process with varying degrees of success and failure, this book builds on histories of colonial medicine that have questioned the primacy of physicians in pursuit of the "alternate rationalities" shaping the development of modern Western medicine.⁴⁶ Most recently, Claire Edington has characterized psychiatry in colonial Vietnam as a "process of daily negotiation and exchange" that exposes far more than the "shortcomings of a hegemonic European science," highlighting the central role of local beliefs, practices, families, and legal professionals.⁴⁷ For colonial Spanish America, historians have identified the late eighteenth century as a period marked by medical modernization and nascent professionalization that made important inroads while never fully displacing unlicensed healers and religious specialists. In particular, this book heeds Martha Few's call "that histories of medicine take a more complex view of religion" for this period, recognizing its critical and complex role in the formation of modern scientific modernity.⁴⁸

While the literature on medicine in colonial Spanish America has gained traction in recent decades, it has yet to seriously engage the historiography on madness, which for Europe remains robust. As the discussion that opens this section indicates, one can approach the history of madness in the New World from myriad perspectives. I choose to focus on the case of San Hipólito in part because of the unique set of questions it generates as the New World's earliest mental hospital and also for the richness of its archival record. While I gesture whenever possible to its fascinating sister institution, the Hospital del Divino Salvador, founded in 1698 for poor madwomen, its paltry records have made it impossible to offer a detailed account of its history.⁴⁹ This book makes extensive use of San Hipólito's abundant and largely untapped documentation, which comprises account books, detailed patient admission records, statutes prescribing proper hospital administration and care of patients, correspondences, architectural layouts, medical receipts, and official decrees. I complement this evidence with cases from the Inquisition and secular criminal courts involving some of the hospital's patients. From the trial of a melancholy mulatto charged with bigamy to the scandal provoked by a *castiza* (one-fourth Indian, three-fourths Spanish) seamstress who stabbed the daughter of her former employer in a fit of passionate rage, these cases serve in part as patient itineraries that illuminate the complex scenarios in which certain individuals were charged with crimes, judged to be mad, and involuntarily confined. Together, this evidence confirms a trend toward the medicalization of both madness and hospitals during colonial Mexico's *Ilustración* while revealing complex local politics and contingencies.

In drawing on Inquisition cases as sources for the history of madness, this book builds on the pioneering scholarship of Mexican historian María Cristina Sacristán, who has produced two excellent monographs on the subject.

In *Locura e Inquisición en Nueva España, 1571–1760*, Sacristán unearthed a host of Inquisition cases involving madness, meticulously documenting local attitudes and the surprising leniency of the Holy Office toward allegedly mad criminals, given the doctrine of free will as a necessary constituent for human sin. *Bedlam in the New World* is especially in dialogue with her second book, *Locura y disidencia en el México ilustrado, 1760–1810*, which turned to the late colonial period, adding secular criminal cases to her arsenal of sources. This book accepts many of Sacristán's most significant findings: first, that the late eighteenth and early nineteenth century witnessed the privileging of medical expertise over the testimony of lay audiences; second, that roughly a third of the cases she analyzed (from a total of fifty-eight) sought resolution within the confines of a hospital, particularly San Hipólito, a phenomenon unseen in earlier periods; and finally, that the cases chart a growing divide between lay and elite cultures with respect to attitudes toward madness, with the latter favoring medical interpretations. My work departs from Sacristán in placing the cases in deeper conversation with San Hipólito's archive, in asking how such changes relate to the Enlightenment and the Bourbon reforms, and finally in offering a more critical reading of the Inquisition's vexed place in Enlightenment history and historiography as an instrument of madness's medicalization.

In contrast to Sacristán's comprehensive overview, *Bedlam in the New World* is in many ways a micro-history. It reconstructs the interior life of a single custodial institution dedicated to madness, explores its relationship to the outside world, and offers intimate sketches of the lives of its patients through deep analysis of Inquisition and criminal records. Popularized by Carlo Ginzburg, micro-history has come to refer to a genre of historical writing that aims to reconstruct the worldview of a subaltern subject through deep textual analysis and contextualization of a historical source, usually an Inquisition trial transcript. While historians have criticized Ginzburg and others for uncritical readings of Inquisition sources and problematic characterizations of "popular" culture, I remain attentive, whenever possible, to the manifold layers of mediation determining how Inquisition trials were recorded and preserved for posterity. Here, too, I am mindful of the recent "archival turn" in the humanities and accept Zeb Tortorici's characterization of the colonial archive as an unstable "contact zone" between past and present. Indeed, I would go so far as to claim that states of mind and emotion—much like the carnal desires he analyzes—are "inherently messy, complex, and resistant to categorization," and concede that my sources more sharply capture institutional authority while offering faint if precious glimpses into the lives of the men and women who fell into its apparatus.[50]

The goal of reconstructing the institutional life of a little-known but important colonial hospital in the midst of larger historical developments and changes—of using the "micro" to rethink the "meta"—has shaped this book. Although it prioritizes the eighteenth century, Bedlam in the New World begins two centuries earlier, examining the hospital's precocious foundations against the backdrop of Iberian systems of social welfare and their transfer and adaptation in the New World as part of the consolidation of Spanish rule. Between 1521 and 1524, following the collapse of the Mexica Empire and destruction of the city of Tenochtitlán, the conqueror of Mexico himself, Hernán Cortés, founded a hospital in a gesture that signaled both a desire for spiritual atonement and the beginnings of a system of medical charity in New Spain rooted in the proliferation of hospitals. He would not be the only conquistador to found a hospital as an act of redemption. In 1567, a native of Andalusia named Bernardino Alvarez established San Hipólito following a spiritual transformation that inspired him to dedicate his life to the Christian virtue of *hospitalidad*, or charitable service to the sick and the poor. Chapter 1 recounts Alvarez's career, chronicles San Hipólito's evolution from a convalescent hospital to an institution focused exclusively on caring for *pobres dementes*, and reconstructs the hospital's inner life and activities. It argues that in both its charitable mission to shelter mad paupers and its varied services, the hospital functioned as a limited tool of colonial governance that lent legitimacy to Catholicism and the Habsburg model of paternal rule.

Beginning in the late seventeenth century, the hospital would launch itself on a slow but steady downward path, a process propelled by financial hardship, patient overcrowding, and internal disarray and conflict within the Order of San Hipólito. In the decades that followed, it would undergo a number of changes: In the 1740s and 1750s, the brothers of San Hipólito, like other monastic orders throughout the Spanish Empire, would become the targets of a reform movement aimed to spiritually reinvigorate the order, rein in its autonomy, and impose a more disciplined and austere lifestyle on its members. In the 1770s, the viceroy and municipal government would join forces to reorganize and strengthen San Hipólito's finances and rebuild what was a deteriorating building, compromised by centuries of wear and tear, seasonal flooding, and two violent earthquakes. In 1777, San Hipólito reopened its doors, flaunting a much improved and amplified facility, as well as a modified institutional mission that couched its charitable activities in terms of a utilitarian service to the state and society. What did these changes signify?

Chapter 2 examines these transformations, framing the hospital's history as a microcosm of the Hispanic Enlightenment in all its aspirations, paradoxes, and limitations. In particular, it places these changes in conversation with the Bourbon reforms—a series of political, economic, and social policies that drew on Enlightenment ideas to augment state authority and instill a new colonial order. It argues that while the hospital in many ways came to embody the Spanish crown's ambitions to create an orderly and economically viable colony, it also reproduced the myriad limitations and failures of imperial rule during its touted era of enlightened reform. Moreover, efforts at state centralization did not necessarily signal the hardening of views toward the *pobres dementes*, or the hospital's transformation into a mechanism of state repression. If anything, the hospital's transformation disclosed uneven efforts to modernize hospital care and medicalize mental illness.

The remaining chapters move beyond the hospital's walls to the *salas* (interrogation rooms) of the Inquisition and the secular criminal courts to consider cases in which colonial magistrates were called on to make judgments about mental states. The emphasis here is on the challenges—practical, moral, and epistemological—that madness posed to colonial authorities concerned with the maintenance of public order or the enforcement of religious orthodoxy; the diverse (and often diverging) perspectives of expert and nonexpert witnesses; the growing persuasiveness of medical expertise alongside the instability of achieving an accurate diagnosis; the ad hoc implementation of the insanity defense; and the varied uses of the hospital as an institutional strategy for dealing with the predicament of criminals who were not in their full senses.

Chapters 3 and 4 approach the hospital's history from the vantage point of the Inquisition. While the late eighteenth and early nineteenth centuries witnessed a noticeable spike in the number of inmates who arrived at San Hipólito via the Holy Office, these chapters argue that this outcome was not part of a deliberate attempt to mass confine, discipline, or punish the mentally disturbed. Rather, it reflected a wider process of medicalization, a process in which the Inquisition played an integral if unexpected part. In particular, chapter 3 sets out to complicate the notion of the Inquisition as an anti-Enlightenment institution staunchly opposed to the forces of rationalism and secularization. Drawing on a series of cases in which the suspect's sanity was in doubt, this chapter maintains that due to its fixation on matters of human interiority and conscience, the Holy Office unwittingly found itself at the forefront of devising new modes for understanding the complexities of human reasoning and the nuances of intent. While such methods of discernment drew in no small part on theological concerns and practices, they also helped pave the way for the medicalization of madness and the growing use of the insanity defense as justifiable, indeed compelling, grounds for exonerating criminal liability.

Chapter 4 continues this line of inquiry but pays closer attention to the role of medical expertise and medical discourse within the inquisitorial courts. It demonstrates that while medical professionals equipped inquisitors with a more refined set of tools for gauging interiority—such as empiricism and a rational, theoretical framework for understanding mental disorder—they were but secondary agents in a process of medicalization that was ultimately propelled by the Inquisition and its religious motives. The final sections of the chapter examine the hospital's growing alignment with the Inquisition to demonstrate that confinement was not necessarily punitive; rather, it was the practical, imperfect, and at times creative outcome of the Holy Office's willingness to insist on madness's physiological underpinnings.

Chapter 5 turns to the secular criminal courts, contextualizing cases involving criminal insanity within the broader context of state efforts to expand the colonial judiciary, fortify the police force, and combat growing levels of crime, especially among the racially mixed poorer classes. But as this chapter demonstrates, the Bourbon concern with law and order falls glaringly short of explaining why the criminally insane were sent to San Hipólito. Colonial magistrates sent criminals to mental hospitals not as acts of punishment but as gestures of paternalistic leniency, informed by an eclectic combination of enlightened rationalism stimulated by the views of reformers like Beccaria and Lardizábal, age-old medieval laws protecting the insane from unwarranted punishment, and practical concerns about containing violent and dangerous individuals. Moreover, this chapter stresses that San Hipólito was far from an appendage of colonial law enforcement, and cases involving the criminally insane—including efforts at hospital escape—show how the hospital often reproduced in microcosm deep-seated tensions and vulnerabilities in Spanish rule on the eve of the empire's collapse.

The book's conclusion discusses San Hipólito's fortunes and misfortunes during the closing decades of Spanish rule and the turbulent transition to nationhood. The 1808 overthrow of the Spanish monarchy by the French invader Napoleon triggered the humiliating collapse of the Spanish Empire, creating a political vacuum for the establishment of a liberal *cortes* (parliament) in Spain that would ultimately curb the monarch's absolute power once he was reinstated. This legislative body would also decree a dissolution of the hospital orders, including the Order of San Hipólito, and the abolishment of the Inquisition, an icon of Old Regime decadence, its futility ever more manifest in the face of escalating secular crime.[51] As Mexico consolidated its independence from Spain in 1821, San Hipólito began its transformation into a wholly secular state-run institution. Nevertheless, members of the Order of San Hipólito remained in the hospital they had once governed for another two decades, witnessing the steady infiltration of a handful of ambitious medical men, armed with the latest psychiatric theories emanating from Europe. In the end, the drivers of *locura*'s medicalization ultimately lost control of a process they had helped to unleash.

The Language of *Locura*

Throughout this book, I widely use the terms "madness" and its cognate "insanity." Though modern psychiatrists shun these terms because they are technically imprecise, historians embrace them for their methodological value. "*Madness*," writes H. C. Erik Midelfort, "is so general, so vague a term that we find ourselves forced to ask what it meant in any given time or place, and so it well serves the purposes of an empirical historian who aims . . . to convey some of the flavor and strangeness of a forgotten culture."[52] The very ambiguity and malleability of the term, in other words, underscores the historicity of mental disorders — bounded in time, space, and culture.[53] This is not, of course, to deny the reality of mental illnesses and the very real suffering they inflict on their victims but to prioritize society's role in defining the bounds between reason and unreason. Furthermore, I do not hesitate to use the word "mental" in conjunction with illness, incapacity, disorder, or impairment. In doing so, I wish to make the point, as Elizabeth Mellyn has done for early modern Italy, that colonial people in Mexico understood that certain diseases and impairments influenced a person's brain functioning and cognitive faculties, albeit in ways strikingly different from our own understandings.[54]

While I keep my own language purposefully vague, whenever possible I try to privilege the specific words used by contemporaries. Not unlike today, colonial people in Mexico employed a broad range of terms and phrases to convey mental, behavioral, and emotional states that resided outside the bounds of what was considered natural or usual. In the most general sense, contemporaries referred to a mad person as either *loco* or *demente*, and to states of madness as *locura* and *demencia*. They further demarcated whether a mad person was feebleminded and thus harmless (*loco inocente*) or uncontrollably violent and dangerous (*loco furioso*). According to Sebastián de Covarrubias Orozco's 1611 Spanish dictionary, *Tesoro de la lengua castellana, o española*, the category of *inocente* denoted someone who was "without blame" and applied to both children, "who harmed no one," and the simpleminded, who "lacked malice."[55] The *furiosos*, by comparison, could be either insane or extremely "angry and choleric"; either way, he argued, their ire clouded their reason, making it necessary to "hold them in chains or cages," a practice not uncommon at San Hipólito and its Spanish antecedents.[56]

The verbal repertoire for describing disordered mental states did not stop there. Contemporaries also spoke of mad people as lacking sound judgment or reason (*sin juicio, sin razón*); as having "empty" (*bacio*) thoughts; as not being in their *entero conocimiento*, or full senses; and as having their "head" (*cabeza*), or mental faculties—often described as "powers" (*potencias*)— "perturbed" (*pertubado*), "injured" (*lesionado*), or "disturbed" (*trastornado*). Other descriptors, such as *fatuo*, *tonto*, and *simple*, implied foolishness or mental immaturity, while a term like *enagenado* could refer to mental disturbances that arose from demonic possession.[57]

Perhaps surprisingly, the richest repositories for this language are not San Hipólito's institutional records, which mostly document the material mundanities of hospital life, but cases from the Inquisition and criminal courts. These sources not only capture the local flavor of the communities in which madmen and madwomen roamed before they were confined but also the more technical language employed by the medical and legal experts who were summoned to provide expert testimony in specific cases. It is here, in the extensive and occasionally laconic reports of the courts' appointed physicians and surgeons, that we find the medical diagnoses of *mania*, *melancolía*, *frenesi*, and uterine fury (*furor uterino*); symptoms such as *furor*; and transitory states of lucidity called *intervalos*.

That one must turn to judicial cases and not hospital records to find physicians' reports, discussions of patients' symptoms, and diagnostic categories underscores the dissonance between the hospital and the colonial medical establishment. As this book stresses, throughout the period under investigation, San Hipólito was under the administration of a religious order, and it was its members, known as the *hipólitos*, who undertook the majority of the labor involved in caring for the hospital's patients. Physicians were, for the most part, a peripheral presence; they were a luxury the hospital could rarely afford, and when colonial magistrates hospitalized allegedly insane criminals, they always sent their own appointed physicians or surgeons to check up on them and report back. The marginal presence of the medical establishment reinforces the impression that San Hipólito was primarily a religious institution, charitable in orientation and concerned solely with the custodial care and protection of the *pobres dementes*. This was only partially the case, however, and one cannot overestimate the extent to which the brothers themselves were skilled in the art of healing and the ways in which the hospital assimilated medical functions under the broader umbrella of religion and in the name of charity, even despite recurring evidence of limited resources.

It is largely for this reason that I prefer "mental hospital" to "asylum" when referring to my subject institution. While I have seen the latter term occasionally employed in the few English-language studies that reference San Hipólito, I choose to eschew it because of its connotations with psychiatric expertise. Contemporaries did not refer to San Hipólito as a *manicomio*, the modern Spanish equivalent for a psychiatric facility. Instead, they dubbed it a *convento-hospital* (convent-hospital), more disparagingly a *casa de los locos* (madhouse), and occasionally an *hospicio* (hospice). An additional variant that appears, though sparingly, in the records is *loquería*; this was the most medicalized of all the terminology, referring to specific wards within the hospital where the mad patients were treated and confined. Such diversity of terms registers the hospital's varied uses and services, which ranged from charitable to coercive, and combined both spiritual and medical forms of care.

CHAPTER ONE

Bedlam in the New World

It began with a spiritual awakening. Legend has it that the New World's first mental hospital emerged out of a transformative experience, when a reformed conquistador named Bernardino Alvarez returned to the capital of New Spain after more than a decade in exile and vowed to atone for the sins of his past through selfless service to the sick and indigent. Two posthumous biographies, one of them authored by a bishop and the other by a Jesuit father writing in vocal support of Alvarez's beatification, record the events that preceded and followed.[1] In 1534, the native of Andalusia arrived in the viceregal capital of New Spain and embarked on a military career, immediately heading north to Zacatecas to participate in the military campaign to subdue the Chichimecas, a nomadic Indigenous group that posed a strong challenge to Spanish rule on the northern frontier. Following his military discharge, Alvarez returned to Mexico City, where his life took a sharp turn for the worst. The ex-conquistador fell into bad company and quickly earned notoriety as the leader of a gang that frequented taverns, engaged in fraudulent card playing, and took part in public brawls. His moral descent plummeted to its nadir when colonial authorities had him arrested, tried, and ultimately sentenced to forced labor in the Philippine galleys, a fate he narrowly escaped by taking flight to Peru. Settling in Cuzco, he secured anonymity and resuscitated his military career before amassing a sizable fortune through a series of unnamed commercial ventures.[2]

The official, laudatory account relates that Alvarez's spiritual transformation occurred more than a decade later, when he returned once again to Mexico City, now a more mature and wealthier individual. It was then that he received a letter from his mother, Anna de Herrera, informing him of his father's demise and her decision to retreat to convent life. The moving epistle, in which the mother exhorted her son to abandon worldly pursuits and devote himself to the service of God, struck a moral nerve. Suddenly, the former conquistador—"touched by the Hand of God," as his biographer, Juan Díaz de Arce, put it—became penitent, vowing atonement through the "sweetness" of hospital service.[3]

Alvarez's penitential sojourn began at the Hospital de la Concepción de Nuestra Señora, the institution patronized by another repentant conquistador, Hernán Cortés. It was there that Alvarez observed firsthand the troubling inadequacy of the capital's extant welfare institutions, short on space and resources to accommodate the vast number of patients demanding their services. Particularly alarming to his pious sensibilities was the plight of the mentally incapacitated; while the *locos inocentes*, or feebleminded, helplessly wandered the streets—the objects of public scorn and humiliation—those displaying more violent tendencies, the *locos furiosos*, were incarcerated in public jails and treated like common criminals.[4]

According to both biographies, Alvarez was so stirred to compassion by this sorry spectacle that he embarked on a charitable mission to found his own hospital. This enterprise was wholly inspired by evangelical motives. In the words of Díaz de Arce, Alvarez practiced the virtue of *hospitalidad*—that is, hospitality or charitable service to the sick and poor—with "complete perfection" so that "his fellow Spaniards would see him, and see themselves in him, as in a mirror." The penitent conquistador also hoped his altruistic and selfless actions would serve as a model of ideal Christian conduct for the recently converted natives, described metaphorically as *"plantas nuevas,"* or "new plants" prime for spiritual harvesting.[5] Alvarez got to work immediately, obtaining a license to establish the hospital from the archbishop Alonso de Montufar in 1566. Although he originally intended to erect a small building in the center of the capital on the street of Celada, in 1567 he set his ambitions on a more attractive and historically propitious site in the city's outskirts, near the Tacuba causeway.[6] The new location was once the scene of the infamous *noche triste* (sad night), the Mexica uprising following the death of Montezuma that resulted in the military retreat of Cortés and his troops from the capital of Tenochtitlán. When the Spanish forces finally subjugated the Mexica in 1521 and demolished the great city, they erected a church on the premises of the former battleground. Appropriately, the church was dedicated to Saint Hippolytus, the saint whose feast day had coincided with the date of the military victory. On account of its proximity to the historic church, the Hospital of Convalescents, as Alvarez's hospital was originally called, eventually became known as the Hospital de San Hipólito.[7]

While the hospital was still under construction, Alvarez took to the streets. His *caridad* (charity), his biographers emphasized, possessed no limits. He collected the convalescents, the poor, the orphaned, and the old and weary. Then he turned his philanthropic gaze to the most miserable lot: the mad. As the Jesuit father Francisco García recounted in effusive baroque praise, "He [Bernardino Alvarez] gathered all the mad and feeble-minded of New Spain in order to cure and sustain them. He said that these individuals were the most needy because, like reasonable creatures they need food and clothing, but cannot fend for themselves . . . and since they cannot care for themselves, it is necessary that someone else care for them. He would treat these poor individuals, whom everyone else had deprecated, with special affection, seeing in them the image of God, blessed with grace [and] lacking the taint of sin."[8]

THE STORY OF SAN HIPÓLITO'S auspicious beginnings cannot be taken at face value. In medieval and early modern Europe, similar accounts of heroic charity circulated as a way to describe the origins of different welfare institutions. Whether factual or mythic, the plot usually centered on the transformative experience of a benefactor who was stirred to action by the suffering of the sick and poor. These narratives served not just to extol the institution and the exemplary piety of its founder but also to inspire others to bestow compassion and charity on the needy.[9] San Hipólito's foundational story conveyed this message, yet it did so within a colonial framework that yoked Christian beneficence to the paternalism and evangelical agenda endorsed by the Catholic Church and the Habsburg crown to legitimize colonial expansion.[10] The illustration of Bernardino Alvarez (figure 1.1) included in the 1762 edition of Juan Díaz de Arce's *Libro de la vida del próximo evangelico*, originally published in 1652, encapsulates the hospital's religious and colonial origins. Alvarez is represented as a humble supplicant kneeling before an altar on which sits a scourged Christ in a scene from the Passion, crowned with thorns and bound with a rope around his neck. Referred to as a "*siervo de Dios*" (servant of God) in the caption in the banderole beneath the altar, Alvarez clasps his hands over his heart in a gesture of devotion as he utters the Latin phrase, "*Dominus providebit*" (God will provide). The illustration portrays the founder of the Hospital de San Hipólito as undertaking God's work in the Americas. Alvarez's piety is in the foreground, while the beneficiaries of his charity, one of them physically disabled, reside in the distant background.

Fully appreciating the significance of the hospital's foundational story requires us to situate it in its historical context. Although Alvarez's posthumous biographies were published a century after San Hipólito's establishment, they capture a formative phase of Spanish colonization that was marked by the proliferation of hospitals, rooted in Iberian institutional models and religious ideals but reconfigured in the New World to suit imperial designs. This chapter recaps this particular episode in Spanish colonial history and reconstructs San Hipólito's early institutional life, from its precocious 1567 origins to the early eighteenth century. Examining this period of the

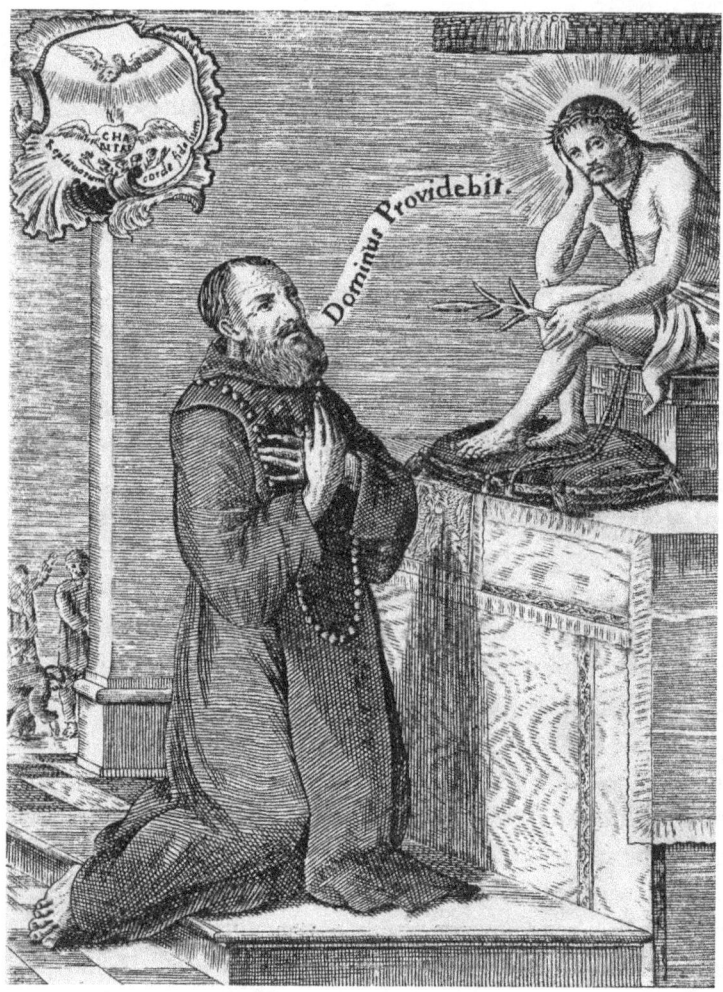

FIGURE 1.1 Image of Bernardino Alvarez, founder of the Hospital de San Hipólito. Source: Juan Díaz de Arce, *Libro de la vida del próximo evangelico, el venerable Padre Bernardino Alvarez* (Mexico, 1762). Courtesy of the John Carter Brown Library.

hospital's history affords an opportunity to consider how Iberian institutions and institutional practices pertaining to madness and its management were exported to the New World, and the degree to which they adapted to their new environment and endorsed a colonizing agenda.

As the earliest "mental hospital" in the Western Hemisphere, San Hipólito was modeled on antecedents located in Spain, where the practice of delivering specialized medical and custodial services to the mentally disturbed under the banner of Christian charity was a time-tested tradition. Its evolution within the Americas, however, meant that both its practices and its spaces, as well as its shifting institutional mission, would be tailored to local circumstances and rehearsed colonizing efforts to reproduce Iberian culture and secure Spanish hegemony in the New World. Specifically, this chapter contends that the hospital functioned as a limited tool of colonial governance whose utility resided less in the forceful confinement of a multiracial, recalcitrant, and vulnerable group of colonial subjects than in the reproduction of charitable practices and ideas that lent legitimacy to Catholicism and Habsburg models of paternal authority. Reconstructing the hospital's origins and activities during the first century and a half of Spanish rule sheds light on the ways in which institutions of madness reconstituted colonial authority in the absence of the biopolitical regimes that figure prominently in scholarly accounts of colonial psychiatry.[11]

This chapter makes its case in three parts. The first section examines the hospital's prescient foundations, showing how its origin story resonated with a formative phase of Spanish colonization in which hospitals figured prominently as aspirational tools of empire that embodied ideals of Catholic charity, community, and Habsburg models of paternal rule.[12] The second section discusses the history of Spanish mental hospitals as a preface to considering the ways in which San Hipólito both reproduced and transgressed Old World paradigms. The final section provides an intimate sketch of hospital life that shows how Spanish colonialism was embodied and reproduced in everyday institutional, religious, and medical practices. Taken together, the early history of San Hipólito and its treatment of *pobres dementes* reaffirms Woodrow Borah's claim that social welfare in New Spain was essentially a "history of transfer, adaptation, and experiment."[13]

Colonization and *Hospitalidad*

There were, to be sure, no hospitals in Mesoamerica until the arrival of Spanish colonizers. When, in the sixteenth century, the Indigenous artists of the Codex Osuna famously depicted a "sick house"—in Nahuatl, *cocoxcalli*—they were representing a colonial institution, not a pre-Hispanic construction.[14] In Spanish America, the establishment of institutions dealing with health and healing began shortly after the initial encounter with the New World and its native inhabitants. In a letter dating to 1502, Queen Isabel of Castile ordered Nicolas de Ovando, Columbus's successor as governor of Hispaniola, "to build hospitals where the poor can be housed and cured, whether Christians or Indians."[15] A century later, well over a hundred hospitals existed in New Spain alone, located in densely inhabited areas near important roads, mostly in the Valley of Mexico and the province of Michoacán, although their reach extended to Central and South America as well as the Caribbean.[16]

The establishment of colonial health-care institutions was an extension of long-standing European practices and attitudes to poverty and poor relief.[17] Within Spain's rigidly ordered society, the wealthy and noble classes, the church, and the monarch were all obligated to extend both justice and physical relief to the poor, provided the latter remained socially subservient and politically compliant.[18] This system of social welfare had religious underpinnings: specifically, it was driven by a Christian view of the poor as Christ-like and innocent and therefore worthy of material assistance. As articulated in the seven works of mercy—feeding the hungry, sheltering the homeless, dressing the naked, giving drink to the thirsty, visiting the sick, ransoming the captive, and burying the dead—the Catholic Church taught its followers that service to the needy was a fundamental part of being a good Christian and a way to salvation.[19] Beyond church and individual aid, charitable organizations such as hospitals and hospices—variously founded and financed by private individuals, the crown, municipal governments, and religious orders or confraternities—addressed the needs of the poor, providing them with shelter, nourishment, clothing, basic medical attention, and custodial and spiritual care.

Fueling hospital development in the New World were pragmatic and political concerns. In pragmatics terms, such facilities addressed the physical needs of the colony's multiracial inhabitants, many of whom were weakened by warfare, social and material displacement, and epidemic disease. In political terms, these institutions worked to further a colonial agenda concerned with enforcing social and political stability, reproducing Iberian culture, and, in the case of hospitals for Indians, preserving a diminishing labor force and fostering evangelization.[20]

Indeed, both church and state took an active interest in the founding of hospitals precisely because they endorsed efforts to spiritually colonize the New World. True to their medieval roots, hospitals were foremost religious rather than medical institutions. Sixteenth-century Spaniards often referred to them as *templos de piedad* (temples of piety and compassion), underscoring their importance as symbols and reenactments of Christian *caridad* (charity).[21] Transplanted to a colonial setting, the hospital's religious mission came to resonate with the agenda to Christianize the natives of Mexico. As the Franciscan friar Pedro de Gante made clear in a 1532 letter to Charles V, the establishment of hospitals for the natives "helped with [their] conversion" because it was through such institutions that sick and needy Indians "came to know the charity that exists among Christians, and thus they are invited to join the faith."[22] Prior to New World invasion and settlement, the Spanish had exploited the hospital's potential to proselytize and assimilate in their campaign to subdue the Moors following the *reconquista* (reconquest).[23] Drawing on these experiences, they founded hospitals in New Spain in close proximity to churches and monasteries, thus bringing patients into contact with Catholic priests and friars who served as models of piety, spiritual counselors, and bodily healers.[24]

The impetus to found hospitals in the Americas was given official endorsement in a number of royal decrees. In 1541, Charles V demanded that hospitals be erected in all towns populated by Spaniards and Indians so that the "poor can be cured and Christian charity be exercised."[25] This order was reissued in the 1573 Ordenanzas de pobladores.[26] Although the physical care of the sick, aged, and impoverished fell under the administrative purview of the Catholic Church, the Spanish crown wielded jurisdiction over social welfare projects in the Americas by virtue of the *patronato real* (royal patronage): a series of papal rulings granting civil authorities control over church affairs in the colonies. Due to this unique arrangement, all hospitals in the New World ultimately embodied the paternalistic philosophies of the Spanish crown, which cast itself as a benevolent protector of the poor and vulnerable—particularly the *miserables* (wretched or unfortunate people), who were the main targets of charitable aid.[27] Traditionally, this category of unfortunates included the disabled (indigent or otherwise), poor widows and orphaned children, and the *dementes*, or the mentally incapacitated. These individuals were, to varying degrees, deemed worthy of assistance and shelter, and minors and the mentally disturbed were accorded some legal protection. In the Americas, this category of unfortunates was necessarily expanded to include people of Indigenous and African descent, who lived on the economic fringes.[28] In particular, Spanish jurists spilled no shortage of ink in expounding on the miserable status of the native population, who were likened to children, bereft of the spiritual tutelage to govern themselves and lead meaningful Christian lives.[29]

When the Hospital de San Hipólito was conceived in 1567, it addressed a void in the colonial health-care system. By the mid-sixteenth century, Mexico City possessed its first general hospital—the Hospital de la Concepción de Nuestra Señora, founded by Cortés—in addition to a number of specialized institutions: San Lázaro (for lepers), Amor de Dios (for syphilitics), and the Hospital Real de los Naturales (for Indigenous patients). Alongside these institutions, the Spanish crown had founded the tribunal of Protomedicato to regulate medical practice in the colony and the Royal and Pontifical University of Mexico to provide medical education.[30] This landscape broadly reflected the structure of medicine and medical charity in Europe, which by the sixteenth century had transitioned from generalized hospitality directed toward the needy to more targeted and increasingly medical care to different sectors of the poor.[31] Still, there was no hospital in the New World to extend succor to the mad poor until Bernardino Alvarez championed their plight.

Spanish Bedlam Travels to the New World

As the preceding paragraphs have shown, colonial hospitals were based on Spanish institutional models but adapted to address the conditions of the New World environment and the political imperatives of the church and crown. The history of the Hospital de San Hipólito provides a case study of this process, documenting the transfer and adaptation of a unique type of institution dedicated to *locura* or madness. Although early records identify San Hipólito as a convalescent hospital, from its inception the institution acquired a unique reputation for sheltering *pobres dementes* and adopted many of the specialized features of Spanish mental hospitals, including the use of physical restraints, and Western categories for framing mental disorder and its management. However, its spaces, varied services, and practices were also shaped by local circumstances and accommodated new visions for social order informed by Spanish colonialism.

In early modern Spain, the practice of delivering specialized welfare and medical services to the mentally incapacitated was a well-established tradition. Evidence suggests that as early as the late fourteenth century, the Hospital de Colom in Barcelona began to admit mad patients, implementing restraints such as chains and shackles on those whose mental disturbances provoked physical aggression or suicidal tendencies.[32] In 1409, the Mercedarian friar Gilaberto Jofré founded one of the earliest mental hospitals not just in Christian Spain but in all of Europe, the Hospital de los Inocentes in Valencia, when he took pity on a poor madman who was suffering abuse and ridicule on the street.[33] This establishment was quite possibly modeled on similar foundations located in North Africa, where Jofré's religious order had long dedicated itself to the rescue of Christian captives. Or it may very well have been inspired by a similar hospital founded in Muslim Granada decades earlier in 1375.[34] As a number of scholars have opined, the legacy of Islamic occupation on the Iberian Peninsula offers a compelling explanation for Spain's active and early involvement in allocating hospital resources to madness. Like their Christian counterparts, Islamic hospitals, which flourished from the ninth century on, took in the mad poor within a larger charitable framework. The inclusion of small but specialized mad wards was an early feature of these institutions, their appearance possibly stimulated by the dissemination of Arabic Galenism, which occurred contemporaneously.[35]

Following the establishment of the Valencia hospital, similar facilities gradually dispersed throughout the Spanish kingdoms, loosely modeled on their Arab predecessors. By the middle of the sixteenth century, the cities of Seville, Toledo, and Valladolid each possessed a hospital exclusively designated for those who were mentally incapacitated, while seven general hospitals situated across the Catalan-Aragonese and Castilian territories contained mad wards.[36] Despite the scattered presence of specialized spaces for the care and confinement of the mad, one must be wary of overstating their significance. Madness during this period was largely a domestic affair, with facilities such as these typically reserved for the most desperate of individuals and scenarios: mad paupers without resources or family to sustain them, and the raving insane, who were deemed a danger to themselves and society.

At least initially, Spain's earliest mental hospitals operated more like hospices than medical institutions. The original hospital in Valencia, for instance, demonstrated little interest in medical treatment even though Galenic understandings of madness as a physiological imbalance had already begun to be reintroduced into western Europe from the Islamic world. It approached madness as a condition of poverty, centering its services on the provisioning of food, shelter, and protection. As Sara T. Nalle has commented, "'Protection' went both ways; the ill needed to be sheltered from the abuse they received on the streets, and the city's residents needed protection from the violently insane."[37] The use of physical restraints for patients with violent proclivities, justified as a method of last resort, was widespread and looms as a reminder of the hospital's more unsavory and coercive aspects. According to the 1522 inventory books of the Hospital de la Santa Creu in Barcelona, it contained, in addition to a modest fourteen beds, "twelve shackles with their manacles, three pairs of handcuffs, five chains with their collars, five pins for the blocks and three chairs for the imbeciles."[38] Interest in "cure"—in the form of purging, bloodletting, emetics, and dietary adjustments to restore humoral equilibrium—came gradually, unevenly, and it complemented rather than overshadowed the hospital's religious and custodial functions. By the mid-sixteenth century, the Hospital Real y General de Nuestra Señora de Gracia in Zaragoza—a general hospital with a spacious ward that annually treated around two hundred mentally ill patients—had acquired a unique reputation for its therapeutics. Here, patients who were not physically restrained were placed into cells, fed a special diet intended to prevent the mind from overheating, and kept occupied with various domestic and manual tasks.[39]

Bernardino Alvarez and his followers would have known of these institutional paradigms for managing mental illness. Tellingly, the brothers of San Hipólito—the religious order inspired by Alvarez's example and tasked with administering the hospital—occasionally referenced the renowned Zaragoza hospital in their documents as a way to exalt their activities and garner official recognition.[40] Alvarez himself might have been personally familiar with the Hospital de los Inocentes in Sevilla, located not too far from his native town of Utrera in southern Spain.

Nevertheless, although Spanish precedent was well in place by the time of San Hipólito's foundation, the hospital only gradually came to be considered as a *casa de locos* (madhouse) that mirrored those across the Atlantic. The official license from the archbishop Montúfar granting Alvarez permission to establish the hospital gave the institution the name Hospital de Convalecientes y Desamparados (Hospital of Convalescents and the Defenseless). As the hospital's origin story related, Alvarez was inspired to establish the hospital while undertaking charitable work at the Hospital de la Concepción de Nuestra Señora, where he observed an urgent need for an institution that would receive patients who had been rejected or prematurely dismissed from other hospitals without a place to convalesce. San Hipólito was thus originally conceived as a general shelter for convalescents and the disabled. It received the mentally ill as part of its broader mission to assist the poor, incapacitated, and defenseless, and only gradually came to concentrate its services on this marginal group exclusively. Its transformation, while clearly indebted to Old World antecedents, was also fueled by colonial processes, local demand, and the improvisational nature of Spanish settlement.

One poignant illustration of the hospital's colonial status resides in its symbolic location. As noted earlier, the choice of location for the hospital's construction, adjacent to the Church of San Hipólito, was historically meaningful, as the church commemorated the triumphal fall of the Mexica to the Spanish conquerors. One contemporary, in fact, referred to the Church of San Hipólito as the "old church of conquistadors."[41] Through its association with the church and its patron saint, the hospital took part in a vast project of symbolic and material appropriation, in which Spanish settlers erected churches, monasteries, and hospitals on former battlegrounds or sites of pagan temples. Patricia Seed has termed these gestures of appropriation "ceremonies of possession." Although Seed's work refers specifically to ceremonial acts and processions, such as giving speeches; planting banners, crosses, and coats of arms; and making maps, these "symbolic acts of possession" can be extended to the founding of religious institutions such as hospitals.[42] The most infamous example of the hospital's role in sanctioning Spanish dominion was the founding of the Hospital de la Concepción de Nuestra Señora by Cortés, which occurred shortly after the military siege of Tenochtitlán and on the very site where the conquistador purportedly first encountered his ill-fated adversary, Montezuma. Like Cortés's hospital, San Hipólito associated the conquest with the introduction of Christian *caridad* to the New World through its foundational story and symbolic setting.

The hospital's auspicious location would also mark it as a prominent site of celebration during major holidays. While it was common practice in Iberia for mental hospitals and their patients to publicly partake in the festivities of Holy Week, in the New World religious and civic celebrations inspired a new range of meanings and contributed to the formation of a Creole culture. This was especially true for the feast day of Saint Hippolytus (August 13), when the city of Mexico honored its anniversary with great pomp and fanfare. The "climax of Mexico City's festival year," the event spanned two days and consisted of a banquet, bullfights, and lasso contests, preceded by a lengthy military-style procession led by a member of the *cabildo* (municipal council). Beginning at the Plaza Mayor, the parade followed a route that deliberately recalled scenes of the conquest and culminated at the shrine of San Hipólito.[43] The following day, the Church of San Hipólito hosted a mass, and the hospital's wards were opened so that citizens of Mexico could visit the *pobres dementes* and make a special contribution to the hospital. Similarly, San Hipólito was accustomed to opening its wards to the public in late December on the Day of the Holy Innocents, which commemorated the martyred children slaughtered by Herod.[44] Such events, central to the hospital's financial survival, indicate that the *pobres dementes* were not entirely shuttered from the public gaze. To the contrary, they remained a visible fixture in the capital's ceremonial life, both through their Old World associations with folly and innocence, and through the hospital's affinity with the capital's patron saint and triumphant vision of the conquest.

Of course, San Hipolito's significance to colonial society was not just symbolic. In its earliest incarnation, it provided an expansive range of charitable and practical services, in addition to extending succor to the mentally disturbed, all of which were critical to sustaining Spanish settlement in the Americas. A 1569 document presented by the brothers of San Hipólito to the Council of Indies outlined the hospital's multifaceted mission and its utility to the broader Spanish colonial project:

> The intention of the founder was to collect the *locos inocentes*, and the simple-minded, and shelter them, and to sustain poor clergyman, disabled elderly people, and the sick, and to help those who had recently arrived from the [Spanish] Kingdom, who are called *gachupines*, and not only has [this practice] continued with punctual observance, but it has grown to great lengths, because [the brothers of San Hipólito] are not content to only receive, and shelter the mad, and simple-minded of the city, but they travel long distances to faraway provinces to gather them, and they bring them to the hospital at their own cost, so that in Mexico they can cure them . . . for which the hospital is highly regarded, like the celebrated Zaragosa [hospital], and it sustains a great number [of patients] on a daily basis [such as] ecclesiastics, and lay people [suffering from] different species of furor and madness [*demencia*], treating them with charity, and [is] an example to all.[45]

In spite of the allusion to the celebrated Zaragoza hospital, San Hipólito resembled its Spanish counterpart partially at best. While both facilities allotted accommodations to the mentally disturbed and convalescent, by the sixteenth century Zaragoza had become highly specialized and medical in orientation, with its expanded premises boasting multiple surgical wards, facilities for the treatment of syphilis and special chambers for pregnant women.[46] By contrast, San Hipólito's occupants, ranging from *pobres dementes* to destitute clergymen, were a heterogeneous lot, and its services, while no less wide-ranging, registered strategies directly aimed at addressing the challenges wrought by Spanish settlement in the New World. For instance, the passage references the highly touted *recua*, an impressive system of transport devised by the brothers of San Hipólito that consisted of seventy to one hundred mules. Serving as a relief convoy, the *recua* was used to transport weak and ill European immigrants from the port of San Juan de Ulúa to the Hospital de San Hipólito and other hospitals en route.[47] Immigrants were provided with food, clothing, and medical attention at San Hipólito, where they remained until they recuperated their health and obtained a livelihood. Potential employers seeking domestic servants or overseers for their haciendas often sought employees from among San Hipólito's sheltered guests.[48] In this way, the hospital functioned as a vital site of transit, facilitating the movement of immigrant bodies throughout the Spanish American mainland.

The hospital's interior arrangement underlined these varied activities. According to García's description of the hospital's original interior, which was completed in the mid- to late 1580s, the finished building contained

> many quarters and rooms for diverse sick and needy individuals; one for convalescents; another for the feeble minded and mad, with cages [*jaulas*], and restraints [*prisiones*] to contain the violent ones [*furiosos*] so that they wouldn't inflict nor receive harm; another to house those who had recently arrived from Spain, until they found their livelihood [*comodidad*], and extra rooms for poor priests, and people of high status [*calidad*] who suffer need, with the necessary offices for the service of the hospital, and enough rooms for the hospital's administrators, everything with great order, and distinction, according to what he [Alvarez] had learned in the ten years at the Hospital of the Marques de Valle [Cortés's hospital].[49]

San Hipólito's expansive charitable project and role in supporting Spanish settlement was thus mapped onto space. One of its quarters was reserved exclusively for the *pobres dementes*—fully equipped with cages and physical restraints to contain the more unruly patients—while other rooms were designated for convalescents and still others for "diverse sick and needy individuals." Some of its rooms were even converted into schoolrooms, where elderly tutors and teachers sheltered within the hospital could offer free schooling to children, teaching them "the Christian doctrine, to read, write, [and] count."[50]

The hospital's finances, which combined both public and private sources, also reflected the transfer of Iberian systems of social welfare while accommodating new arrangements and relationships forged through colonialism. Unlike the Hospital Real de los Naturales (Royal Indian Hospital), San Hipólito was not under direct royal patronage, although it occasionally received limited amounts of viceregal support. Alvarez used his personal wealth, which according to various testimonies amounted to over 30,000 pesos, to establish his hospital.[51] Afterward, the institution relied extensively on charitable donations. An official decree dating to 1589 granted Alvarez license to publicly beg for alms (*pedir limosna*), as the hospital was considered a charitable good work (*obra pía*) that benefited colonial society.[52]

Similar concessions urging the citizens of Mexico City to donate funds to the hospital were issued well into the eighteenth century. The hospital's account books registered a boost in charitable donations on major holidays, when, as discussed previously, the hospital welcomed local spectators.

Limited funds may also have come from native communities, although the evidence here is muddy. In a radical departure from traditional notions of poor relief, the crown required Indigenous villages to pay tribute (known as the *medio real de hospital*) to the Royal Indian Hospital to sustain their own health care.[53] The presence of hospitals designated exclusively for the native population was consonant with the two-tiered model of sociopolitical organization enforced in New Spain, comprising a "republic of Spaniards" (*república de españoles*) and a "republic of Indians" (*república de indios*). However, these institutions lacked the appropriate facilities to accommodate mad patients, making San Hipólito one of the few colonial hospitals to receive a mixed patient population. By the late eighteenth century, the Bourbon government would oblige the Royal Indian Hospital to allocate funds to the mental hospital for each Indigenous patient that was admitted.[54] However, in the sixteenth and seventeenth centuries, such arrangements did not exist, and official documents stipulated only that any charity donated by the natives must be voluntary, stemming from genuine Christian benevolence and not any coercive measure.[55]

Although the care and shelter delivered to the *pobres dementes* was intended to be free, the hospital's records indicate that it occasionally charged family members and even slave owners for its services. In 1697, for instance, the hospital received forty pesos for the care of Pedro de Cacaquatero for his four-month hospitalization. That same year, Captain Juan de Santana paid the hospital sixteen pesos to look after his slave Marco.[56] In a society that legitimized human bondage, the hospitalization of slaves reflected economic motivations as well as a Christian obligation to treat slaves in a responsible and "humane" manner.[57] San Hipólito's statutes indicated that slaves would be admitted on the condition that the respective owner pay the hospital a fee of twenty pesos per month of hospitalization; slaves were refused otherwise. Although the exchange of medical treatment for payment seemed to contradict the institute of hospitality, the statutes contended that such was not the case: the brothers of San Hipólito delivered their labor at no charge, while the money was used to finance the patient's food, clothing, and necessary medications.[58] In other words, the economy of charity only permitted funds collected through alms to be directed to the needy. Since slaves were considered private property, colonial logic dictated that the owner was financially and morally obligated to procure the slave's medical care.

San Hipólito's transformation from a convalescent hospital to an institution focused exclusively on confining the mad was not calculated. Rather, it unfolded in an ad hoc manner, propelled in no small part by a combination of strained finances, local exigencies, and the wider demands of the colonial state. While it is difficult to pinpoint precisely when the shift fully materialized, the nineteenth-century historian José María Marroqui identified the mid-seventeenth century as a critical turning point, citing financial stress as the driving agent.[59] Given its heavy dependence on the charitable impulses of the public, financial hardship was a perennial theme in San Hipólito's history, rendering it an acute barometer of the larger economic and demographic stresses occurring in the capital city. One contemporary observer even remarked that the hospital's ability to sustain its numerous projects on limited funds "seemed like a miraculous thing."[60] In the decades following Alvarez's death in 1589, the brothers of San Hipólito acquired various haciendas, which they transformed into sugar plantations; however, these ventures failed to deliver a steady source of income.[61] Gradually, the once ambitious project initiated by Alvarez became increasingly modest, leaving only the *pobres dementes* as the hospital's principal charge. By the middle of the seventeenth century, the brothers of San Hipólito had abandoned the school for orphans; soon after, they discontinued the practice of using mule trains to transport Spanish settlers, which had been an important hallmark of their hospitality.[62] While economic concerns may have constrained the hospital's charitable ambit, its transformation also reflected the shifting needs of colonial society as the number of newly arrived immigrants declined and the problem of *pobres dementes* rose in precedence.

Responsible for the well-being of those inhabiting its realm and the health of the body politic, the Spanish crown also played a role in refining the hospital's institutional mission. Royal interest in the hospital's unique capacity to confine a vulnerable and troublesome category of colonial subjects was articulated in a 1596 *real cédula*, reinforced by viceregal mandate in 1601, which ordered that "all the *locos* of the kingdom be sent to . . . the Hospital de San Hipólito." The decree also included an important addendum: any patients in possession of *bienes* (property) were required to use their personal wealth to fund their hospitalization.[63] In decreeing thus, the colonial government catapulted the hospital's notoriety, further cementing its association with the care of the mad. The stipulation for accommodating patients of economic means also accounts for the presence of patients who were not *miserables* in the traditional sense, including those who arrived from repressive outlets like the Inquisition. In 1598, for instance, the Inquisition advised for the internment of Luis de Zarate, a convicted *alumbrado* (false mystic) who was poised to be burned at the stake but lost his sanity while awaiting execution.[64] Similarly, in 1620, the hospital received Luis Vázquez after he attempted to kill a secretary of the Inquisition and was suspected to lack "*entero juicio*" (full judgment).[65] Such instances, which transgressed the boundaries of traditional medical charity, would begin to mount in the eighteenth century, as chapters 3 and 4 discuss. Nevertheless, these early cases highlight the extent to which San Hipólito was forced to deviate from its original obligation to shelter *pobres dementes* on account of local demand and for the sake of preserving social order. And they also reveal that the hospital in many ways came to embody the contradictions of Spanish colonialism, which cast the king not only as the benevolent protector of the poor and vulnerable but also as a disciplinary agent.

A close examination of San Hipólito's patient population as preserved in its earliest surviving registers discloses the ways in which it reproduced and reinforced, albeit in unanticipated ways, new forms of social order emerging from the colonial experience. Covering an nine-year period from 1697 to 1706, by which point the hospital was exclusively concentrating its services on insane men, the registers document a total of 140 patients and an average of 14 annual admissions. Table 1.1 provides an overview of the patient population as identified on the basis of race, marital status, and place of origin. Strikingly, the records show that while the hospital's patients were culturally and racially diverse, the largest constituency was identified as *españoles* (Spaniards). These were mostly American-born creoles (criollos), although peninsular Spaniards also figured among the population in small numbers. As illustrated in Table 1.1, *españoles* constituted well over half (59.3 percent) of the hospital's inmates. By comparison, only 5 percent (specifically, 7 patients) were classified as *indios* (Indians), while 18.6 percent were described as *negro* (Black) or belonging to the group of mixed-blood *castas* (specifically, *mestizos*, *mulatos*, and two *moriscos*). Of the twelve Black and mulatto patients, four were explicitly designated as slaves.

While the demarcation of patients in racial terms reflected the *sistema de castas* (race-caste system) that had codified in colonial Mexico, the racial breakdown of the patient population refracted the ideal of racial hierarchy in a distorted way. Given that natives constituted the lowest socioeconomic group, their underrepresentation comes as a surprise. The two-republics

TABLE 1.1 Patient population, Hospital de San Hipólito, 1697–1706

A. Race	Number	%
Español	83	59.3
Indio	7	5.0
Negro	6	4.3
Casta	20	14.3
Unspecified	24	17.1
B. Marital Status		
Single	44	31.4
Married	51	36.4
Widowed	2	1.4
Unspecified	43	30.7
C. Place of Origin		
Mexico City	37	26.4
Other cities/villages New Spain	47	33.6
Spain	16	11.4
Other	4	2.9
Unspecified	36	25.7
Total Admissions	140	100.0

Source: AGN, Tierras, vol. 3082, exp. 8.

model of colonial governance, which allotted Indians their own hospital financed through tribute, partially explains their disproportionately low presence. While San Hipólito, along with the Hospital de San Lázaro for lepers, was one of the few colonial hospitals in the capital city to accept Indigenous patients, it was not until the late eighteenth century, as noted previously, that the colonial government mandated routine coordination with the Royal Indian Hospital for the transfer of native mental patients. To this we must add the potential aversion to colonial hospitals among native subjects, which Gabriela Ramos has widely documented for Peru, as well as cultural factors that may have rendered madness among Indigenous people less accessible within the cultural and medical framework employed by colonists.[66]

Likewise, the staggering presence of Creole occupants defied the ideal of racial order that placed Spaniards and their American-born counterparts at the socioeconomic top. Their overrepresentation was not unique to San

Hipólito and dovetails with patterns observed within contemporaneous hospitals and institutions of poor relief.[67] The willingness of colonial citizens claiming full Spanish ancestry to solicit the services of welfare institutions highlights the fact that racial categories and class divisions never neatly mapped onto each other. It also hints that San Hipólito's patients were not all hopeless indigents and that the category of *pobre demente* was malleable, accommodating gradations in means and status. A small handful even bore the honorific title don or were admitted by family members identified as don or doña in the records. The overabundance of white patients may have reflected targeted preference on the part of the hospital's personnel and a tendency in colonial society to view poor whites as more deserving of charitable aid. Or perhaps it was citizens of Spanish ancestry who were more willing to view hospitals as legitimate outlets for managing the twin problems of poverty and sickness. Either way, in keeping demented whites off the streets of the capital, San Hipólito functioned, wittingly or not, to uphold the colonial racial order.

A Portrait of Hospital Life

What did hospital life look like, and how did San Hipólito's charitable and medical practices reproduce Spanish colonialism? Answers to these questions can be partially addressed through a close analysis of the Order of San Hipólito's earliest statutes, dating to 1616. Although the statutes represent an idealized portrait of hospital life, there is no reason to suspect that the brothers of San Hipólito did not strive to conduct themselves and administer the institution according to the rules and procedures laid out in this document.[68] Moreover, when supplemented with other archival records, such as the hospital's account books and what appears to be its earliest existing ground plan (Figure 1.2), an even more coherent depiction of the hospital's activities and interior life surfaces. Taken together, this evidence suggests that San Hipólito's role as a tool of empire resided not so much in its repressive capabilities, which, on a numerical scale, were always minimal. Rather, the hospital operated as an instrument of colonial governance through the reproduction of Iberian charitable and medical models that supported Spanish hegemony and lent legitimacy to the ideal (if not necessarily the reality) of benevolent colonial rule.

While the layout shown in Figure 1.2 cannot be confirmed as belonging to San Hipólito, or one of the other institutions administered by the brotherhood, San Hipólito likely followed a similar design.[69] The spatial configu-

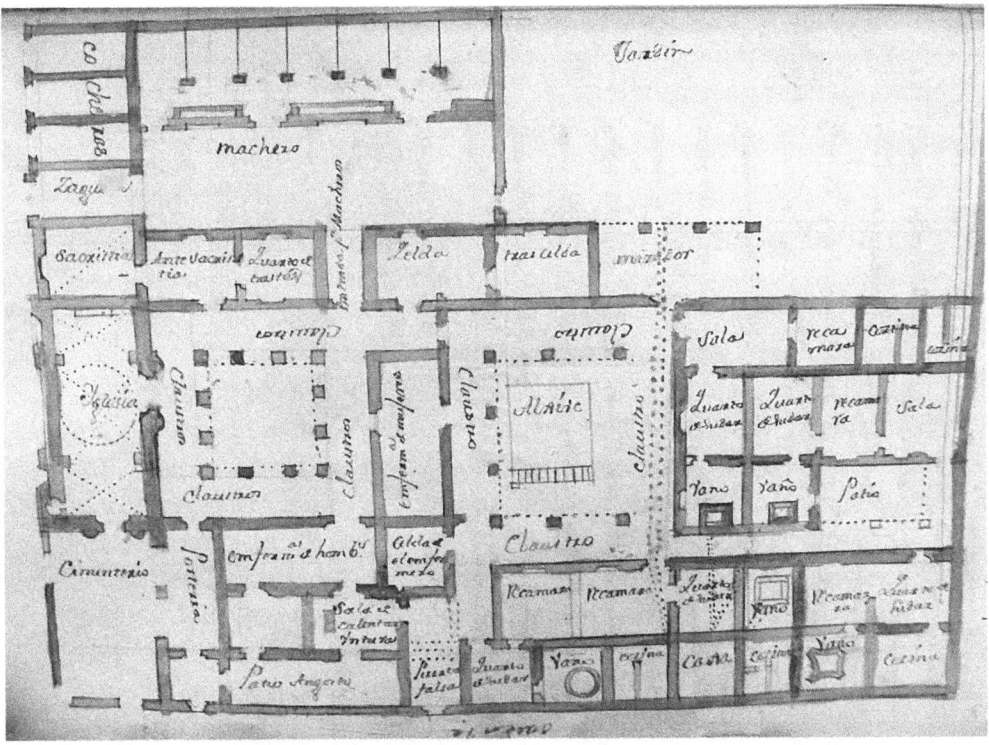

FIGURE 1.2 Potential ground design of the Hospital de San Hipólito, c. 1690s. Source: AGN, Tierras, vol. 3082, exp. 8.

ration illustrated in the figure was typical for a hospital of its place and time, underscoring the interdependence of religion and medicine and ensuring that the imposition of Catholicism and the salvation of souls remained a central facet of its function. While it deviated from the popular cruciform plan adopted by larger Spanish hospitals and exported overseas, it adhered to a traditional monastic model in combining the cloister and the infirmary into a single architectural unit.[70]

The hospital's main entrance, located adjacent to the cemetery, led directly to one of the main cloisters and to the hospital chapel, which would have been frequented by ambulatory patients and the public at large. The infirmary was located to the north of the chapel; it comprised two patients' wards (one for men, one for women), a smaller fevers unit (*sala de calenturas*) for treating patients stricken with frenzy (*frenesí*), and the nurses' quarters. The presence of a women's ward is striking. While hospital documents make no reference to the gender of the *pobres dementes*, the inclusion of the women's ward in the layout, coupled with stipulations on the treatment of female mental patients in the order's statutes, suggest that San Hipólito may have admitted women well into the middle of the seventeenth century.[71] The infirmary was located in close proximity to the chapel, following a pattern documented for the Hospital de los Inocentes in Valencia.[72] This enabled patients who were too ill to attend church or, under physical restraint, to listen to the mass and thus receive the spiritual sustenance that was considered vital to the healing process. In this way, the hospital's design united spaces of healing and spaces of worship, materializing in the most literal sense the hospital's dual function to "cure the body" and "cure the soul."[73]

In comparison to the hospital in Zaragoza, San Hipólito was a humble establishment. Nevertheless, its statutes attest to a relatively developed system of care and an elaborate division of labor, organized along racial lines. The hospital, in short, was meant to embody an orderly institutional space that in many ways would mirror the world beyond its walls, at least in theory if not necessarily in practice. Overseeing the hospital's daily operations was the chief brother, or *hermano mayor*. Appointed through a special election process for a three-year term, this individual directed the activities of a spiritual and manual workforce that included an official alms seeker (*demandante*), a doorman (*portero*), a cook (*cocinero*), an apothecary (*boticario*), the head nurse (*enfermero mayor*) and his assistants, the sacristan who safeguarded the chapel and the instruments of worship, the *refitolero* who looked after the table linens and dishes, the *procurador* who purchased supplies, and a number of servants.

Like its patients, San Hipólito's personnel reproduced racial hierarchies. While the brothers of San Hipólito were primarily Iberian in origin, the hospital's servants were usually *indios*, *negros*, or of mixed race.[74] Local vendors, such as the *atolera* who sold *atole* (a drink derived from cornmeal) and the "yndio" (Indian) who delivered beef, would have also infiltrated the hospital's spaces on a routine basis.[75] In addition, the brothers of San Hipólito may have collectively owned a small number of slaves. For instance, a 1675 record shows that Alonso de Arellano y Ocampo willed his slave Blas to San Hipólito. (However, Blas appears to have fled shortly after his owner's demise.)[76] Indeed, it was not uncommon during this period for slave owners to will their slaves to a hospital or monastery as an act of Christian beneficence. The statutes in fact made reference to the potential for wealthier patients on their deathbeds to bequeath money or goods—including slaves—to the hospital in gratitude for its services.[77]

The onus of caring for the sick and mad was primarily undertaken by the brothers of San Hipólito, who delivered both spiritual and physical medicine.[78] Given the dearth of university-trained physicians in the Spanish Americas, the role of the religious in the care of *pobres dementes* was accentuated.[79] Membership into the brotherhood could in fact grant access to a career in medicine, as the *hermano general* (the brother who oversaw the entire congregation) was given instructions to choose from among members those that seemed the most "suitable and inclined to this ministry so that they may practice and study medicine and surgery." Brothers with appropriate training could then serve as hospital nurses, with the most experienced and skilled among them acting as the *enfermero mayor*.[80]

The head nurse's duties and obligations were minutely detailed in the statutes. One of the head nurse's responsibilities was to ensure that patients confessed and took Communion within three days of their arrival, for only once the "cure of the soul" was addressed, the statutes stipulated, was the patient poised to "best receive the medicines of the body." Patients who resisted confession and Communion were admonished and eventually expelled from the hospital. In addition to confession and Communion, the nurse was instructed to provide the patient "with spiritual nourishment through good counsel and doctrine." If time permitted, he was encouraged to "read some spiritual book" while "consoling and uplifting" the patient's spirits; these services were especially critical in situations of life-threatening illness. When a physician was available (a rare occurrence), the head nurse was supposed to accompany him on his routine rounds through the hospital's wards, recording notes concerning each patient's condition and the corresponding method of treatment to ensure the proper management of the patient's diet and medications.[81]

The treatment of the mad patients continuously oscillated between benevolence and coercion. Upon admission, the *pobres dementes* usually had their feet washed, which was not only a hygienic measure but also a symbolic one, which recalled Christ's washing the feet of the disciples.[82] Their entire bodies were washed as well, and then they received a haircut. Once their feet and bodies were clean, the patients were issued a new set of hospital clothes, which consisted of a jacket and gown made of sackcloth, a shirt, stockings, and shoes; the clothing was to be changed on a weekly basis.[83] The harmonious characterization of hospital life depicted in the statutes would have been punctuated by moments of chaos as patients engaged in fits and violent outbursts. According to friar Francisco López—a member of the brotherhood of San Hipólito who testified on its behalf in 1645—although the *"pobres inocentes y faltos de juico"* (feebleminded poor and those without judgment) were given two sets of clothing to ensure "cleanliness," many ran around topless, having torn their own clothes out of "excessive fury."[84]

While all colonial hospitals engaged in the inculcation of moral and religious rectitude, San Hipólito partook in the use of physical force, marking it as a distinct space that dramatized the forceful and contradictory nature of colonial charity. Following Old World precedent, it enforced sharp distinctions between the *furiosos* and *inocentes*, reserving harsher treatment for the former. During especially aggressive episodes, the *furiosos* were usually placed into physical restraints called *prisiones*. The statutes stressed that placing the restraints should be accomplished with the greatest "charity and docility" possible, "although on the exterior, in order to intimidate [*atemorizar*] and domesticate them, one should demonstrate roughness [*aspereza*] and appropriate rigor, enclosing and punishing them in the form that was necessary." In the most extreme cases, in which the patient's fury proved too much to handle, the patient was to be locked inside a cage (*jaula*) or a special chamber (*aposento*) with "great care and precaution." Because they did not pose any real danger to themselves or others, the *inocentes* were treated less forcefully. It was even customary for the most harmless patients to accompany the *hermano demandante* (alms seeker) as he begged for charity throughout the city.[85] Thus, whether through harsh or gentle tactics, the hospital was implicated in the production of docile and pious colonial subjects.

The treatment of female patients was essentially supposed to follow the procedures outlined for the men, except that women were to be looked after by "*mujeres negras, o españolas*" (Black or Spanish women) of "age, virtue, and honesty." The brothers were expressly forbidden from entering the women's ward because it was thought that such close contact with female patients, who were exposed and vulnerable, challenged not only the limits of decorum but also the brothers' vow of chastity. To ensure that the brothers remained faithful to their vows, the statutes required that the door to the women's ward stay shut with two locks and two sets of keys, one in the possession of the head female nurse and the other belonging to the *hermano mayor*. The only exceptions permitting male access into the ward were to assist in pacifying violent patients or to address a medical condition that required the attention of a skilled physician or surgeon. The doors were also permitted to remain open on Sundays and holidays so that the female patients could hear the mass.[86] While the hospital appears to have ceased to admit women in the mid-seventeenth century, these practices possibly extended to its sister institution, the Hospital del Divino Salvador, which was founded in 1698 to address the problem of *pobres mujeres dementes* (poor madwomen) wandering through the streets of the capital.[87]

It is difficult to discern the precise types of treatments that were performed on the patients of San Hipólito and the degree to which humoral theories of madness—more precisely, melancholy, mania, and frenzy—were put into daily practice. Certainly the fevers unit, outlined in the hospital's layout, indicates knowledge and engagement with the learned medical consensus of the time. Medical writers working within the humoral framework inherited from the Greco-Roman world identified frenzy (*frenesi*) as an acute form of madness signaled by the onset of fever, and it was customary in Spanish hospitals to place patients stricken with this condition into special rooms designated exclusively for fevers.[88] The most common malady of humoral origin that would have been treated within San Hipólito's wards was *melancolía* (melancholy), an illness associated with the superfluity of black bile, which resulted in prolonged bouts of sadness along with symptoms such as irrational fear, anxiety, and clouded or distorted judgment, including delusions. However, beyond the allusion to the hospital's spaces for the treatment of frenzied patients, references to medical theory are evasive.

It is likewise difficult to determine the extent to which Indigenous beliefs about health and illness, and madness specifically, informed medical practice and treatment. It is possible that the medicines that were concocted by the hospital's *boticario* may have incorporated local plants and herbs as well as Indigenous knowledge about their healing properties.[89] As a number of scholars have discussed, while the Spanish tended to dismiss Indigenous healing beliefs and customs as superstitious, they demonstrated keen interest in native knowledge of botany and pharmacy, widely assimilating Indigenous materia medica into European categories and paradigms. Moreover, the hospital's location on the outskirts of the capital, away from the "hustle and bustle" (*trafago*) of the city where patients could be exposed to the salubrious effects of the clean *ayres* (airs), reflected not only European understandings of the role of air in the transmission of disease but also pre-Hispanic views of air's potentially curative effects.[90]

These speculations aside, therapeutics at San Hipólito reflected the imposition of Iberian medical models that stressed the centrality of regimen (diet, rest, exercise, and other practices) to health and recovery, complemented by spiritual counsel and medicines derived largely from both local and imported substances.[91] Hospital medicine during this period made no sharp demarcation between care and cure, placing preventive measures and spiritual services on par with medical intervention. The hospital's earliest account books, all dating to the late seventeenth century, generally confirm this characterization of hospital life. Specifically, the account books indicate that San Hipólito's expenditures were modest and overwhelmingly devoted to liturgy (church-related expenses such as incense, wine, candles, and hosts); food, shoes, and clothing for the patients; firewood and carbon (for heating and cooking); minor repairs to the building; and occasionally extra hospital beds. Patients were generally fed a local diet that consisted of a ration of beef, bread or tortillas, beans, and atole.[92] They were fed three times a day, and their diets were sometimes tailored to address their individual medical needs.[93] On the feast days of Saint Hippolytus and the Holy Innocents, hospital life transcended its routine: the cook prepared an elaborate feast, and patients were given an extra helping of food. On these days, the brothers also ensured that the *inocentes* were properly dressed and presentable to greet the citizens of Mexico City who paid the hospital and its occupants a visit. On the feast day of the Holy Innocents in 1673, for instance, the hospital purchased sixty pieces of sackcloth in which to dress the *inocentes*, along with stitching supplies, twenty handkerchiefs, and twenty pairs of shoes.[94]

Taken together, these sketches of hospital life highlight the ways in which San Hipólito functioned to sanction the colonial enterprise. Through its therapeutic, religious, and quotidian practices, the hospital was meant to highlight the bounty and benevolence of the Habsburg state toward its *pobres dementes*, who were viewed as deserving of charitable care and assistance. Of course, the cloak of charity and religion, no matter how heavy its fabric, could never fully mask the hospital's more coercive and disciplinary aspects, manifested in the physical use of restraints and cages to pacify, domesticate, and shut away its most unruly inhabitants. Confinement and force perpetually sullied San Hipólito's reputation and dramatized the contradictions, tensions, and outright violence central to the colonial project writ large.

AS THE EARLIEST HOSPITAL of the New World to specialize in the care and confinement of the mad, San Hipólito was part of the transfer and adaptation of practices, ideas, and institutions from Spain to the Americas. From its attention to mad paupers as a special type of *miserable* to the forceful measures it employed to subdue madness, the hospital embodied an Old World prototype in a New World setting. Yet while it preserved core features of Iberian mental hospitals, its deployment in the Americas within a colonial context produced a new range of meanings and implications. For one, its evolution from a convalescent hospital with an expansive charitable agenda to a *casa de locos* that rivaled those across the Atlantic was driven by the shifting needs of a colonial society in flux and the improvisational nature of Spanish expansion and settlement.

As it developed into a full-fledged mental hospital during the following century, the hospital came to register the influences of its surrounding environment in a variety of ways: through its multiracial patient population and personnel that variously reproduced, distorted, and reinforced racial hierarchies; through its affinity with the capital's patron saint and participation in the formation of a Creole culture; and through its charitable and religious practices, which served a legitimizing function. Although the hospital functioned as a tool of colonial governance, it hardly did so according to Foucauldian models of discipline and repression, and there was never a "great confinement" of the mad in the New World, a fact paralleled by scholarship on early modern Europe that has exposed the phenomenon of mass internment as misleading.[95] Instead, the hospital's utility to the colonial project resided in its charitable, medical, and custodial services, which reinforced Catholicism and attested to the benevolence of the Spanish king toward its most vulnerable and marginal subjects. However, the degree to which it succeeded in legitimizing colonial rule warrants skepticism. Certainly, when it came to the Indigenous population, its charitable message and institutional reach fell stunningly short.

By the late eighteenth century, Habsburg models of charity would fall into full decline and San Hipólito would plummet into a state of misery, driven by limited finances and monastic indiscipline among the brothers of San Hipólito. Under the broader umbrella of "reform" initiated by the Bourbon monarchs, the hospital would undergo a series of transformations, including physical amplification of its premises to accommodate a larger number of patients and a redefinition of its charitable mission in terms of a utilitarian service to the state and the greater public. Chapter 2 examines the details of this transformation.

CHAPTER TWO

An Enlightened Madhouse

On January 20, 1777, Antonio María de Bucareli y Ursúa, viceroy of New Spain, attended a solemn ceremony commemorating the Hospital de San Hipólito's much anticipated reopening. For two years, the hospital had been closed while its building underwent wholesale remodeling. In his correspondence with the Bourbon bureaucrat and visitor-general of New Spain, José de Gálvez, Bucareli described the "pious demonstration" that took place during the hospital's debut as the *pobres dementes* were transferred from their provisional accommodations to the "new magnificent house."[1] The redesigned facility was a definite upgrade; simple but sturdy, functional but aesthetically pleasing, it was considerably larger and more accommodating than its predecessor. The viceroy commented to Gálvez, somewhat exaggeratedly, that it far outrivaled any hospital he had ever seen in Europe.[2] No longer attached to the convent, the infirmary alone consisted of two stories, boasting individual private cells for the patients. Each equipped with its own window facing inward, the small rooms were tightly flanked around spacious interior patios that showcased freshwater fountains and classical arcades (figure 2.1). Juan de Viera, the Jesuit priest who visited the hospital shortly after its inauguration, was also awestruck, remarking on the building's beautiful "construction" and "symmetry." The new San Hipólito was, in his words, a "marvel" to behold, with its "magnificent" patios that, when aligned with those of the adjacent convent, offered a perspective that resembled the ancient theaters of Rome or a grand Spanish bullfighting ring.[3]

San Hipólito's renovation could not have occurred at a more pressing moment. By the time the viceroy had endorsed the reconstruction project in earnest, the original building had deteriorated to the point of ruin. The building's walls were in such battered condition that they displayed the visible imprint of the repeated bangs and blows made by the *locos furiosos* who had vented their maddened rage.[4] The torrential rains that characterize Mexico City during the months of May through August had likewise left their deleterious mark: scattered leaks infiltrated the roof, while the building's floors and fragile foundation were dank, sunken, and moldy on account of periodic flooding.[5] Furthermore, recurring earthquakes—one in 1754 and another in 1773—had accelerated this slow decay; windows had shattered, floors had cracked, and the hospital's adobe walls had begun to crumble.[6]

Like an insidious malaise, the building's physical corruption was symptomatic of a deeper disquietude rumbling within the hospital's walls. Although San Hipólito's origins were auspicious, since the late seventeenth century the hospital had launched itself on what would become a long period of decline. As the building withered, so too did the hospital's finances; the number of inmates steadily mounted while charitable donations slowly but surely dwindled. Suspicions of maladministration appeared to reside at the root of the problem. In the decades that followed their elevation to the status of a full religious order in 1700, the brothers of San Hipólito became the targets of a series of attacks waged by state and church officials who complained that the *hipólitos* were growing spiritually lax and negligent. Aside from dreadful accusations of malfeasance and patient mistreatment, one of the principle charges directed against the order's members was that they pilfered the alms intended for the patients' medicines and daily sustenance, a shocking affront to the system of medical charity. Such criticisms bore a grain of truth—the *hipólitos* had indeed lost sight of their commitment to the cherished ideal of hospitality. However, accusations of corruption and lapses in vocation overlooked deeper structural issues, ranging from demographic shifts to personnel shortages that posed serious challenges to effective hospital management. By 1774, San Hipólito had come to embody the misery of its patients, a sentiment that was expressed in the prior general's desperate and impassioned appeal to the viceroy for financial succor, in which he lamented the "urgent and grave necessity" of the inmates—referred to as *estos infelices* (these unhappy ones)—who were confined, much to their discomfort and contrary to their physical and mental well-being, in a "ruinous house" without sufficient food and proper clothing.[7]

The renovation was therefore nothing short of an attempt to resuscitate, and even reinvent, a dying institution. It followed closely on the heels of a protracted and collaborative effort by church and state authorities to curtail the autonomy of the Order of San Hipólito and reform its members. Moreover, it coincided with the Bourbon king's aggressive campaign to modernize Spain and its colonies and garnered much of its momentum from the crown's targeted encroachment in matters of *salud pública* (public health). While reform-minded clerics fought to improve the hospital from within, they succeeded in attracting state sponsorship. The Spanish monarchy provided the philosophical buttress in reasserting its benevolent paternalism toward its poor insane subjects with renewed dedication and zeal.[8] On the home front, viceroy Bucareli championed the hospital's reconstruction, enlisting the support of Mexico City's municipal government (*ayuntamiento*) and the tribunal of the *consulado* (merchants' guild). Validating their efforts in terms of the hospital's utility and benefit to the greater public, royal and local authorities paved the way for a stunning resurrection: San Hipólito was granted a much-needed face-lift, its physical size was amplified to house a larger body of inmates with greater efficiency and order, its status was catapulted throughout the viceroyalty, and its finances were bolstered to ensure its future growth and prosperity.

Taken together, these developments incarnated critical aspects of the Hispanic Enlightenment in all its aspirations, contradictions, and limitations. More concisely, they can be viewed in concert with the so-called Bourbon reforms—sweeping changes instituted to the imperial administration, economy, and military that dramatically reconfigured the relationship between the metropole and the colony.[9] The reforms were formulated to address the political and economic weaknesses that had set the Spanish Empire back during the last century of Habsburg rule. They incorporated a French model of absolutist authority and drew on the Enlightenment discourses of efficiency, order, rationalism, and public happiness (*felicidad pública*) to justify state expansion.[10] Under the aegis of enlightened administration, the colonial government undertook varied measures to strengthen welfare services, promote better sanitation and hygiene, and advance the study of science and medicine to the benefit of the empire.[11] The state also brought its enlightened agenda to bear on the colony's hospitals as part of a broader campaign to subordinate the church to the royal bureaucracy.[12] On account of these developments, studies have identified the late colonial period as a pivotal early stage in the modernization of hospital care and the period that witnessed the shift from "traditional notions of charity to modern ideas of secular social welfare."[13] Most recently, Adam Warren has characterized this process as a chaotic and contested one, with colonial hospitals often serving as sites where the "politics of secularism and sacred" were played out to their fullest discord among patients, agents of the state, professionalizing physicians, and entrenched lay and ecclesiastical entities.[14] "The hospital," he writes, "became a site of conflict over new visions of modernization and reform."[15] Warren's view of hospital reform dovetails with more recent interpretations of the Bourbon period, which emphasize the uneven and often failed outcomes of the reform efforts and the contributions of local populations, who variously resisted, reshaped, and coopted its rhetoric and policies.[16]

In what ways had San Hipólito become an "enlightened" madhouse? While the transformation of its building constituted the most obvious indicator of change, enlightened reform arrived earlier, and more quietly, as a series of efforts to curb the independence of the Order of San Hipólito and impose a more rigorous and austere lifestyle on its members. Echoing developments taking place throughout Spanish American convents and monasteries, the reforms spoke to the religious tenor of the Hispanic Enlightenment, in which the reform of Catholicism—its institutions and personnel—was a critical aspect of the empire's embrace of modernity. However, rehabilitating the Order of San Hipólito and reprising the hospital's building necessarily entailed a fragile alliance between church, state, and society, with tensions thinly concealed at the level of rhetoric. When San Hipólito reopened its doors in 1777, it launched an updated institutional mission that couched its activities in terms of utilitarian service to the state and society. The utilitarian mission was in keeping with the Enlightenment ideals of progress, social improvement, rational order, and public happiness, while its redesigned building implied a more rational and efficient approach to the management of mental disease.

And yet continuity lurked. Despite the new look and layout of San Hipólito, and the new mandates and decrees, deep-set notions and practices still haunted its halls. In this way, the hospital constituted a microcosm of the Hispanic Enlightenment. From the crises that sparked the hospital's decline, to the first efforts of church and state to address it, to the new language of utility and physical reorganization, to the hospital's sincere attempt at but uneven transition to modern medicine, the history of San Hipólito during the late colonial period replicates the occasional successes and many failures, as well as the contradictions between traditional Christian practices and rising secularism, that crackled through the Hispanic Enlightenment like a live wire.

The Crisis in Hospitality

The first murmurings of a potential crisis at San Hipólito began in the middle of the seventeenth century, when the hospital fell into serious economic hardship. By the turn of the century, there were palpable hints that the decline had expanded way beyond finances to include concerns of a more existential variety: Could San Hipólito, much like the Catholic Church itself, weather the demands of a shifting age and its call for a society structured according to the ideals of secular and rational order? As the number of *pobres dementes* steadily crowded the hospital's cramped quarters, taxing its limited resources, San Hipólito seemed to epitomize the shortcomings of traditional medical charity and religious medicine to address the problem of mental illness and the stresses it unleashed on colonial society.

A major facet of the hospital's decline—and one that left a hefty paper trail—centered on the Order of San Hipólito itself and widespread complaints about its members' lack of spiritual rigor and discipline. As chapter 1 discussed, since the sixteenth century, the brothers of San Hipólito had dedicated themselves to the daily drudgery of administering to the mentally disturbed, delivering both physical and spiritual medicine. Unlike the learned Jesuits, the *hipólitos* were a humble order that had earned its reputation through the mundane nursing of ailing bodies and minds, rather than lofty philosophical reflection.[17] By the early 1700s, the order had expanded its nursing enterprise to become one of the most visible and active hospital orders in all of New Spain. While it operated a total of twelve hospitals, only the Hospital de San Roque in Puebla, in addition to San Hipólito, specialized in the care of the mentally incapacitated, although the scope of its operations was considerably more modest. By the 1730s, all the institutions under the *hipólitos*' administration suffered varying degrees of financial distress and steady deterioration such that their collective plight warranted church and state intervention. In 1739, Juan Antonio Vizarrón y Eguiarreta, jointly occupying the office of viceroy and archbishop, vociferously sounded the alarm when he issued a report on their "deplorable" condition, describing them as little more than "sites where [patients] go to die, and the poor to have their afflictions worsen."[18]

While the source of the crisis in hospital care was manifold, both church and state authorities concentrated their criticisms on the brothers' alleged moral turpitude and growing worldliness. And in an unprecedented move that highlighted the growing encroachment of governmental authorities in the brothers' affairs, Vizarrón proceeded to call for the order's permanent extinction. This appeal to extreme action, shocking as it may seem, must be situated within the context of shifting church and state politics, as the Bourbon dynasty, which ascended the throne in 1700, sponsored campaigns to subject the regular clergy—the nursing orders included—to greater royal and diocesan authority. While these religious bodies had enjoyed considerable independence under the decentralized rule of the Habsburgs, the Bourbon crown, under the principles of enlightened absolutism, sought to render them more compliant and accountable to secular authority. In this endeavor, they enjoyed active, if at times uneasy, collaboration with progressive clergymen who were dedicated to reforming Catholicism in response to the growing threat of Protestantism and the anti-clerical elements of Enlightenment thought. Only an "enlightened piety" (*la piedad ilustrada*) that stressed inward devotion and strict observance over baroque excess, religious reformers argued, could counter these challenges. Thus, accusations of decadence and spiritual laxity waged at the *hipólitos* (similar complaints were leveled at nuns) accentuated larger fears that the Catholic Church had lost its way and that the regular orders, in particular, begged reform and greater supervision. That said, there is ample reason to believe that Vizarrón and his allies did not exaggerate solely for political effect; a lapse in spiritual vocation, in addition to fierce quibbling among the order's members, had indeed contributed to a veritable crisis in hospitality.

Ironically, the earliest indication of a slackening in spiritual zeal within the brotherhood is revealed in documents pertaining to their glorious and much sought after elevation in rank. In 1699, friar Juan de Cabrera presented a memorial before the Council of Indies, requesting permission to approach the pope with a petition to elevate his congregation to the status of a religious order. His stated main motive was the hardening of monastic discipline. As members of a congregation and not a full-fledged religious order, the brothers of San Hipólito were only required to pledge solemn vows to obedience and hospitality, not the additional monastic vows of chastity and poverty, which would have imposed greater internal discipline.[19] Cabrera's petition maintained that the brotherhood suffered from a preponderance of members whose commitment to hospital service was at best lukewarm. Many of these disingenuous members had fully deserted their posts and obligation to assist the poor, the medically skilled among them opting to pursue secular, and thus more lucrative, careers in medicine instead, "in grave harm to Hospitality, and scandal to the republic."[20] Cabrera reasoned that the elevation in status would initiate a reform within the brotherhood, obligating its members to profess all four solemn vows and follow the rigid monastic regime of Saint Augustine. His petition proved persuasive and, in 1700, Pope Innocent XII acceded to the request, promulgating his approval in a series of decrees.[21]

The ascension in status did little to halt, much less reverse, the order's continuing decline. This is unsurprising, since the promotion in rank did not address a major source of the problem: limited revenues. The lapse in monastic discipline notwithstanding, economic hardship, coupled with issues of overcrowding and a shortage of nurses, posed a serious challenge for the *hipólitos*, rendering effective and efficient hospital administration and care extremely difficult. Throughout the eighteenth century, this was more or less true for all of Mexico City's hospitals, as urbanization and a spike in population exacerbated public health problems and taxed hospital resources.[22] Traditional forms of healing, heavily reliant on palliative treatment and spiritual solace, were both ineffective and cost prohibitive.[23] There were simply too many people requiring hospitalization to be housed for extended periods of time and under direct, scrutinizing care.

Moreover, a series of calamities ranging from epidemics to earthquakes convulsed the capital, transforming an otherwise latent problem into an immediate public health crisis. San Hipólito was often struck, undermining its ability to attend to the *pobres dementes*. In 1722, for instance, when a large fire severely damaged the building of the Royal Indian Hospital, San Hipólito was flooded with additional patients (none of whom were insane), and the brothers were obligated to care, clothe, and feed them while the Royal Indian Hospital underwent reconstruction. A 1725 *visita* (visitation or inspection) conducted by Nicolas Rodriguez Moreno lucidly captured San Hipólito's dire conditions as the influx of new patients strapped its resources thin. Entrusted with the task of reporting on the state of the Indigenous patients that had been transferred over, Moreno, a royal secretary, documented a disconcerting spectacle: "I saw many sick Indians who it was said suffered from different ailments, and they also seemed to be suffering with great discomfort and without clothes; some were on beds with the greatest discomfort and others were on the floor, and all of them were on mats or bedrolls instead of mattresses, without more clothing than underwear made of ordinary linen, some with pillows and others without."[24]

Twelve years later, San Hipólito's wards were once again swamped with a deluge of patients when, in 1737, an outbreak of *matlazahuatl*, or typhus, ravaged the colony. One of the deadliest epidemics to strike New Spain since the conquest, the scourge claimed more than forty thousand people in the capital alone. The relief effort was robust, involving the spiritual and manual labor of both the secular and the regular clergy and all nine of the city's hospitals. As the epidemic ultimately served as the catalyst for the surge in popularity of the cult of Our Lady of Guadalupe, its disastrous effects and valiant public response were richly documented in Cayetano de Cabrera y Quintero's panegyric, *Escudo de Armas de México*. Befitting the text's genre and lofty subject matter, Cabrera celebrated the *hipólitos*, emphasizing their tenacity and dedication in caring for those stricken with the malady even while many of their own took sick and died from contagion. Their "great care" and "fine charity," he lauded, was "incomparable."[25] San Hipólito, too, figured prominently in Cabrera's account. Transcending its traditional role as a "receptacle" for the colony's mad paupers, Cabrera reported, the institution provided refuge to approximately 1,477 ill men and women; of these, 464 died.[26] The hospital's success in treating an abundance of patients depended greatly on the fact that it received viceregal support in the form of twenty pesos daily for the sustenance of the patients and extra money for medical expenditures.[27] However, the standard of care extended to the *pobres dementes* no doubt suffered during the calamity. Cabrera reported that given the staggering number of patients and a shortage of manpower, the brothers of San Hipólito recruited the help of the mentally ill patients, who, in their limited capacities, could assist only in the burial of corpses.[28]

Cabrera's characterization of the relief effort, while informed by immediate events, nonetheless looked nostalgically to the baroque charity of earlier times, marked by its lavish rituals, effusive displays of piety, and communal spirit. That hospital service had deteriorated to inadequate standards is demonstrated by the fact that just two years after the epidemic that earned the *hipólitos* praise in Cabrera's eyes, the viceroy-archbishop Vizarrón had penned his scathing report to the Council of Indies decrying the brothers for their vices and negligence and portraying their institutions as the most inhospitable of places.

Called in to settle a protracted dispute among rival members within the order, Vizarrón depicted a brotherhood that was plagued by factionalism and corruption, and on the brink of collapse. With palpable ire and disdain, he denounced many of the order's members, accusing them of sins ranging from apostasy to sodomy.[29] Of the *hipólitos*' four monastic vows, the most violated, according to Vizarrón, was the cherished vow to hospitality. He minced no words in portraying the appalling conditions of the San Hipólito hospitals, stating that "the patients in the hospitals are very poorly assisted that a great number of them die because they receive little to no care from these brothers, [and] lack nourishment and medicines to treat their illnesses." Poverty was endemic, mostly because the careless brothers squandered the hospital funds in "games, foolish activities, [and] idle pursuits," leaving the institutions bereft of money to properly feed, clothe, and medically treat the ill. Further, with the funds dissipated, the order lacked any means to repair the hospital buildings, which showed signs of "much deterioration." The patients suffered neglect and in the saddest of situations died unassisted, without witnesses and spiritual comfort. Once dead, the brothers stripped them entirely of their possessions, often to such extremes that they buried the dead completely naked. If the hospitals had fulfilled a spiritual mandate in the sixteenth century, now their wretched conditions "endangered the soul"—and certainly the body—of the suffering.[30]

Vizarrón's report represented a turning point in the history of San Hipólito and its religious personnel. His call for the order's abolishment revealed the extreme actions church and state authorities were willing to take in their resolve to revitalize Catholicism and its institutions. It also disclosed fissures within the order itself. While certain members wholly resisted mounting church and state oversight, a faction led by members José Balbuena and Felipe Barberá devised a plan for reform that was ultimately approved by both crown and papacy.[31] The Bourbon period is often portrayed as a time when church and state antipathy intensified as the crown pursued policies that undermined the composite monarchy that had granted the church considerable power over local affairs. The church, however, was not necessarily resistant to change and fashioned reform projects of its own to regenerate religious life, welcoming the muscle of the state when it suited these designs.[32] In New Spain as in the Spanish Empire more widely, the path to enlightenment would entail a serious rethinking of Catholicism, both its institutions and its practices, which extended to the domain of religious nursing and medical charity.

The reform of the Order of San Hipólito constituted part of what some scholars have characterized as a "Catholic Enlightenment"—that is, a concerted movement on the part of church thinkers and officials to "reconcile Catholicism with modern culture."[33] In keeping with the tenor of eighteenth-century Catholic reformism, the reform looked backward to the Council of Trent and its call for strict observance and greater austerity. It sought to root out worldly vice among the brothers and restore the order to the "vows, statutes, and rules of the *vida común*," or the communal way of life.[34] Eighteenth-century religious reformers aimed to revitalize many of the ideals of Trent, especially those concerned with moral rigor and spiritual discipline, while ridding the church of the sensual excesses that had become a hallmark of Counter-Reformation piety and a major target of the Enlightenment critique of Catholicism.[35] In 1743, Benedict XIV entrusted Vizarrón with the task of overseeing the reform, along with Balbuena and Barberá. However, due to Vizarrón's death in 1747, his duties were eventually assumed by the visitor-general, Francisco Javier Gómez de Cervantes.

Aside from reinforcing monastic discipline and punishing brothers who strayed from its strict lifestyle, the reforms targeted the order's finances and introduced a system of surveillance and accountability. One of Cervantes's first acts was the appointment of an official bookkeeper (*procurador conventual*) to oversee the order's income, including the rent accrued from its dwindling estates, the contributions collected during mass, and especially the activities of the public alms seekers (*demandantes*). Confirming an accusation made earlier by Vizzarón, Balbuena and Barberá had unearthed widespread abuse surrounding the tradition of soliciting alms and accused many brothers of hoarding money for personal profit through "false devotion."[36] These accusations echoed the Bourbon critique of begging and its associated vices, reflecting widespread fears that traditional forms of collecting and distributing charity had fallen into rampant corruption.[37] Since the reformers could do little to increase the returns from the order's investments, they focused their energies mostly on restoring integrity to this much-abused system. Thus, Cervantes ordered that the number of *demandantes* be reduced to four "to avoid the nuisance caused to the public by the multiplicity of beggars, and the disorder and idleness of these [individuals]."[38] He specified that the *demandantes* be chosen from among the order's most virtuous members and demanded they circulate in pairs—never alone—on the streets, in plazas and other public venues, and door to door. They would also carry a license with them at all times, thus identifying themselves as legitimate beggars in a society where begging was becoming increasingly suspect. The reformers also took care to preserve a tradition long ago introduced by Bernardino Alvarez whereby the religious solicited charity in the accompaniment of San Hipólito's mad patients, whose presence was supposed to elicit both the sympathy and the generosity of the public. Reviving this practice, they appointed two *pobres dementes*, Joseph Zedillo and Manuel Villegas, to accompany the *demandantes* and carry a special collections box decorated with the sacred image of Our Lady of Charity.[39]

Ultimately, these reformist efforts, which unfolded over a fifteen-year period, achieved only modest success. Although Cervantes, like Vizzarón before him, cited stubborn impiety and deeply rooted vice as the source of the problem, the reforms failed to enact dramatic change for more pragmatic reasons, such as the failure to generate additional sources of income and prohibitions placed on the admittance of novices, which had resulted in a diminution of nurses and consequently inferior hospital care.[40] However, San Hipólito's fortunes took a serious turn for the better in the 1760s with the appointment of friar José de la Peña, who succeeded Barberá as the prior general of the Order of San Hipólito. Peña's ascension to the office followed close on the heels of the crown's decision to reinstate the admittance of novices into the order, thus ensuring a future generation of nurses. Fueled by this positive momentum, Peña enforced stricter adherence to the monastic codes of conduct. In particular, he was rigorously attentive to the brothers' mode of dress, ensuring that it was modest and without any superfluous adornment, and expressly forbid the brothers from owning possessions. Furthermore, he encouraged the study of surgery among the order's members as the "most useful exercise" to facilitate hospitality, a move that would make the hospital less dependent on outside practitioners whose salaries it could rarely if ever afford. Finally, Peña concentrated his energies on organizing the hospital's finances by establishing a syndicate in 1768 to oversee all economic matters.[41]

In many respects, Peña was more effective in his first four years in office than his predecessors had been in over a decade. But even for Peña, who scrutinized every aspect of the order, there were limits as to what he could achieve. And as he strained against them, he looked outside the order, and even the church, to the colonial state for help in rebuilding and even transforming San Hipólito.

The Prior's Plea

Peña's tenure as prior general of the Order of San Hipólito coincided with the reign of Charles III (1759–88), who implemented some of the more aggressive and extreme policies of the Bourbon reforms. Influenced by Enlightenment rationalism, financial expediency, and a desire to return the Spanish Empire to its former glory, Charles III and his successor, Charles IV (1788–1808), oversaw a wholesale reorganization of the empire with the goal of governing with more efficiency and centralizing secular rule. As Adam Warren has discussed, the political rhetoric of the Bourbon crown—its emphasis on efficiency, rationalism, and the utility of scientific and medical knowledge—coupled with its growing intrusion in church affairs, created an opportunity for enterprising physicians to enhance their professional authority and penetrate the religious space of the hospital.[42] However, here it was Peña, the most powerful and respected spokesperson for religious traditions for managing madness, who carefully latched on to the rhetoric and logic of state expansion in a strategic bid to ameliorate the hospital's financial distress and enact larger transformational change.

Reform-minded clerics like Peña knew their institutions needed dire rejuvenation but they could not enact compelling long-term change without the financial muscle of the state and private sector. Peña's first line of defense on the path to revive San Hipólito was the *ayuntamiento* (city council). In

1764, he tactically approached the council for financial succor. His plea emphasized San Hipólito's parlous financial situation, the pitiful conditions of hospital life, and the shortcomings of traditional medical charity. Charitable donations were "limited," barely covering half of the hospital's total expenditures; meanwhile, the number of patients consistently exceeded eighty. To exacerbate the situation, the hospital had suffered a shortage of personnel, due not only to the (only recently lifted) prohibition against admitting novices but to the fact that many of the servants had fled San Hipólito "fearing the risks" associated with caring for the mad, which he admitted was a "very laborious, dangerous, and hazardous" task. Attending to the *locos furiosos* was particularly trying, for their "fury wreaked the greatest havoc," he claimed, and "many brothers had died at their hands." He added that dressing *furiosos* was financially onerous because they often tore their own clothing to shreds during violent episodes.[43] Moreover, the furiously insane damaged the already deteriorated hospital building more than any other group, imposing an additional financial burden and health hazard.[44]

The prior general also voiced frustration that San Hipólito had come to be stigmatized and viewed by the general public as an institution of last resort. "It has been observed," he stated, "that for those individuals who fall into the dreadful state of demencia, and have the resources to maintain and support their treatment, they are placed by relatives in other hospitals where they are received until all their possessions are consumed, or their relatives stop their contributions, and then they are abandoned as a last resort in this [hospital]."[45] The prior's main concern here was money: only by admitting wealthier patients could San Hipólito ensure that its services were self-sustaining. Peña thus beseeched the municipal government to issue an order prohibiting other institutions in the capital from accepting mad patients so that, he stated, "they must come to *this* [hospital] be they poor or rich." He went further, requesting that he be entrusted with the privilege of managing any personal possessions belonging to wealthier inmates to "ensure that their preservation or distribution was to the benefit of the patient."[46] Assuaging anxieties about the social and racial mixing of the rich and poor inmates, he asserted that patients of higher status would be treated, clothed, and fed with "corresponding distinction."[47]

In many ways, Peña's requests were unprecedented, but he couched them in terms sure to appeal to the *ayuntamiento*. In particular, he latched on to the Enlightenment rhetoric of utility, articulating the numerous ways San Hipólito contributed to the *beneficio común* (public good). For instance, he emphasized the hospital's role in keeping not just the city but the entire kingdom orderly—or "clean," as he put it—as the institution was the "only receptacle" where the mentally ill were sent "by mandate of the justices, or by the willingness of their dependents, parents, wives, brothers, or relatives."[48] The hospital performed an invaluable service to the state in confining violent patients who were, in the prior's words, potentially poised to commit "many atrocities without the remedy of punishment, since [they] lacked *culpa* [guilt]." Here Peña alluded to San Hipólito's growing use as an outlet for the criminally insane, an attractive alternative to prisons, yoking these services to the *ayuntamiento*'s desire for social stability and order. Moreover, it was not just that the hospital took in problematic citizens poised to commit violent crimes; San Hipólito was the city's best hope for curing the insane.[49] As Peña noted, when the hospital had possessed the necessary funds to afford daily visits from a physician, it had achieved remarkable success in "restoring certain [inmates] to perfect sanity."[50]

As Peña's appeal elucidates, the move to modernize traditional health care stemmed not only from reform-minded state bureaucrats or physicians but from the religious themselves who reenvisioned the hospital's role and purpose in colonial society. Whether the prior's plea reflected genuine sentiment or tactical jockeying for money is hard to say. Nevertheless, his efforts to attract greater state funding necessitated negotiations over the hospital's institutional mission. Skillfully, he reframed the hospital's mandate to shelter and care for *pobres dementes*, originally conceived in purely religious terms, as a necessary public service that the government should provide. Moreover, in seeking to attract a higher number of paying clients, he aspired to extend the hospital's reach to the public at large, extract greater profit, and rescue the hospital's reputation from its association with wretchedness and destitution. In referencing San Hipólito's potential to cure patients, he deviated from traditional notions of *curar* (to cure) as encompassing caring and nursing for the sick to the eighteenth-century idea of "cure" as employing medical ideas and technologies to achieve recovery.[51] The prior general's vision was ambitious—perhaps too ambitious—but as with the Hispanic Enlightenment more broadly, he sought a compromise between tradition and innovation, and a greater collaboration between church and state in the name of progress.

The prior's plea was ultimately compelling. While the hospital technically lay outside the *ayuntamiento*'s jurisdiction—which included only financial responsibility for the repair and maintenance of the Church of San Hipólito and monetary contributions for its annual festivities—Peña had succeeded in stretching the limits of the city council's role to encompass a civic obligation to the "miserable *pobres* who needed their support."[52] In 1766, the *ayuntamiento* agreed to assign the hospital a *tabla de carniceria* (a tax on the butchering of cattle), which would yield 1,000 pesos annually to help finance the food and care of the hospital's poorest patients. In addition, it granted the institution four employees to begin working on the most critical repairs to the hospital's main building. Most importantly, it was the *ayuntamiento*, in collaboration with Peña, that rediscovered the 1601 mandate that decreed that all mad individuals in the kingdom who needed hospital care be brought to San Hipólito, including propertied patients who would be compelled to use their own wealth to support their hospitalization.[53] The city council agreed on the urgency of bringing this discovery to the viceroy's attention, as the decree would no doubt catapult the hospital's reputation and shore up its finances.

Despite these achievements, Peña's lobbying with the city had little to show for itself in the end. The city contributed only a small token amount, far too little to alleviate San Hipólito's financial woes. It was not long before money was once again stretched thin; and although Peña had established a syndicate to oversee the hospital's income and prevent the pilfering of alms, members of its governing board frequently resigned their posts, finding the implicit obligation to donate their private wealth in order to keep the hospital afloat onerous.[54] Moreover, the four construction workers allotted to the hospital by the city government could only introduce the most minimal of improvements to the building, which showed the devastating signs of nearly two centuries of wear and tear, as well as the 1754 earthquake that had convulsed its floors and foundation.[55] Peña was far from defeated, however, and began targeting an even more powerful ally: viceroy Bucareli.

Remaking the Colonial Mental Hospital

San Hipólito's renovation materialized through a complicated alliance between church, state, and society and their variously shared and competing agendas. In appealing to the municipal government and then to the viceroy for greater involvement, the prior general had not only reframed the hospital's spiritual mandate in secular terms but also, wittingly or not, signaled San Hipólito's alignment with the Bourbon crown's agenda to solidify its rule over its overseas possessions and govern colonial society according to the ideals of order, efficiency, and rationalism. From its reordered finances to its finished and expanded building, the remaking of San Hipólito in many ways mirrored the successes and limitations of enlightened state reforms to modernize and rationalize the distribution of charitable and medical resources.

A major actor in the unfolding saga was viceroy Bucareli. A peninsular Spaniard who pledged loyalty directly to the king of Spain, Bucareli implemented many of the crown's reforms during his tenure as viceroy. Significantly, around the time Peña alerted him to San Hipólito's plight, he was also overseeing the establishment of Mexico City's Poor House (Hospicio de Pobres), a project that epitomized the crown's investment in overhauling traditional forms of charity. When the Poor House opened in 1774, three years before San Hipólito's reopening, it represented a radical attempt to desacralize poverty and secularize the culture of almsgiving. Accompanying the Poor House establishment was draconian legislation that outlawed begging and categorized paupers according to their "worthiness," with the "unworthy" beggars (*mendigos falsos*) forced into labor, and the "deserving" ones (*verdaderos pobres*) confined inside the Poor House. Bourbon officials optimistically believed these extreme measures would combat perceived levels of escalating vagrancy, eradicate poverty, and render the colony more economically viable.[56] To be sure, San Hipólito never formed a direct part of the campaign to institutionalize paupers—nor were *pobres dementes* singled out as vagrants in need of discipline—but the viceroy did see fit to expand and rebuild its edifice anew, seeing its resurrection as essential to restoring order and grandeur to the capital city, and improving public health services.

Plans to renovate the hospital were already under negotiation when a second earthquake in the summer of 1773 dealt its main building a disastrous blow. Although none of the patients were harmed, the quake violently shook the hospital's walls and foundation. The architects, Idelfonso de Iniesta Bejarano and Lorenzo Rodriguez, surveyed the premises shortly after the quake and warned of the institution's imminent ruin.[57] Spurred by the persuasive pleas of Peña, Bucareli took the warning to heart and used the authority of his office to expand and accelerate the hospital's remodeling. In his letter to the minister of the Indies, he emphatically stated that it would be of great service to "this opulent city and even all of the kingdom for the ill of this class to have a secure hospital to facilitate their relief, assistance, and cure."[58]

The utility of the project could not be denied, but how to finance it was a thornier matter. Although the crown renewed its interest and paternalistic concern for the plight of the *pobres dementes*, readily granting royal approval of the reconstruction, it lacked the resources to fund a complete rebuild alone.[59] The *ayuntamiento* had agreed to supply the 7,000 pesos needed for the repairs to the church and sacristy, plus up to 2,000 pesos for the hospital's rebuilding, which it had estimated would amount to 40,000 pesos. To cover the bulk of the costs, the viceroy solicited the support of a wealthy private party, the capital's merchants' guild (*consulado*). On August 29, 1773, the *consulado* voted unanimously to sponsor San Hipólito's renovation "to its complete perfection," describing the venture as a worthy "contribution to the happiness of the monarchy." Two of its most esteemed members, Don Ambrosio Meave and Don José González Calderón, were appointed to guide the project into completion.[60]

Deliberations over finances did not stop there. A rejuvenated building would simply not be enough to revive San Hipólito; what the hospital desperately needed was a strengthened and durable financial infrastructure that would enable it to sustain its daily activities without dependence on desultory charity. Although the brothers of San Hipólito would continue the time-worn tradition of soliciting alms on the streets of the city, the viceroy and municipal government negotiated further arrangements to secure more stable funding. The *tabla de carnicería* assigned to the hospital by the *ayuntamiento* would continue to provide an annual sum of 1,000 pesos. In addition, the hospital could rely on the support of the Congregación de la Purísima, which had earlier created an endowment in honor of the *pobres dementes*. On top of that, the city proposed allotting the hospital proceeds from two additional sources: the *temporalidades*, assets formerly belonging to the Jesuits but confiscated by the state during their 1767 expulsion, arguably an exercise in enlightened state power; and the *gremio de panaderos* (public granary). In his 1776 *instrucción* (instruction) to the viceroy regarding the particulars of San Hipólito's renovation, Charles III voiced his approval of these funding strategies, which in truth were not totally new but rather a continuation of a long-standing tradition whereby institutions of charity enjoyed mixed sources of income from public, private, and ecclesiastical bodies.[61]

The novelty resided in a formerly derelict and bankrupt institution receiving heightened public awareness of its utility and financial demands. The remodel—or, more precisely, rebirth—of San Hipólito also brought out new ideas and sources of support, as when the city council proposed that the other cities, villages, and pueblos of the jurisdiction should be required to contribute a fixed annual pension toward the patients' food and clothing, since the hospital's services extended well beyond the capital's limits.[62] In 1776, the viceroy, backed by royal endorsement, enforced this stipulation through an official document that circulated throughout the neighboring municipalities, reminding local officials of their vested interest in supporting an institution that promoted the peace and order of their respective communities.[63] While these new funding strategies did not eradicate the hospital's dependence on alms, the collection of pensions from neighboring areas marked a concerted attempt to "rationalize the distribution of assistance."[64]

Finally, these efforts to bolster and reorganize San Hipólito's financial apparatus targeted the hospital's Indigenous patients. Since its inception, San Hipólito had welcomed Indigenous patients into its facilities, as the Royal Indian Hospital lacked appropriate accommodations for the insane. However, no specific provisions existed to finance the care of this small but growing minority of inmates, even though the Royal Indian Hospital possessed solid funding from the crown and Indian tribute. Everyone involved in San Hipólito's remodeling and reorganization agreed that this was a problem that could be easily remedied: either the Indigenous patients of San Hipólito should be promptly transferred to the Royal Indian Hospital, or San Hipólito should be duly compensated for these services, which lay outside the traditional economy of charity. The administrator of the Royal Indian Hospital favored the latter option, citing not only the hospital's lack of cages to restrain unruly patients but the comfort and security of the other occupants. Thus, from then on, the administrator of the Royal Indian Hospital would be required to keep a monthly tally of the number of Indigenous patients hospitalized at San Hipólito and pay the institution approximately one and a half reales per inmate per day.[65] It was not much, but it signaled that the days of sloppy accounting, unwritten understandings, and relying solely on Christian charity were over. After 1776, medical care would begin to have a clear (or, at least, clearer) price associated with it, at least for certain patients.

Although deliberations over funding were protracted, the hospital's physical remodeling was relatively quick, taking just two years. Significantly, the hospital celebrated its debut on Charles III's birthday. Whereas earlier festivities centered around the feast day of St. Hippolytus had recounted the conquest and the triumph of Christianity over paganism, here the hospital tied its renovation and reopening directly to the Bourbon king's bounty. After the celebration, both the viceroy and visitor-general Gálvez sent letters to the king that described the "fortitude" of the new building and applauded the efforts of the *consulado* in erecting an institution that, in their opinion, far surpassed the hospitals of Europe.[66] In truth, the *consulado*'s donation of 14,000 pesos was modest when compared to the total cost of the renovation, which had exceeded the initial estimate of 40,000, totaling instead 61,832. Don José González Calderón furnished the remaining sum out of pocket and was subsequently reimbursed by the viceroy, who extracted the funds from the *avería*, a tax imposed on merchant-convoys.[67]

Given the original building's dismal condition on the eve of its renovation, any repairs would have amounted to an improvement. However, this was no small touch-up but rather a reimagining of what the hospital could be. The municipal government, which had commissioned the surveying of the original building, found it to be wholly inadequate. In addition to structural issues, it was far too small, barely accommodating sixty-six wooden *jaulas* (cages) to confine the *furiosos*.[68] While this number may have been acceptable in earlier times, it was now ill-suited for an institution whose operations had expanded and were growing each day.

Bigger and more spacious, the new hospital addressed this chief concern. Mexican historian Josefina Muriel has suggested that the main architect, whose identity remains unknown, took the inmates' comfort and humanity into consideration when he redesigned the facility.[69] He did away with the large wards that kept inmates chained to their beds and the *jaulas* that caged them like animals and, in their place, introduced small rooms that granted the inmates not only the luxury of privacy but the freedom of movement.[70] But benevolence and humanistic concern alone do not explain the new layout of the private cells; financial motives also came into play. Given the prior general's ambitions to admit patients of higher social standing, the individual rooms were also meant to temper misgivings about the mixing of clients of different social and racial classes. Moreover, though the private cells were certainly an improvement over earlier wards, how much of an improvement is unclear. Juan de Viera, in his firsthand account of the hospital, referred to the rooms as "cages," and one could imagine that these cramped and dark quarters would come to evoke the oppressiveness of prison cells. Viera further noted that while the rooms flaunted doors of the "finest cedar," they also possessed tiny prison-like windows (*troneras*) used to deliver food to the *furiosos*, thus sparing the nurses the danger of direct contact.[71]

The private cells constituted a novel development that implied a new approach to the management of mental disease. However, the building itself, with its emphasis on the interlacing of sacred and medical spaces, did not signal a radical departure from traditional forms of hospital care and architecture. Although the new design severed the infirmary from the convent, both structures nevertheless remained connected through a small hallway, which granted the brothers easy access to the patients and enforced the traditional linkage between monastic and hospital life. A ground sketch of the remodeled facility originally submitted by the viceroy to the king of Spain (figure 2.1) illustrates that the new building was a single two-storied rectangular structure that unfolded around two large airy patios, which were

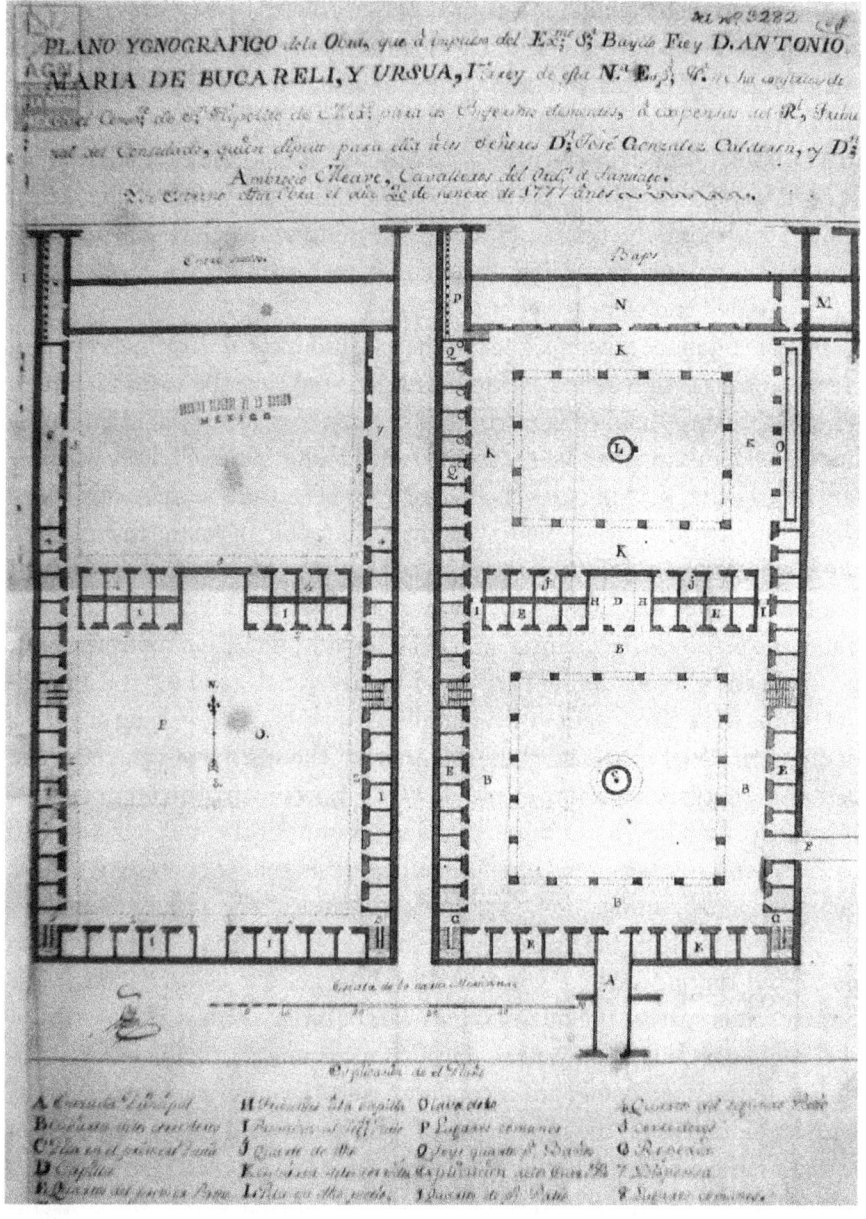

FIGURE 2.1 San Hipólito's remodeled ground design, ca. 1777.
Source: c de Virreyes, 1a serie, vol. 96, exp. 1.

Key to plan:

A Main entrance
B arched hallway
C fountain in 1st patio
D chapel
E individual rooms
F hallway to convent
G stairs
H platform to chapel
I passageways to second patio
J individual rooms
K arched hallway
L fountain in 2nd patio
M kitchen
N dining room
O laundry room
P communal spaces
Q six bathrooms
1 individual rooms
2 walkway
3 stairs
4 individual rooms
5 walkway
6 closet
7 pantry
8 communal spaces

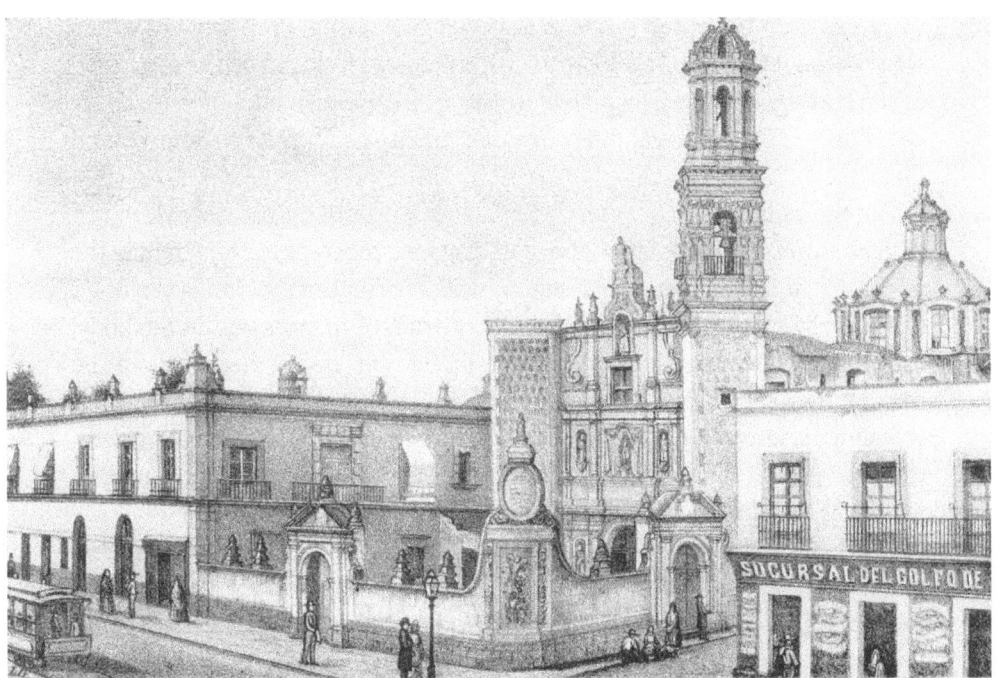

FIGURE 2.2 Nineteenth-century lithograph of Church and Hospital de San Hipólito. Source: Manuel Riveras Cambas, *México pintoresco, artístico y monumental* (Imprenta de la Reforma, 1880–83). Courtesy of the Getty Institute.

flanked by classical archways. The private cells filled both stories, with their small *troneras* facing inward toward the patios; the patios displayed freshwater fountains at their centers. Both floors of the building were lined with ample corridors that enabled the nurses to efficiently feed and care for the inmates. While the building's design (like that of its predecessor) did not adopt the popular cruciform plan that was common in hospitals of Roman Catholic countries, its layout unfolded according to a similar logic: namely, the central positioning of the chapel between both patios, whose convenient location enabled patients who were confined to their cells to hear the mass.[72]

Contemporaries lauded the renovated edifice as a pleasing sight that enhanced the beauty and grandeur of the viceregal capital. Figure 2.2, a nineteenth-century lithograph of the church's and hospital's facade, shows that the exterior of the remodeled building betrayed little indication of its status as an institution designed to confine the insane. Instead, its simple but elegant architecture blended seamlessly into the urban tapestry of the capital, marked by ubiquitous churches, palatial buildings, and active commerce; in fact, the ground floor exterior contained several *asesorías* (offices) that were meant to be rented out to artisans or businesses, the profits of which would benefit the hospital.[73] The main entrance was located on the south end of the building. To the far north were the dining room and kitchen (both located on the ground level) and the common areas (on the first and second floors).

But the building was not merely aesthetically pleasing; it had been designed with an emphasis on hygiene. Above all, hygienic concerns were evident in the building's large and open construction, which permitted the circulation of air and thereby prevented the harmful putrefaction of humors within the body; its numerous bathrooms (a total of six, located on the northeast side of the building); and, opposite the bathrooms, its large *lavendera* (laundry room) for washing the inmates' soiled clothes and bed linens. Even the two patios, with their glistening fountains and verdant gardens, served a therapeutic function, providing ambulatory patients with comfort and solace.[74]

Taken together, the hospital's design and spatial arrangement all bore testament to a reformed and revitalized institution. This was certainly the impression of San Hipólito provided by Juan de Viera, priest and director of the Colegio de San Idelfonso, when he visited the newly reopened institution:

> On the first floor it has a curiously tidy and devout chapel, with a railing that serves as a door so that the *dementes* that are experiencing fits can hear the mass from outside.
>
> It possesses a refectory where with great comfort it can hold up to two-hundred *dementes*, with sturdy tables and benches to eat and dine, and it is pleasing to attend lunch or dinner there, for although only those who are tolerable and not violent can attend, [the patients] are usually very grateful. The brothers serve them food with great humility and modesty, and while they consume lunch or dinner one brother sings the Christian doctrine in a very somber tone, having a catechism at hand. The kitchen is a gorgeous room with all its conveniences, and before entering it there is another room that serves as a bakery with a semi-circular coffered ceiling and many shelves of crockery for the service.[75]

At the time of Viera's visit, the hospital comfortably housed over 140 inmates. The way the *dementes* "subjected themselves with such care and respect" to the orders of the religious *niño* (boy), who apparently looked after them the day Viera visited, was truly a "marvel," Viera claimed with palpable admiration.[76] Its orderly spaces and novel luxuries captivated the Jesuit priest, who, downplaying the *furiosos* locked inside their cells, portrayed the institution in the most flattering terms: as a model of Bourbon order and enlightened piety.

After 1776, the state invested itself in the mental care of its colonial subjects like it never had during the previous two centuries. This was in many respects a monumental shift that marked the incipient secularization and modernization of hospital care. In spite of these efforts, however, straitened circumstances in terms of finances remained a serious problem for San Hipólito. For all its lofty ambitious and grandiose rhetoric, the pecuniary crown was never fiscally strong enough to support the hospital in full, and San Hipólito persisted to struggle financially in the decades that followed, beholden to the culture of almsgiving to sustain its activities.

Evidence of continued fiscal stress comes from a 1794 exchange between viceroy Revillagigedo and Peña's successor as prior general, friar José de Castro. In the previous year, the viceroy had ordered the hospital to discontinue the practice of welcoming spectators into the hospital's infirmaries on the feast days of the Holy Innocents and Saint Hippolytus for the purpose of soliciting charitable donations. Such spectacles, he reasoned, only served to disrupt "good order," "irritate" the hospital's patients, and turn them into the laughingstock of the city.[77] However, the following year the prior general begged Revillagigedo to reconsider, his persuasive plea hinging on an issue of deep importance to both the hospital and viceroy—money. According to Castro, the act of shunning visitors on both the day of the Holy Innocents and on the feast day of the hospital's own patron saint had the effect of "hardening" (*resfriar*) the charitable goodwill of the faithful citizens of Mexico, who were not able to behold the "sight of the objects worthy of their compassion such as these poor miserable [patients]," for whom he also claimed the festivities served as a healthy form of distraction and respite.[78] Clearly aware of the financial burden San Hipólito posed to the state should it fail to stay afloat, Revillagigedo ultimately rescinded his previous decree, condoning the hospital's participation in the public festivals on the condition that its personnel exercise the utmost "zeal and vigilance" to avoid any "disorder."[79] As was the case in many aspects of the Bourbon reforms, when new half-hearted practices stumbled, tradition was the only available safety net.

The Patients of San Hipólito: The View from the Admissions List

It is difficult to gauge how and to what extent the hospital's physical reordering mirrored the reordering occurring within the hospital's walls. However, evidence of shifting institutional practices—as well as striking continuities—can be gleaned through close analysis of a remarkable source: a richly documented leather-bound notebook that comprises San Hipólito's most expansive surviving register of patient admissions (figure 2.3). Spanning the dates 1751–86, the register covers the critical decades before and after the hospital's renovation and physical expansion. In contrast to the registers discussed in chapter 1, these records cover a wider period and are far more sophisticated and standardized. In their depiction of the sheer effort taken to quantify and systematize the patient population, they embody the rationalism at the heart of the hospital's transformation and the Enlightenment project writ large.[80] And yet they also disclose how San Hipólito made an incomplete shift to more modern forms of hospital care with evidence of incipient medicalization.

A cursory perusal at the register showcases comprehensive bookkeeping that bears witness to greater attempts at systematic surveillance and accountability. The *enfermero mayor* (head nurse) who monitored patient admissions, identified as friar Felipe Ruiz, was an assiduous, detailed notetaker. Owing to tighter administrative organization and a proliferating body of patients to manage and account for, he recorded a host of information, including the patient's name and surname and date of arrival, with marginal notations on the date of death or release. He judiciously documented deaths by drawing a cross next to the name of the deceased, though he was largely reticent on recording the cause. He also remarked when a patient took flight—a not uncommon scenario. More sporadically, the *enfermero mayor* jotted down characteristics specific to each patient, such as his race, age, parentage, marital status, and place of origin. With respect to the patient's racial identity, at times he felt compelled to speculate ("*al parecer mulato*" [he appears to be a mulatto]). When the information was relevant or available, he also alluded to specific circumstances that provoked hospital confinement, mentioning, for instance, that an inmate had arrived at the recommendation of a local priest, with a medical certification, or by order of a law enforcement official. Finally, on an annual basis he dutifully tallied total admissions, deaths, and exits. Table 2.1 reproduces these calculations, plotting the flow of patients in and out of San Hipólito.

The registers confirm that the hospital's patient population did in fact swell. Yearly admissions remained consistently elevated both before and after its remodeling, with an all-time high of forty-two new admits in 1779. However, it is difficult to glean shifting or enduring institutional practices from

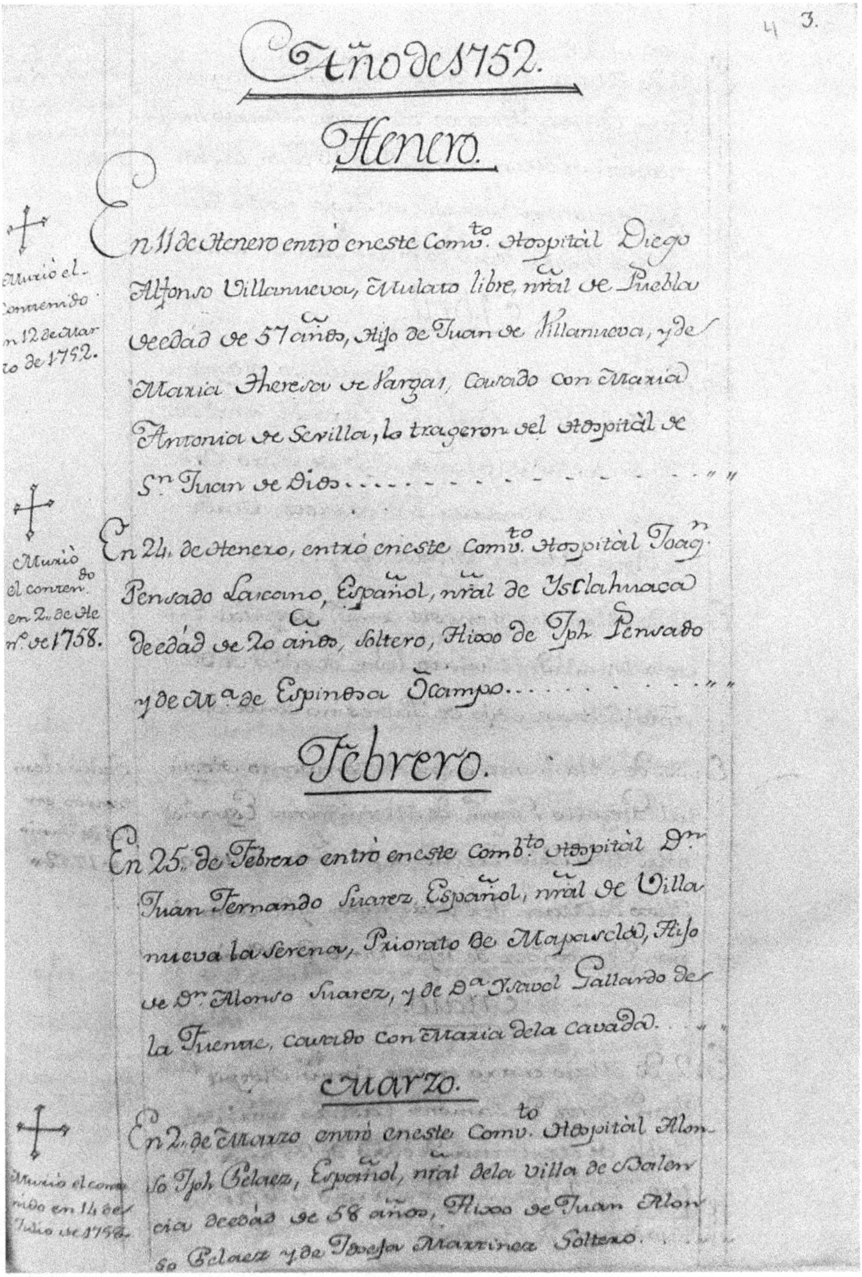

Año de 1752.

Henero.

† En 11 de Henero entró en este Comv.to Hospital Diego
Murió el Alfonso Villanueva, Mulato libre, n.ral de Puebla
contenido de edad de 57 años, Hijo de Juan de Villanueva, y de
en 12 de Mar-
zo de 1752. María Theresa de Vargas, Casado con María
Antonia de Sevilla, lo trageron del Hospital de
S.n Juan de Dios..................."

† En 24. de Henero, entró en este Comv.to Hospital Joaq.n
Murió Pensado Lascano, Español, n.ral de Ystlahuaca
el conven-
to en 2. de He- de edad de 20 años, soltero, Hixo de Joph. Pensado
n.o de 1758.
y de Ar.a de Espinosa Ocampo............"

Febrero.

En 25. de Febrero entró en este Comb.to Hospital D.n
Juan Fernando Suarez, Español, n.ral de Villa
nueva la Serena, Priorato de Magascela, Hijo
de D.n Alonso Suarez, y de D.a Ysavel Gallardo de
la Fuente, Casado con María de la Cavada..."

Marzo.

† En 2. de Marzo entró en este Comv.to Hospital Alon-
Murió el conte- so Joph. Pelaez, Español, n.ral de la Villa de Balen-
nido en 14 de
Julio de 1752. cia de edad de 58 años, Hixo de Juan Alonso Pelaez y de Josefa Marrinea Soltero.

FIGURE 2.3 Representative patient register, January–March, 1752.
Source: AGN, Indiferente Virreinal, caja 4951, exp. 47.

TABLE 2.1 Records of admissions, discharges, and deaths at the Hospital de San Hipólito, 1751–1785*

Year	Admitted	Discharged	Died
1751	15	7	0
1752	19	3	8
1753	28	12	7
1754	39	15	16
1755	37	20	12
1756	27	13	8
1757	20	11	8
1758	18	8	8
1759	19	7	10
1760	27	12	11
1761	26	7	9
1762	22	5	6
1763	11	3	6
1764	21	8	9
1765	22	12	7
1766	15	4	10
1767	23	8	10
1768	20	8	9
1769	21	13	6
1770	34	22	6
1771	21	10	9
1772	18	8	10
1773	18	6	4
1774	21	1	7
1775	29	10	10
1776	30	15	12
1777	30	14	13
1778	36	15	10
1779	42	15	17
1780	23	5	13
1781	26	6	8
1782	34	14	16
1783	34	10	13
1784	35	4	11
1785	25	1	4

*1786 is not included because its records are incomplete.
Source: AGN, Indiferente Virreinal, caja 1005, exp. 5; caja 4951, exp. 47.

the expanding size of the patient population alone. One must look to other factors.

To begin with, while more patients entered San Hipólito, many also left—with the brothers' blessing. Higher rates of patient turnover offer circumspect proof of the order's ability to treat madness as a medical condition and potentially even cure it. While it is difficult to gauge discharge rates from earlier registers, it is patently observable that long-term hospitalization had been the norm, and that for two centuries San Hipólito had been less a site of therapy than an eternal reclusion for the hopeless and forlorn—or the extremely dangerous—whose madness was incurable. By contrast, the later registers reveal that by 1750, the hospital had released a substantial fraction of patients within a couple of years to a few months—and, in some cases, even weeks or days—after admittance. For instance, Indigenous patient Lázaro Guzmán, admitted in the summer of 1751, resided at San Hipólito for only one month.[81] Francisco Gonzalez's 1754 internment was even shorter, lasting just twenty days.[82] Short-term hospitalizations can be interpreted in a number of ways. In part, they reflected the hospital's growing therapeutic capabilities and a shifting preference to admit milder or curable cases in greater numbers. Such a view is supported by the fact that, starting in the late 1770s, annotations recording exits began to remark that a particular client left the hospital in "good health" (*salio bueno*) and was reintegrated into society. In 1778, San Hipólito's most successful year in therapeutic terms, the hospital discharged fifteen patients; approximately eight were demarcated as leaving in "good health," most having been hospitalized between two years and less than one year.

Medicalization had its limits, however. If San Hipólito could make a modest claim to therapeutic efficacy, it continued to house the incurably mad for the long duration. The admissions records demonstrate that the pattern of chronic, extended internment endured well into the 1780s (and probably much later), even as certain patients were rapidly discharged. In 1768, Pablo de Aguilera, an *español* originally from Irapuato, was admitted to San Hipólito and died there seventeen years later.[83] Admitted in 1755, Indigenous patient Vicente Rafael spent a staggering forty-four years in confinement—from the age of thirty to seventy-four—before fleeing the hospital's premises in 1799.[84] Similar entries documenting the demise or exit of inmates who had been hospitalized for decades are scattered throughout the registers.

Moreover, while the discharge of recovered patients marked an important therapeutic milestone, not all who left San Hipólito may have done so in good health. Short-term hospitalizations may have been symptomatic of an institution strapped for resources and space and therefore driven to expel inmates prematurely. Rapid turnovers may also speak to the specific needs of the families of mentally disturbed kin who came to rely on the hospital's services intermittently. While the perspectives of spouses and relatives remain difficult to access from this terse document, marginal notations left by the *enfermero mayor* indicate that certain patients were often discharged at the behest of a relative. In addition, the *enfermero mayor's* varied scribblings disclose additional patterns. For instance, patients were sometimes discharged only to be readmitted later. Indeed, recidivism was common, with patients reentering San Hipólito up to five times, further casting a shadow of doubt on the hospital's therapeutic achievements. Finally, in addition to formal discharges, a number of exits recorded in the registers (roughly 11 percent) referred to inmates who had taken flight from the hospital clandestinely, an issue explicitly addressed in chapter 5.

The hospital's high mortality rate also adds complexity to this evolving portrait of hospital life. From midcentury on, an average of nine to ten mental patients died in the wards of San Hipólito each year (table 2.1). While it might be tempting to interpret this information as proof of poor conditions and rudimentary medical attention, resorting to age-old stereotypes of premodern medical institutions as unsanitary cesspits, high mortality was also a reflection of the type of patient San Hipólito admitted. Although the hospital appears to have made an effort to attract curable cases that could be efficiently treated and discharged, and while its rate of turnover certainly mounted, the institution still took in the severely debilitated and moribund as part of its utilitarian enterprise. This is illustrated by the surprisingly brief time span between date of admission and date of death in many of the entries, indicating that lots of patients reached the hospital in truly dire condition. On July 4, 1782, for example, Manuel Trinidad—a twenty-five-year-old Black slave—was transferred from the Hospital del Espiritu Santo to San Hipólito; he died just a week later.[85] Moreover, on at least two occasions, the *enfermero mayor* marked specific deaths as suicides. Next to the entry for Leandro Muñoz Montero, a *mestizo* of forty-five years of age, he wrote on August 29, 1760: "*Murió degollado por su propia mano*" (He died by cutting his own throat).[86] Similarly, in 1774 he noted that inmate José Antonio Robles, an *español* of twenty-one years of age, took his own life (*el mismo se mato*).[87] Brief but troubling references of this sort recall the intransigent nature of madness and the suffering it inflicted on its victims. By and large, however, most deaths were not suicides but chronically ill patients who died of natural causes.

However faltering San Hipólito's steps toward medicalization were, and however hard it was to shake off the practices of the past, change was coming—particularly from the outside. During the period the notebook covers, patients began to arrive with certificates of mental illness from trained medical practitioners—usually a licensed physician or surgeon, although one patient entered with a "plea of the apothecary."[88] This was a truly novel development that underscores the medicalization of both madness and the hospital. The earliest reference to a medical certificate appeared in 1755, when a Creole patient, Manuel Castil de Oro, was admitted and discharged just three months later.[89] Similarly, in 1773 José Cervantes arrived at the hospital with a certificate penned by the physician Bernardo Cortes, "who had been treating him of the madness he suffered."[90] The appearance of the medical certificate highlights an important new trend: namely, a nascent shift to define the criteria for admission in medical terms rather than by poverty or need alone.

And yet, as was the case with rates of turnover, older habits carried on. For all the patients who arrived with medical certificates, many more did not. The requirement for medical certification seems to have applied only to non-pauper candidates, or patients transferred from other hospitals or institutions, who bore the greater burden of demonstrating an urgent reason for internment. By that same token, not all formal endorsements came from medical men. Many patients arrived with letters of recommendation from local priests, judges, or esteemed members of the community. These letters of recommendation have not survived, so their contents remain a mystery, but they likely attested to a potential patient's personal background, family and financial circumstances, and mental state, presenting a compelling case for internment. For instance, in September 1779, the patient Nicolas de Olivares arrived with two *cartas* (letters): one from the local magistrate of the pueblo of Huamantla, located in the present-day state of Tlaxcala, and another from Franciscan friar Francisco José Rangel.[91] Similarly, in June 1762, the hospital received the mulatto patient Luis with a recommendation from the priest of Orizaba.[92] That the majority of recommendations came from parish priests is hardly surprising given the central role they played within the parish community, both as collectors and distributors of charity, and as practitioners of "spiritual physic"—that is, the use of prayer, confession, communion, and even exorcism as tools for alleviating a range of afflictions of the mind, body, and soul.[93] Letters from priests may very well have affirmed that the candidate in question was a good Christian who had recently confessed as well as disclosed more intimate details concerning the candidate's personal and emotional life. However, as with the medical certificates, not all patients appeared to have furnished these documents—or at least the *enfermero mayor* did not record that they had. Nevertheless, these references to accompanying letters of support indicate that the process of admitting patients was not arbitrary but based on the careful assessment of personal need and the severity of the condition. And at a time when the medical profession had not yet achieved a monopoly on madness and certainly lacked control over the hospital, a range of authorities held sway over who was admitted.

A closer look at the complex composition of the hospital's occupants further underscores the hospital's incomplete transformation. Table 2.2 provides an overview of the patients of San Hipólito, as identified on the basis of the various variables the head nurse provided. Taken together, this evidence underscores an important continuity noted in chapter 1: that the hospital's patient population was not homogeneous. However, by the late eighteenth century, the category of *pobre demente* had become even *more* malleable, accommodating diversity in status, means, age, occupation, and race. Indeed, it would appear from this evidence that the hospital's population was slowly shifting from *pobres dementes* as a socioeconomic group to *dementes* as a more expansive population defined in medical terms.

Put differently, nascent medicalization allowed for the expansion of the category of *pobre demente* without erasing its traditional connotations with poverty and the status of *miserable*. While one can reach this conclusion in a number of ways, it is difficult to do so on the basis of the racial composition of the patient population alone. While the *casta* system had crystallized in the eighteenth century in the form of the famous *casta* paintings, in social practice class and race no longer neatly mapped onto each other.[94] As with the earlier registers, *españoles* (mostly Creoles) continued to make up the largest constituency. Patients identified as *negros* made up a small minority, followed by Indigenous patients. The number of native patients more than doubled when contrasted to the registers from the earlier period, the outcome of tighter coordination between the Royal Indian Hospital and San Hipólito. Records from the Royal Indian Hospital (see table A.1 in the appendix) confirm this trend, indicating that San Hipólito housed anywhere between nine and twenty-eight Indigenous patients per month for the period between 1774 and 1799, with the highest concentration occurring between 1784 and 1786. Individuals of mixed racial background were a sizable minority comprising the following taxonomies: *mestizos, mulatos, moriscos, castizos*, a handful of light-skinned *mulatos* known as *pardos*, and one *coyote*.[95]

TABLE 2.2 Overview of San Hipolito's patients, 1751–1786

A. Race	Number	%
Español	493	54.9
Indio	99	11.0
Negro	8	0.9
Casta	147	16.4
Unspecified	151	16.8
B. Marital Status		
Single	361	40.2
Married	339	37.8
Widowed	53	5.9
Unspecified	145	16.1
C. Place of Origin		
Mexico City	221	24.6
Other cities/villages in New Spain	454	50.6
Spain	71	7.9
Other	8	0.9
Unspecified	144	16.0
D. Age Group		
14 and under	7	0.8
15–29	234	26.0
30–44	331	36.9
45–59	141	15.7
60 plus	39	4.3
Unspecified	146	16.3
E. Parentage		
Cited both parents	640	71.2
Cited one parent	25	2.8
Unspecified	233	26.0
F. Title		
Don	96	10.7
Untitled	802	89.3
Total Admissions	898	100.0

Source: AGN, Indiferente Virreinal, caja 4951, exp. 47.

Further evidence underscoring the social and economic diversity of the patient population can be deduced from other factors. For instance, the hospital admitted *huérfanos* (orphans) alongside patients who cited their parentage. A large portion of its occupants, which spanned all racial classes, made no mention of their parents whatsoever (*no dio razon de sus padres*) or claimed to be of "unknown parentage" (*padres no conocidos*), which was possibly a means to camouflage illegitimacy.[96] The *enfermero mayor* occasionally specified the patient's *oficio* (occupation), which included petty merchants, artisans such as carpenters, humble laborers like gardeners and mule drivers, and a substantial number of soldiers admitted at the behest of a military superior or by viceregal command. The register also documents the continued presence of patients who bore the honorific title "don." While patients bearing this title appeared sparingly in the early registers, by the eighteenth century their numbers had markedly increased.[97]

Alongside more respectable patients, San Hipólito continued to admit the city's most destitute and vulnerable inhabitants, *pobres dementes* in the most traditional sense. Scattered entries attest to their anonymity and helplessness, as the *enfermero mayor* admitted patients whom he referred to as "*este pobre*" (this poor one) or "*asimplado*" (this simpleton). Concerned citizens brought in some pauper patients after finding them ambling aimlessly through the streets. In 1772, for instance, the Indian Quintero Moreno was delivered to San Hipólito after he was spotted distastefully begging for alms near the Hospital de San Roque in Puebla.[98] Some came willingly or even by accident. On July 31, 1755, the *enfermero mayor* recorded the admission of a poor Spaniard named Juan Ballejo. "This poorman," he wrote, "was wandering through the streets, and by accident came to this hospital; moved by his cries and [out of] charity he was received."[99] Many were deposited by local priests or members of the regular clergy. In 1759, for instance, an *español* named Francisco Mora was admitted to San Hipólito for the fourth time at the request of the deacon of the Mexico City cathedral for provoking "inquietude" in church.[100] On another occasion, in 1786 the *enfermero mayor* recorded the arrival of four unnamed *pobres*, who were transferred from the Hospital de San Roque in Puebla by the brother Juan de Charola.[101]

Finally, to the hospital's expanding population one must add the inmates who arrived as prisoners accused of serious crimes or who had at least fallen afoul of colonial authorities in some capacity. Table A.2 in the appendix provides an overview of the inmates who were recorded to have entered the hospital through correctional outlets and any available details about their internment and identities. It shows that San Hipólito received offenders from all the major colonial institutions concerned with policing crimes, both religious and secular, and administering justice and order: namely, the Holy Office of the Inquisition; the high criminal court, or Real Audiencia (also listed as the Real Sala del Crimen); and the Tribunal of the Acordada, the latter being a law enforcement agency established in the eighteenth century to patrol highway banditry and regulate crime within the capital city. In addition, the *enfermero mayor* made numerous references to the arrival of inmates directly from public or royal jails and by mandate of the viceroy or any one of the array of lesser judicial officials operating at the district or local level, including *alcades mayores, alcaldes ordinarios, corregidores, tenientes*, and constables (*aguaciles*). The remaining three chapters more closely examine this phenomenon, showing a complicated process of the medicalization of mental disorder at work and the hospital's growing role as a site not only of medical attention but of confinement and protection.

SAN HIPÓLITO'S 1777 REOPENING represented its zenith. In many ways the hospital had come to embody the ambitions of the Enlightenment project as it was embraced by the crown and its agents who practiced enlightened administration in the name of progress, social utility, and rational order. So too did it reflect the church's desire to preserve traditional Catholic values and practices while adapting to a changing world marked by the growing threat of Protestantism and the anti-clerical sentiments of more radical Enlightenment thinkers. Under the aegis of church and state reform, the hospital enjoyed an unprecedented renovation that enabled it to serve a broader colonial population and survive well into the following century. However, beneath the surface of its pristine new edifice were abundant signs of continuity, of the hospital's intractable commitment to traditional forms of medical charity—a bond likely reinforced by the colonial population it served—and of persistent economic hardship as Spain fought a failed war with England.

Notably, San Hipólito carried all this out without the figures most commonly associated with the medical Enlightenment: university-trained physicians. Rather, it was clergy who reshaped, reinvented, and managed the madhouse. If the hospital could make a modest claim to therapeutic efficacy, it was at the hands of the religious, who practiced both medicine and pastoral forms of spiritual and custodial care. From the wards of San Hipólito, medicalization was incipient and incomplete, with physicians as marginal if not invisible actors. While doctors had begun to play a greater role in diagnosing sicknesses of the mind, their impact was felt most profoundly within the courts, but even there they had to contend with entrenched religious and legal institutions.

CHAPTER THREE

It Is Easy to Mistake a Heretic for a Madman

On a November afternoon in 1776, a mulatto miner named Teodoro Francisco de Aspe y Aguirre appeared before the headquarters of the Holy Office in Mexico City to formally declare himself a victim of *hechicería*, or witchcraft. During the span of five months, Aspe had experienced a series of unusual and perturbing "accidents," which a local physician in Taxco had assured him were the products of *hechisos*, or evil spells, rather than natural causes. To begin with, the tormented miner claimed to hear voices—these, he specified, were not verbal utterances but rather "internal locutions." He further complained of an "oppression," or tightness in his chest, and of suffering headaches every time he looked at a holy image. The headaches were intense—indeed, so much so that he could not help but wonder if there was "some living thing" residing inside his head, "impeding the use of [his] *potencias*," or mental faculties, and causing clouded judgment and "much confusion." Aspe also reported episodes of piercing bodily pain so agonizing he sensed himself being "stabbed by many lances." The corporeal symptoms of his bewitchment were accompanied by hallucinations; he recalled how he was startled from sleep one evening by the sound of a screaming cat and was horrified to find a "very formidable dragon" in the middle of his room. The demon "seemed to come from hell," he proclaimed, "and then it suddenly transformed into a turkey, and disappeared." When questioned by the friar and commissary of the Holy Office, Antonio García Navarro, about whom he suspected of evildoing, the distraught miner readily accused his estranged brother- and sister-in-law, Joaquín and Josefina Montoya, as well as a handful of neighbors, who would often appear before him in "imaginary" form, eerily whispering to him, "Save yourself, we are all condemned; condemn yourself, and we are all saved." By this, Aspe understood that his tormentors wanted him "to become a witch just like them" or else he would "pay with his life."[1]

In spite of the severity of his symptoms and his palpable anguish, the mulatto miner's denunciation was not taken seriously and abruptly dismissed within a month, his allegations reduced to little more than the "fantasies of a melancholic imagination."[2] Swaying the commissary's opinion that Aspe suffered from mental disturbance rather than bewitchment was a letter from a reputable source: Joseph de la Borda, Aspe's former employer in the mining district of Chontalpa, where he resided. De la Borda informed the Holy Office that Aspe was a devout Christian who regularly attended mass and took the sacraments, but he had unfortunately suffered a breakdown in health that previous summer. His deterioration began with a bout of jealousy directed toward his wife, Getrudis, whom he wrongfully suspected of infidelity. Gradually, his thoughts and actions became more extreme and erratic, to the point that he became fixated with the idea that a group of men were out to kill him. De la Borda blamed a "lack of reason" (*falta de juicio*) for the miner's unusual conduct, a sentiment echoed by a local physician summoned by Aspe's relatives who affirmed that the miner's "illness was madness, not *maleficio*." De la Borda went on to speculate that Aspe's condition was hereditary, inherited from his mother, a reputed madwoman who was tolerated by her community because she was not *furiosa*, or violently insane.[3]

With the case thus dismissed, the troubled miner slips from the historical record, leaving us to ponder his fate. Although inquisitors sometimes placed suspects deemed to be mentally disturbed into confinement at San Hipólito, in this particular instance they made no specifications for how Aspe was to be cared for. Beyond his misdirected allegations, he had committed no real crime and most likely returned home to Chontalpa with little comfort to assuage his addled and unpleasant thoughts. One might further speculate that given the gravity of his condition, he struggled to maintain steady employment and was in all likelihood cared for by relatives, including his alienated and allegedly adulterous wife, the original source of his ire and mental decline.

INQUISITION CASES HAVE LONG served historians well. Like Aspe, countless inhabitants of Spain's colonial possessions, faced with communal pressure to denounce religiously suspect behavior, flocked to the headquarters of the Holy Office in the capital city or to their nearest local representative, thus generating a hefty paper trail replete with denunciations that, when deemed legitimate, spawned elaborate trial transcripts and correspondence that traversed the Atlantic. These documents not only offer insight into the inner mechanisms of one of the empire's most notorious institutions but shed precious light on various aspects of the daily lives of colonial subjects, from religious beliefs to community relations to sexual practice. More generally, as Carlo Ginzburg long ago pointed out, these "archives of repression" capture, albeit imperfectly, the voices of the most humble and marginalized, individuals who otherwise would have been absent from the historical record.[4]

Inquisition documents also have plenty to say about madness as it was experienced by its victims and perceived by observers. Indeed, where hospital records fall short, Inquisition cases go the extra mile: Aspe's witchcraft denunciation almost approximates a patient's narrative, as he describes his symptoms in vivid detail, from his stinging bodily pain to his debilitating and confusing headaches and harrowing visions. In the absence of medical casebooks or personal memoirs capturing individual struggles with states of mental distress, documented testimonies of the kind provided by Aspe offer some of the most intimate glimpses into the coveted "patient's perspective" that has long eluded historians. Of course, here one must also be mindful to ways in which Inquisition documents consist of mediated accounts, produced for the purposes of investigating, regulating, and ultimately punishing unorthodox thoughts and practices, and likewise to their role in upholding Spain's "textual imperial power"—that is, the paperwork of the crown, judiciary, and church that maintained colonial rule.[5]

The lessons do not end there. From this brief case, which never made it to trial, we also learn a great deal about the wider social context in which San Hipólito operated: the networks of people affected by Aspe's condition, from his employer to his relatives and wife; the conflicting opinions of physicians, one believing him to be bewitched, the other confirming madness; the community's tolerance for his mad but nonviolent mother; and existing notions of mental disorder as an inherited condition. Finally, while the mulatto miner adamantly deemed himself bewitched, we can see that eighteenth-century inquisitors exercised a healthy dose of skepticism and could recognize the distinction between mental impairment as a physical disease and instances of bewitchment or diabolical possession.

This last point may come as a surprise given commonplace assumptions of the Holy Office as a vehicle of intolerance utterly enmeshed in an enchanted worldview infiltrated by satanic forces bent on corrupting the souls of vulnerable believers. However, it was precisely because they were in the business of interrogating the complexities of human interiority that the magistrates manning the Holy Office in New Spain were no strangers to madness in all its sundry variations. Occasionally they stumbled upon troubled minds, when individuals like Aspe appeared before them to denounce others—and sometimes themselves—for crimes they had only imagined. But this was the rarest of scenarios. More commonly, members of the community came forward to report religiously aberrant speech and behavior committed by others whom the Inquisition eventually came to suspect were not heretics but mentally unsound. It was generally custom for the inquisitorial courts to treat such suspects with leniency, as church doctrine held that all sin was voluntary. By this logic, the mentally impaired were virtually blameless, since they lacked the consciousness—or *juicio* (judgment)—to willfully attack the faith.[6] In an equally common albeit more complicated scenario, prisoners of the Holy Office charged or convicted of crimes committed in states of reasoned lucidity frequently lost their wits while detained in the dreaded and insalubrious secret prisons. Here, the circumstances provoking the loss of sanity are not difficult to fathom. Suspects could find themselves languishing in prison without knowing the charges against them, and interrogations could last for days, months, even years. Fear of punishment, infamy, the sequestration of property—to say nothing of the threat of torture—weighed heavily on the accused's mind and emotions. Faced with numerous instances in which suspects suffered altered mental states, inquisitors clearly understood that sanity was a slippery spectrum on which the accused resided and demonstrated a responsiveness to this complicated reality. Once they deemed someone who had formerly been sane to be insane, they extended to them all the protections of that designation, even though it inevitably complicated—stymied even—judicial proceedings.[7]

By the eighteenth century, the Inquisition increasingly dealt with the presence of *locura* in its courts by shipping allegedly mad suspects to hospitals, especially San Hipólito, for medical treatment and custodial surveillance. This outcome was not part of a deliberate effort to mass confine, discipline, or punish the mentally disturbed, as some might contend. Instead, it reflected a process of medicalization taking place in Enlightenment Mexico—a process in which, I argue in both this chapter and chapter 4, the Inquisition played an integral, if unexpected, part. The medicalization of *locura* in Mexican society—that is, the appeal to medical frameworks to explain irrational thought and behavior—has a long and complex history. Its origins can be traced to medieval Spain and the adoption of humoral medicine as a dominant paradigm, and its trajectory spans well into the late nineteenth century, when new theories of human cognition rooted in the modern science of psychiatry began to gain purchase among Porfirian positivists.[8] In this expansive timeline, the eighteenth century, especially the closing decades, looms large as a critical turning point. This period was marked not only by the expansion of hospital care for the mentally disturbed, as described in chapter 2, but also by greater appeal to medical expertise and medical theory within judicial settings to explain aberrant, offensive, or harmful actions. Thus, returning to the case of the tormented and allegedly bewitched mulatto miner, while perhaps a century earlier inquisitors might have accepted Aspe's accusation and version of events at face value, by the late eighteenth century they were more inclined to attribute such afflictions to an underlying medical cause—in this instance, the condition known as *melancolía* (melancholy).

How and why did the Inquisition, long considered the most backward and anti-rational of institutions, become a driving agent for the medicalization of madness in eighteenth-century New Spain? This chapter and chapter 4 set out to address this question. While chapter 4 delves more deeply into the complexities of medical diagnosis and the uses of San Hipólito for the purposes of treating and studying mental disorder, this chapter looks more broadly at the problem of *locura* within the inquisitorial courts, especially in light of the tribunal's long-standing preoccupation with human interiority as the key site for gauging guilt and sin.

More specifically, this chapter aims to complicate the notion of the Inquisition as an anti-Enlightenment institution staunchly opposed to the forces of rationalism and secularization.[9] To be sure, as a bastion of Catholic orthodoxy in the Americas tightly allied with state imperatives, the Holy Office operated in many ways as an "enemy of the Enlightenment," to borrow Darrin McMahon's coinage.[10] Indeed, many of the individuals that populate the following pages had fallen under the grip of the Holy Office precisely for spouting Enlightenment viewpoints that were not only religiously unorthodox but politically seditious. Nevertheless, as this chapter contends, when it came to identifying and managing *locura* in colonial subjects, it was the Inquisition that unwittingly found itself at the forefront in devising new modes for understanding the complexities of human reasoning and the nuances of intent. While such methods of discernment drew in no small part on theological concerns and practices, they also helped pave the way for the medicalization of madness in eighteenth-century New Spain and the growing use of the insanity defense as justifiable, indeed compelling, grounds for exonerating criminal liability.

The Inquisitor's Quandary: The Challenge of Madness in the Inquisitorial Courts

In recent decades, studies of the Inquisition, both in Spain and its American colonies, have challenged its characterization as the despotic institution of social repression that formed an integral part of the *leyenda negra* or "black legend."[11] While the Inquisition was certainly a force to be reckoned with, its activities were far more mundane than its reputation implies, operating "not [on] the presumption of heresy, but the conviction that the faithful needed instruction, correction, and discipline."[12] This was especially true of the Inquisition as it developed in the Spanish American colonies. Although the early tribunals that accompanied the so-called spiritual conquest persecuted natives—often quite ruthlessly—who were unwilling to convert or blended Christian and pagan rituals, the Holy Office that was established in 1571 was a much more sober version of its predecessors.[13] For one, it lacked jurisdiction over the Indigenous population, who were, by the mid-sixteenth century, considered neophytes in matters of religion, concentrating its authority instead on Old World Spaniards, their Creole and mestizo offspring, as well as Blacks and mulattos.[14] Only a fraction of the cases it tried involved formal heresy, and even fewer elicited the use of torture. For the most part, the tribunal in New Spain remained occupied in less severe instances of social disciplining centered on crimes involving offensive speech, sexual impropriety, and practices labeled superstitious, such as *hechicería*.[15]

Furthermore, unlike the medieval Inquisition, which was under papal jurisdiction, the early modern equivalent was an appendage of the state. As such, it was arguably more powerful, making no demarcation between the enforcement of Catholic orthodoxy in the Americas and the expansion of Spanish political and cultural dominion. Consequently, as Irene Silverblatt has emphasized, the Holy Office constituted a vital component of the imperial apparatus, functioning very much like a "modern bureaucracy," and was "larded with procedures, protocols, and regulations."[16] Although the accused were severely disadvantaged in that they carried the presumption of guilt, the inquisitors tended not to make arrests without studiously examining the evidence first, questioning witnesses—more was better—and ratifying their testimonies. Moreover, inquisitors rarely pursued an investigation out of their own initiative. Instead, they conducted their inquiries largely on the basis of denunciations made by members of the community or self-accusations by individuals seeking to divulge their troubled consciences. Once an accusation was lodged, the tribunal voted on whether to proceed. If the case went forward, they would conduct a preliminary investigation, the findings of which would result in a lengthy official summary called a *sumaria*. In theory if not always in practice, only once the *sumaria* was carefully scrutinized by theological evaluators or consultants known as *calificadores*, and only if the *calificadores* determined that the evidence was sufficient to warrant prosecution, would the suspect be apprehended and summoned for questioning, his goods confiscated. When a case went to trial, it was usually a long drawn-out affair, consisting of a series of interrogations of the accused carried out in the presence of an *escribano* (notary) and formal hearings called *audiencias* in which the prosecution and the defense respectively pursued and refuted the charges.[17]

In spite of its rigid rules and procedures—or perhaps because of them—the Holy Office did not issue foreordained verdicts.[18] Indeed, cases involving defendants whose sanity was in question call attention to the indeterminacy of Inquisition *procesos*, exposing inquisitors not as rabid fanatics bent on burning and torturing bodies but as concerned (albeit forbidding) judges and churchmen who worried intensely about matters involving evidence, motive, and the possibility of wrongfully punishing an innocent offender—or, by that same token, of letting the guilty go free.[19]

Far more than any other phenomenon, *locura* placed inquisitors in a state of heightened moral and legal quandary as they waded through the intricacies of inquisitorial protocol and struggled to make sense of the behavior that confronted them. Sin, after all, had to arise willingly from an unencumbered mind, and inquisitors became adept at asking questions that allowed them to probe mental states. In policing the realm of belief and understanding, the Inquisition differed markedly from the secular criminal courts, where the magistrates proved far more concerned with criminal acts and their corresponding retribution. Inquisitors, by comparison, had staked their jurisdiction over matters of religious conviction and were thus keenly interested in the mental, moral, and spiritual universe of the countless suspects who slipped into the toils of the inquisitorial machinery. As Laura Lewis has written, "Secular judges were more interested in what a defendant might have done, while inquisitors were more concerned with the defendant's moral world and motivations."[20] Inquisition *procesos*, in other words, hinged on the intense and thorough interrogation of reasoning and belief in a way that was unparalleled within the secular criminal courts. This was because for heresy to occur, it was insufficient for the suspect in question to religiously err; he or she had to embrace ideas that were contradictory to Catholic doctrine with total awareness or cognizance and, on top of that, fully reject the possibility of being corrected once their errors or misunderstandings were made manifest.[21] Such stringent requirements meant that questions of volition, understanding, and gradations of intent were a routine facet of inquisitorial investigation, and that those deemed mentally incompetent were, by definition, incapable of committing heresy and therefore innocent. This mode of inquiry not only necessitated deep appreciation for the nuances of human reasoning but made medical explanations for irrational thought and behavior heuristically useful if not highly seductive.

The insanity defense, to be sure, was not an invention of the Catholic Church, even though the Inquisition came to employ some of its most sophisticated uses. While canon law made conscious will a necessary precondition for sin, the notion that the criminally insane should be exempt from punishment, even for heinous crimes like murder, stemmed back to Roman jurisprudence, which reiterated the adage that "madness was punishment enough."[22] *Las Siete Partidas*, a widely cited medieval Spanish legal compendium, echoed similar views, stipulating that while a mad person may have "committed an offense for which another man would be imprisoned or put to death, the same person . . . did not commit the act with intelligence, and the same guilt cannot be imputed to him as to another in possession of his senses."[23] The Inquisition's contribution was to put the law into early action and likewise to elaborate and debate the criteria that would establish whether a suspect was indeed mad and thereby innocent of the charges brought against him or her or fully competent and thus capable of facing trial and punishment. Despite the pretenses of civil law codes, madness was rarely an easily identifiable state for the inquisitor. Instead, it needed to be corroborated through the thorough questioning of witnesses—friends and family of the accused, bystanders who had witnessed the crime in question, priests, lawyers, prison inmates, and, increasingly, medical experts—in conjunction with the inquisitor's own judiciary discretion, informed by close observation of the suspect in question (though not always) and with the aid of interrogation manuals and learned philosophical and theological tomes. The stakes were high. The confirmation of madness or, for that matter, any mitigating factor thought to dull judgment—ignorance, excessive emotions, drunkenness, youth—could be viewed, at the inquisitor's discretion, to justify more lenient treatment.[24]

While medieval canonists began to delve into the intricacies of intent and legal responsibility as early as the thirteenth century, insanity as a practical defense before the courts of the Holy Office in the Hispanic world does not appear in the archival record with any routine recurrence until the sixteenth century.[25] For Spain, Dale Shuger has traced its rise to the 1530s, while in New Spain the earliest case appeared in 1573, just two years after the tribunal's establishment.[26]

What accounted for the willingness to view certain heretics as ill and harmless? The Reformation and its complicated aftermath hold some answers. The eruption of Protestantism and the surge in religiosity across the confessional divide created a climate for the heightened regulation of interiority and the discernment of spirits. Prior to that point, the Spanish

Inquisition had concentrated its energies almost exclusively on persecuting crypto-Judaism among New Christians, a crime that could be proven largely on the basis of external trappings, such as circumcision, genealogy, and diet.[27] However, following the Council of Trent (1545–63), the Inquisition spread its tentacles to the wider masses as the defender of Catholic orthodoxy in both Europe and the Americas. Moreover, as new forms of spirituality and mysticism took root—especially among women—it became more keenly engaged in diagnosing the interior, proclaiming "who was possessed, who was a saint, who was a fraud, and who was insane."[28]

Within this context, an early arena for the evolution of the insanity defense centered on the overlap between the symptoms of madness and those of spiritual possession, both divine and demonic. Moshe Sluhovsky has emphasized the "morphological similarities between divine and demonic possession," arguing that in the early modern period, spiritual possession constituted a "powerful hermeneutic challenge" in Catholic nation-states. As inquisitors, theologians, physicians, and exorcists debated the etiology of spiritual possession and its psychosomatic symptoms—convulsions, contortions, visions, pain or ecstasy, incoherent speech—they came to redefine the boundaries between the divine and the demonic, the supernatural and the natural.[29] In this process, the Christian tradition that had attributed disease to the influence of demons and humoral paradigms for explaining illness became increasingly intertwined. Theologians "bent upon 'empiricizing' the demonic" drew increasingly on medicine; meanwhile, medical texts propagated views that demonic spirits could infiltrate the body and provoke hallucinations identical to those of melancholy and mania.[30] These conversations provided an early forum for lengthy and erudite reflections on the medical underpinnings of altered mental states; however, to the extent that physicians and inquisitors strove for greater collaboration, their achievements remained largely theoretical. In practice, the preternatural etiology of disease proved difficult to displace with naturalistic models except in extraordinary situations.[31]

In the early modern Hispanic world, the quest to preserve Catholicism in the face of new religious threats and popular religiosity appears to have generated especially skeptical views toward extraordinary phenomena and psychosomatic forms of spirituality. As Andrew Keitt has discussed, sixteenth- and seventeenth-century inquisitors looked to medical models because they equipped them with a way "to destabilize uncritical belief in supernatural phenomenon by constantly reiterating the potentially limitless list of natural causes that could simulate the miraculous, and thereby deceive the overly credulous."[32] This "naturalizing tendency" often gave way to charges of fraud and feigned sanctity among aspiring visionaries, with mystics occasionally dismissed as ill.[33] In New Spain by the late seventeenth century, inquisitors came to exhibit growing contempt for popular diabolism, their skepticism fueled, as Fernando Cervantes has argued, by a "defensive spirit" to preserve the devil as a worthy antagonist to God's grace. "Diabolism," he claims, "was played down or ignored not because it was too credulous but, on the contrary, because it might lead to incredulity."[34] Unlike northern Europe, in New Spain, as in other parts of the Spanish Empire, witches—especially Indigenous, Black, and mixed-race women—were not viewed as threatening agents of the devil. To the contrary, as long as they proved willing to repent, inquisitors readily dismissed these women as superstitious, ignorant, and sometimes even mad.[35]

In short, the aftermath of the Counter-Reformation provided religious authorities with a growing impetus to seek out naturalistic causes for a wide range of embodied spiritual experiences and practices with implications for how madness was to be perceived and approached. Arguably, the eighteenth century witnessed a continuation and accentuation of these trends, as religious women claiming prophetic visions and heavenly communion were increasingly diagnosed by both clerics and physicians as mad, hysterical, or epileptic.[36] However, this in no way implies a teleological process whereby naturalistic paradigms came to evenly supplant supernatural ones.[37] Despite its entanglements with the history of spiritual possession and witchcraft, the Inquisition's use of the insanity defense constituted a phenomenon unique unto itself and unfolded on its own distinct trajectory. From its inception in New Spain, inquisitors recognized that suspects judged to lack their full senses deserved leniency and compassion rather than punishment, and they willingly extended these when the evidence merited it. The majority of cases in which madness surfaced did not involve women claiming access to the divine; instead, they centered on more minor crimes, such as blasphemy committed mostly by men, with the inquisitors demonstrating little concern for the role of preternatural powers to impinge on the faculties of the mind. This was as true for the late sixteenth century as it was for the eighteenth. What made the eighteenth century distinct was the increase in the sheer volume of insanity cases and the growing recourse to medical language and expertise—even in marginal cases—and the use of San Hipólito as an outlet for confining and treating mad suspects.[38] Here it is worth further exploring the larger moral, epistemological, and practical factors at play in this shift.

In investigations into the mental state of the accused, no issue loomed larger than that of feigned madness. Concerns with the simulation of madness echoed fears over feigned sanctity, which intensified during the Counter-Reformation and persisted into the eighteenth century. A popular Inquisition manual written by Nicolau Eimeric, a fourteenth-century Dominican friar from Aragon, warned against the cunningness of heretics, who would often fake ignorance or pretend to be ill, physically weak, or deranged to skirt punishment for their crimes. Eimeric even advocated for the implementation of torture as a legitimate means to determine if the madness was authentic or fraudulent, emphasizing that torture should be administered only in situations where the inquisitor possessed compelling doubt and that it should not "result in the danger of death."[39] Ample evidence suggests that inquisitors rarely acted with the kind of vehemence and bloodlust advocated by Eimeric, opting in favor of a more humane and cautious approach. Nevertheless, like Eimeric, the overriding issue for eighteenth-century inquisitors was not the distinction between madness and diabolical possession but how precisely to differentiate between *locura* that was "real" and that which, to their minds, was guilefully crafted for the purposes of duping authority and evading punishment.[40]

This was tricky, complicated business. While concerns about feigning also surfaced in trials involving mystical phenomenon, the mystic's performance required more elaborate staging through rapture, seizures, visions, stigmata, and even levitation. In contrast, by the late eighteenth century, with diseases such as *demencia parcial* ("partial madness," or what would later become monomania) in vogue, the learned elite had come to recognize that *locura* did not just express itself in the most extreme and obvious ways; it could also be manifest through more subtle and, to the untrained eye, almost indecipherable behavior.

Tellingly, so nebulous was the terrain demarcating madness from heresy that in 1768 the Inquisition's staff physician, Juan Gregorio Campos, frankly admitted that "it was easy to mistake a heretic for a madman." While both essentially espoused truths that were contradictory to reality, the madman issued false claims on account of a defective "imagination." By contrast, the devious heretic advanced erroneous assertions with full volition and unrepentantly in the face of ample evidence to undermine his beliefs. The former suffered from a "mysterious alteration of the brain"; the latter possessed "dark motives" that "moved his will" and swayed his *entendimiento* (understanding).[41] In other words, while on the surface the madman and the heretic appeared astonishingly similar, the inner workings of their mind and conscience betrayed radically different motives, such that one merited compassion and leniency while the other deserved condemnation.

Campos's musings on the fuzzy distinction between madness and heresy were delivered in the context of the trial of Franciscan friar Felipe Antonio Alvarez, a case that shows just how far the Inquisition was willing to stretch the definition of insanity to render heretical ideas not just sinful but the product of sickness. A repeat offender notorious for a life tainted by countless vices, from gambling to promiscuity, as well as several successful attempts to flee imprisonment within his monastery, Alvarez's name had appeared among the Inquisition's daily files on at least three prior occasions. In 1761, he was hauled to the secret cells of the Holy Office a fourth time to stand trial for heresy. By this point, the case against the deviant friar was stacked high: among his numerous offenses, he was accused of lambasting papal authority, calling the pope and church officials "usurpers"; belittling the sanctity of the sacraments, labeling them "ridiculous ceremonies"; and questioning the doctrine of free will in refuting the existence of the biblical Adam and declaring that original sin had not been committed by any "particular or individual man" but was the conjuring of a "community of priests."[42]

These were grave offenses that challenged key articles of Catholic doctrine, and rather than seek penitence, the recalcitrant friar held steadfast to his convictions. Adding insult to injury, he continued to advance heretical arguments during what ultimately amounted to eight years of imprisonment, replete with regular rounds of interrogation. On numerous occasions, Alvarez himself would request hearings just to dispute issues of faith as a matter of sport and to push forth heterodox claims, such as that Christ was a *morisco*—that is, the "son of a black woman and Spanish man"—and therefore possessed dark skin.[43] Given the stubborn tenacity with which he voiced his beliefs and the unabashed lack of reverence for authority or fear of repercussion, the inquisitor Julian Vicente González de Andia began to doubt the suspect's sanity and marshaled in the expertise of four *calificadores* as well as the services of the staff physician, Campos.

Herein lay the inquisitor's quandary: how to gauge the innermost recesses of human interiority to determine if heretical assertions stemmed from a defective brain or a deceitful and spiritually sullied conscience. Resolving this conundrum was no mere intellectual exercise. At stake was both the sanctity and the authority of the church in the Americas during a moment of dwindling power and, equally urgent, the friar's soul and eternal salvation. Increasingly, medicine would be taken to task to resolve the issue of who was mad and who was a heretic. Given their investment in matters pertaining to both soul and psyche, inquisitors raised questions about human cognition and its connection to the production of heretical belief, questions that certainly mattered to theologians but that could also be addressed through the appeal to more rational and scientific forms of knowledge.

In the case of Alvarez, theology and medicine came to different but complementary conclusions that ultimately worked in concert to grant the friar the insanity defense. While all *calificadores* were in agreement in affirming the friar's sanity, they did express concern that Alvarez appeared to lack the mental acumen of a true heretic. Heretics, they claimed, were notorious for their mental agility, for displaying *potencias* that were "alive" and "awake," and for flaunting profound knowledge and a nuanced grasp of canonical texts. By comparison, the disgraced friar espoused discourse devoid of the clear and concrete "connection" of ideas and demonstrated what was at best superficial erudition.[44] The physician Campos came to a different, if somewhat tentative, conclusion in diagnosing the friar with *demencia parcial*, an illness in which the sufferer was mentally sound except with regards to one particular arena—in the friar's case, all matters pertaining to religion. While the two interpretations of the friar's conduct seemed to contradict each other—indeed, deliberations dragged on for another year—the diagnosis of partial madness ultimately gained ground, as it helped to explain how the friar could engage in lofty discourse and expound at length on delicate matters and yet pursue arguments that were so outlandish as to call into question his capacity to reason. Indeed, the insanity defense worked here not only to discredit the friar's unorthodox views but to protect the Catholic Church from growing attack. Implicit in this case was the assumption that no *sane* individual, let alone a friar, could utter such irreligious claims and behave in such a morally reprehensible manner.

Indecent Tongues, Ridiculous Speech, and Defective Minds

In granting Felipe Antonio Alvarez the insanity defense, the Inquisition ultimately rendered his religiously hostile statements nonsensical. These were not the dangerous assertions of a devious heretic but the meaningless chitter-chatter of a medically confirmed madman. Facing the serious charge of formal heresy, Alvarez's case was in many respects the exception rather than the norm. Here was an educated cleric expounding at length on intricate theological matters and refusing to recant his convictions, much to the dismay and consternation of inquisitors, who invested years in their quest to arrive at the authentic source of the friar's heretical productions. Nevertheless, his case resonated with others from the period in raising questions about the relationship between speech acts and inward cognitive and spiritual states. What words constituted senseless babble, and which verbal outbursts represented veritable affronts on the Catholic Church?

Disordered mental states frequently begat troublesome, offensive speech. In eighteenth-century Mexico, the majority of instances in which the insanity defense was invoked originated in the unconscious spewing of remarks that rang sacrilegiously to the ears of friends and neighbors. These criminal speech acts ranged from blasphemy to the more ambiguous category of "propositions" (*proposiciones*), or "statements which potentially indicated thoughts that were in error in matters of faith and were thus sinful."[45] The crime of propositions ran the full spectrum, from the unequivocally heretical, such as the statements issued by friar Alvarez, to the "simply erroneous, blasphemous, offensive, scandalous, or ill sounding (*malsonante*) to pious ears."[46] In reporting these sinful utterances to the Holy Office, the denouncer fulfilled his or her imperative to report behavior that was religiously reprehensible—an imperative that was enforced through local preachers and the publication of the Edict of Faith during Lent—leaving the more thorny task of determining whether these insults had been hurled during a moment of sanity squarely on the shoulders of inquisitors.[47]

It should be stressed that *locura* exacerbated long-standing concerns about the causal relationship between cognition and speech acts. Early modern moral and religious authorities attributed great importance to the spoken word, not only for its ability to convey matters of spiritual belief but for its capacity to make legible the inner workings of the psyche. As Maureen Flynn writes with respect to blasphemy, "Speech gave access to the moral center of the human being, to the mind, the seat of logical reasoning and critical reflection."[48] Speech acts were what most approximately mirrored the speaker's intentions and beliefs, "as if language always referred to pre-existing categories contained within the human mind."[49] For inquisitors, a suspect's personal confession constituted the most unadulterated form of evidence (even if extracted through torture), testifying to the heuristic value they accorded to language as the most immediate and intimate gateway into the opaque interiors of the human conscience and psyche.

That said, inquisitors also encountered in their daily practice numerous situations in which speech was severed from intent, or mediated by factors such as inebriation, emotion (especially anger), and even ignorance. Particularly in cases of blasphemy, defendants frequently objected to the literal interpretation of their remarks, claiming to have not been fully cognizant of their meaning at the time they had uttered such profanations.[50] Words, in short, possessed the power to injure, but inquisitors proved willing to consider the context in which verbal assaults were delivered, recognizing that speech could sometimes be at variance with the speaker's genuine intentions. Madness only accentuated these dilemmas, driving a deeper wedge between thought and its articulation. Because the mad suspect possessed what was at best a dubious relationship to his or her speech faculties, the normal tools of interrogation and confession for arriving at the motive behind a verbal assault simply did not work.[51]

For example, in 1771, Josefa Manuela Leiba denounced Juan de la Vega to the Inquisition after she heard him call the Virgin Mary a *puta cambuja* (swarthy whore) and Christ a *maldito cambujo* (damn dark-skinned person), among other shocking insults.[52] The inquisitors immediately launched a preliminary investigation into Vega's mental state at the time he issued the profanities. The denouncer confidently asserted that the suspect appeared to possess "sane judgment and full reasoning" (*sano juicio y entero conocimiento*), adding that he never drank.[53] Other witnesses also judged him to be mentally competent; even Andrea Valdes, who suggested that Vega's offensive utterances might have been elicited by the "movement of the moon," still agreed that Vega was of sound mind. Likewise, Maria Alvina, the Indigenous servant who had witnessed Vega senselessly throw rocks at sacred images, confirmed that the suspect "was in his full reasoning," showing no signs of excessive passion nor of being demonically possessed (*enagenado*).[54]

Unlike friar Alvarez, whose trial dragged on for nearly a decade and recruited the active participation of both theological and medical experts, the inquisitors wasted little ink in deliberating the case of Juan de la Vega. His trial never made it past the preliminary stage of investigation, and he was never apprehended or made to appear before the tribunal for interrogation. Instead, the inquisitors based their verdict largely on the testimony of one key witness. Although all other witnesses firmly denied Vega was *demente*, his brother-in-law, Joseph Juarez, contended otherwise. When summoned, Juarez informed the tribunal that for the past six years Vega had suffered from *locura* and "injury" (*lesion*) to his mental faculties. Because of this, he was prone to shout, act compulsively, and do "other ungodly things" (*intempestivas*). Juarez related how, at one point, his brother-in-law had even attempted to strangle a servant in a maddened frenzy, leaving him and his wife, Vega's sister, with no option but to temporarily hospitalize him at San Hipólito, where he was diagnosed with "incurable madness." Apparently the inquisitors were not yet fully satisfied that Vega was mad, for they immediately contacted the hospital to corroborate Juarez's testimony. It was San Hipólito's head nurse, friar Felipe Joseph Ruíz, who provided the deciding testimony, informing the tribunal that Vega was indeed suffering from madness and fatuity (*fatuidad*).[55]

In 1773, two years after the Inquisition excused Vega for his foul and blasphemous language, an even more theologically heretical case came to its attention in the form of Diego Mendoza, a native of Andalusia and a soldier turned vagabond. That year, Mendoza had boldly declared in public "I am God, better than God, I command and govern Him," and "Christ is my nephew." When witnesses reprimanded him for his irreverent assertions and threatened to denounce him to the Inquisition, he defiantly retorted that he "shit on the inquisitors, and on the Inquisition!"[56] Mendoza's verbal affronts were soon brought to the attention of the Holy Office, and inquisitors quickly learned that he was a rumored madman. Labeled by his community as "El Loco," he was often seen wandering the streets of Mexico City, hollering improprieties and styling himself as the "Archbishop and Viceroy of Mexico and Cousin of God."[57]

Like Vega's case, Mendoza's illustrates the difficult balancing act the Inquisition had to perform. On the one hand were masses of uncomfortable even irate, witnesses who demanded that religious—and, by extension, social—order be enforced. On the other hand was a clearly insane mind. Which way should justice lean? In Mendoza's case, the inquisitors amassed testimony from a total of twenty-two witnesses, nearly all of whom judged him to be sane. Pedro de Lomber, who was the first to bring Mendoza's impious outbursts to the attention of the tribunal, maintained that he was in his "full judgment [*entero juicio*]," although he did concede that "some people were of the opinion that he was mad."[58] Pablo de las Revillas y Villamor also believed that Mendoza was sane because, aside from his blasphemies, he was able to speak cogently on many matters.[59] How could, Villamor implicitly asked the inquisitors, a person be fully cogent on all matters *except* religion? Other witnesses argued that Mendoza's madness was feigned—including Joaquín Hermosa, who described the suspect as "mad by convenience."[60] Of the nearly two dozen witnesses, only three expressed misgivings about Mendoza's sanity, and even within this tiny minority there were hesitations. Santiago Trelles, who had known the suspect since he had arrived from Spain sixteen years earlier, told inquisitors he suspected that Mendoza's *juicio* was in all likelihood "perturbed," although he too voiced uncertainty.[61] Pedro Gonzalez referred to Mendoza as a "true madman," although he had many years ago observed him to be "rational, moderate, and modest," showing no indications of "stupidity" (*lerdo*).⁶² Finally, Miguel Gonzalez testified to the suspect's bizarre conduct and wayward moods and related how neighbors once inquired into having him admitted to San Hipólito, only to be discouraged when one of the friars informed them that a medical certificate was necessary for internment.⁶³

Cases like those of Mendoza and Vega were not aberrations but struck to the heart of justice. Should the Inquisition assuage the anger and discomfort of the witnesses who were sure that a sane man had attacked some of their most cherished ideals, or should it extend compassion to a disordered mind? In Mendoza's case, the inquisitors punted, opting to suspend the charges—notably, not exonerate him—and transfer him to San Hipólito for a period of two months. In so doing, they reached what Dale Shuger has characterized as "'compromise' verdicts with little theological or judicial coherency," but certainly with pragmatic value."⁶⁴ Temporary confinement at San Hipólito ensured that Mendoza would receive proper medical attention if he was indeed ill and that his egregious utterances (intentional or not) would at the very least remain behind closed doors, albeit for a limited stretch of time.

Mendoza's case also underscores the limitations of witness testimony when dealing with *locura*, suggesting one of the motives fueling the turn toward the greater reliance on expert—especially medical—testimony. Local witnesses proved most insightful and effective when providing information about the suspect's conduct and personal history, noting drastic changes in behavior and stressful life circumstances that might explain shifts in mental health. They could also be expected to offer faithful accounts of the offensive claims the suspect had delivered; or, at the very least, inquisitors could, with confidence, reconstruct the specific details of the crime in question through the accumulation and comparison of multiple testimonies. Beyond that, however, ordinary men and women simply lacked the tools to offer more concise renderings of the activities taking place within the suspect's psyche. In other words, they lacked the technical terminology and theoretical foundation on which disease categories were based to properly identify states of mental disorder.⁶⁵ While colonial witnesses could agree that certain individuals fit within broad terms like *loco* or *demente*, their testimonies rarely achieved consensus, and conflicting opinions inevitably threatened to spiral into indefinite deliberation. By bringing in and privileging expert witnesses, the Inquisition tried to address this problem. There was still space in the proceedings for the voice of ordinary people to express themselves, but their testimony—partial as it often was—was then clarified, classified, and made coherent through the language of trained physicians. It was they, and not the inquisitors, who might then shoulder the responsibility for pardoning what many witnesses surely must have thought was shocking—perhaps even grotesque—words and actions.

Tebanillo's Sketches

If the spoken word often proved an inadequate, slippery means for accessing interiority in situations of alleged madness, in a fascinating case from 1789 inquisitors stumbled upon an even more frustrating and impenetrable form of evidence: a bundle of papers brimming with risqué, troubling images and accompanied by salacious text. The papers in question belonged to José Ventura Gonzalez, a native of Toluca who was known throughout his community as Tebanillo.[66] An embroiderer by occupation, Tebanillo frequently drew embroidery designs and related sketches in his spare time. When inquisitors thumbed through the documents at the conclusion of an investigation against Tebanillo for heretical propositions, they encountered a series of innocuous illustrations of flowers and animal scenery clearly intended for stitching, but they also found more reprehensible and dangerous material. Tebanillo had produced crude etchings of people and animals with pornographic overtones and pages upon pages of written text commenting, often incoherently, on various themes, especially matrimony and illicit sexual acts and carnal desires. Here inquisitors literally had evidence they had to weigh in their hands. Were Tebanillo's shocking sketches and writings a testament to his troubled and disordered mind? Or did they simply expose in material form his perverted and morally debase character and conscience?

Inquisitors not only kept records of eighteenth-century madness; in crucial ways they also shaped the way that madness was manifested and archived.[67] As the previous cases illustrate, the Holy Office's interest in interiority, and the centrality of intent to determining guilt or innocence, fueled its engagement with *locura*. That the inquisitors preserved Tebanillo's images and writings in his file for posterity—albeit with little written mention of their reaction—suggests that they deemed them central to the case. In one a sense, Tebanillo's sketches and incoherent prose were not too different from the disrespectful and scandalous musings of the blabbering madman. The former quite literally materialized the ambiguous nature of evidence inquisitors routinely encountered—and were forced to decipher—when dealing with cases whose central culprits were suspected to be mentally unsound. And yet on another level, the documents were even more dangerous than transitory speech; written and made permanent, Tebanillo's drawings and text had the potential to circulate among a large audience without context—in other words, without knowledge of the madman's condition to mitigate their impact.

Tebanillo had been denounced to the local *comisario* (commissary) of Toluca by José Piña and his wife, María, for a slew of irreverent claims and gestures, including denying the existence of purgatory and hell and disparaging the Virgin Mary by reducing her sanctified status to that of a *muñeca vestida*, or a "dressed-up doll."[68] Although the inquisitors, like many of Tebanillo's neighbors in Toluca, were fully aware that he had formerly resided in San Hipólito after a bout of madness, they nevertheless granted the *comisario*, Mariano José Casasola, permission to proceed with a preliminary investigation.

As he rounded up witnesses, the *comisario* specifically inquired about the outward *señales* (signs) of Tebanillo's mental unrest. Most witnesses accordingly testified to the suspect's strange and wild antics. By far, the most colorful account of his behavior came from his neighbor, Andrea Josefa Estrada. She reported that Tebanillo habitually carried an image of the Virgin Mary, which he casually referred to as *"su muger"*—literally, "his woman," meaning wife—and that he would often sleep with it. Estrada also claimed to have witnessed him take cigarettes and fruit to the image of Mary, but upon seeing that she would not accept the offerings, he would become irate and smack the picture. Estrada believed Tebanillo was a *verdadero loco* (true madman) based on his odd comportment, "the extravagance with which he ate," and his eccentric mode of dress.[69] Another witness, María Tomasa de la Luz, described the suspect as childlike and informed the *comisario* that she frequently saw him dig ditches in the ground, which he would fill with dirt and then claim were graves for his deceased wife.[70] Indeed, the investigation revealed that his wife had died four months following his release from San Hipólito and that since then, his mental health had steadily deteriorated under the weight of his grief. All of Tebanillo's neighbors understood this about him except, as Casasola noted in this report to the tribunal in Mexico City, for the "vulgar" folk, who believed he was *endemoniando* (demonically possessed).[71]

In July 1790, more than a year and a half after the initial denunciation was filed, the inquisitors concluded that Tebanillo was most likely mentally unsound and ordered that he be promptly returned to San Hipólito. As ill as he was, he was not completely divorced from reality, and they specified that the process of transporting the mad embroiderer from Toluca to Mexico City should be undertaken with the utmost "caution," such that even those tasked with the feat of relocation must "remain ignorant of the goal of their mission," lest Tebanillo learn of his impending hospitalization and attempt to flee.[72]

Coerced hospitalization may seem like an excessive, even harsh, choice given that by virtually all accounts, Tebanillo was a harmless and at times amusing madman. It is possible that the outbreak of revolution in France and the social and political tensions it generated prompted inquisitors to come down sternly on the mad embroiderer. In the summer of 1789, as Tebanillo's case was pending, Spanish authorities had established a cordon sanitaire to prevent the influx of revolutionary propaganda into Spain and its imperial domains. For the Inquisition, religious and political heresy were one and the same, and it was around this time that the tribunal oversaw a resurgence in activity against heretical propositions of the kind espoused by the mad embroiderer.[73] In this context of heightened censorship, the contents of Tebanillo's notebook would have done little to help his case. Shortly after he was admitted to San Hipólito, Casasola informed the tribunal in Mexico City of the existence of an *envoltorio* (bundle of papers) brought to his attention by Tebanillo's sister-in-law. Casasola scrutinized the contents of the papers over the course of three days, finding them too copious and unintelligible to thoroughly read, much less interpret. Nevertheless, he emphasized that certain passages and images were clearly "very obscene," "incorrect," and "indecent," while others displayed unequivocally heretical content. Rather than summarize his conclusions regarding their meaning, he had the papers delivered to Mexico City, where the inquisitors added them to Tebanillo's file.[74]

Beyond Casasola's comments, the Inquisition left no written reaction to Tebanillo's sketches and writings. With Gonzalez hospitalized and his documents confiscated, he no longer posed a threat. Yet if there were any misgivings as to the unorthodox nature of Gonzalez's disordered thoughts and proclivities, the papers erased all doubt. In one sketch (figure 3.1), he illustrated various human and animal couples with the caption on the right reading "casamiento" (marriage). An Indigenous figure is shown on the left urinating or masturbating into a small basin. Almost front and center is a large fountain surrounded by phallic imagery. There are references to love magic, specifically women's use of bodily fluids and matter to ensnare husbands. On the lower left, a woman is shown receiving liquid from the fountain, possibly urine or semen, on a metate, while on the lower right, another woman brushes her hair into a large pot. As Martha Few has noted, it was not uncommon for women to incorporate bodily parts and effluvia into food and drink, which they then used in magic rituals that targeted specific men.[75]

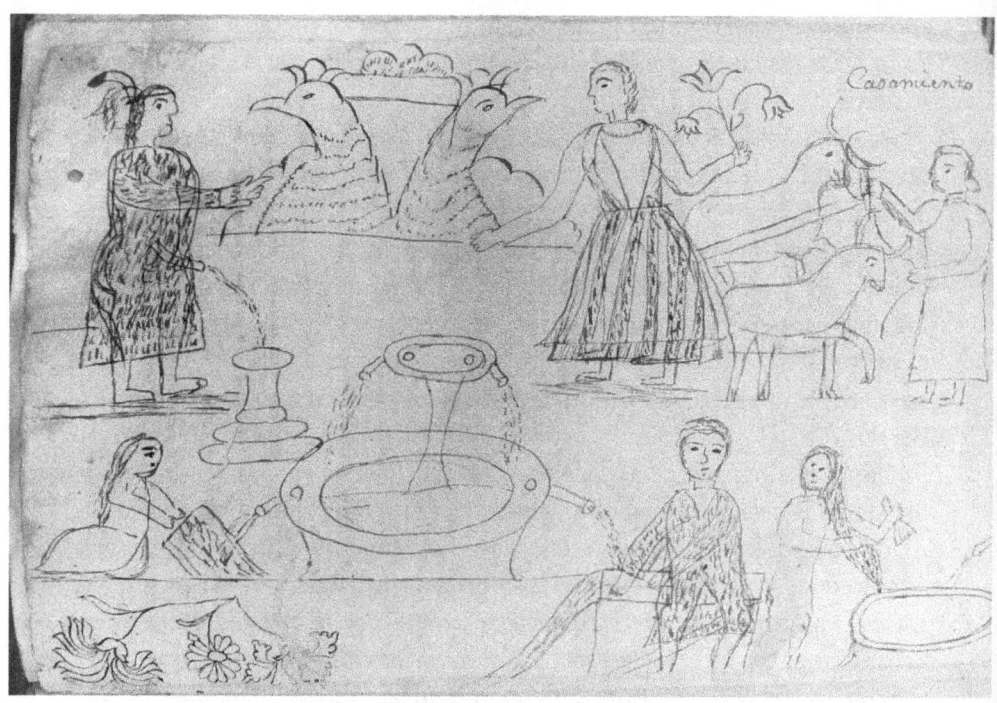

FIGURE 3.1 Salacious sketch by José "Tebanillo" Ventura Gonzalez, ca. 1789. Drawing presents a fountain scene, replete with phallic imagery. The caption on the upper right-hand side references *casamiento* (marriage), while an Indigenous figure is shown in the upper left-hand corner peeing or masturbating into a fountain. Source: AGN, Inquisición, vol. 1505, exp. 3.

The theme of love magic also surfaces in another image (figure 3.2). Here, Tebanillo depicted what appears to be a tonsured priest ejaculating into a cup held by a woman who is on her knees. The speech bubbles all reference *potencias* (powers) bestowed by the priest to the woman in order to choose a husband.

Other drawings were even more sexually explicit. Tebanillo had more than one image of a man masturbating a woman as she sits in a chair (figure 3.3), as well as couples fornicating while a voyeur watches. Indecent by eighteenth-century standards, Tebanillo's drawings became shockingly licentious in places. In one picture (figure 3.4), ostensibly a depiction of purgatory, he drew groups of figures engaged in sexual acts, including bestiality, beneath their gowns. In two other images (figures 3.5 and 3.6), Tebanillo crafted some of his most compelling—and disturbing—imagery around the theme of *pecado nefando* (sodomy). In one (figure 3.5), he has several figures expound-

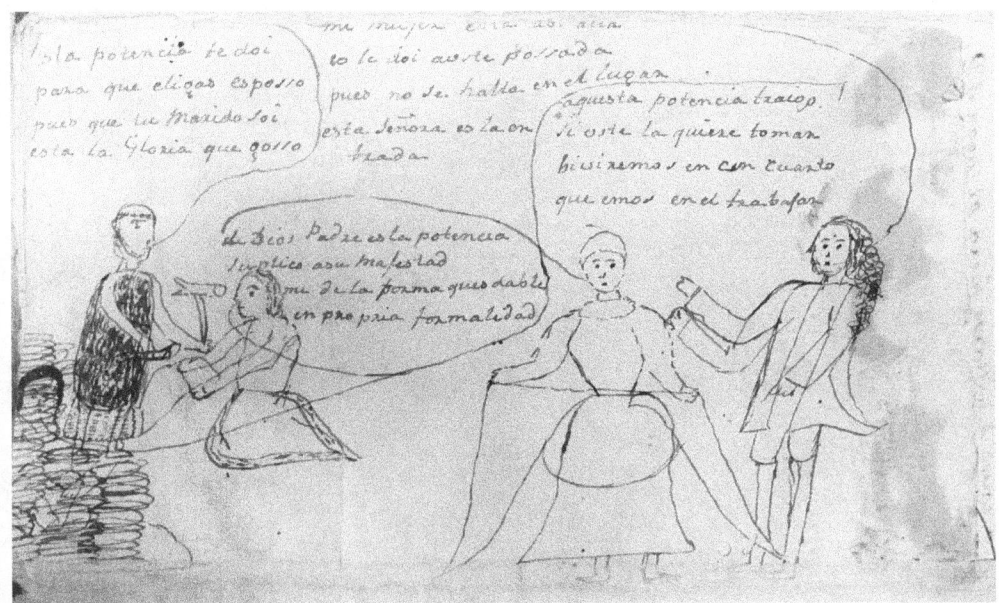

FIGURE 3.2 Salacious sketch by José "Tebanillo" Ventura Gonzalez, ca. 1789. Illustration of two couples. The couple on the left consists of a tonsured priest with a woman kneeling before him. The speech bubbles reference *potencias* (powers) bestowed by the priest to the woman in order to choose a husband. Source: AGN, Inquisición, vol. 1505, exp. 3.

ing at length on the subject, with references to figures having two *partes* (body parts) and being neither men nor women. In another (figure 3.6), there are much fewer words but far more powerful pictures. What appear to be same-sex couples engage in sexual acts, while another couple stands stabbed in the heart and genitals while a corpse lies beneath them.

It is impossible to say what the images meant to Tebanillo other than that the feelings behind them were undoubtedly powerful. However, whether grief had unleashed repressed feelings, urges, and memories was as opaque to the inquisitors in 1790 as it is to modern viewers. What the inquisitors made of the images also mystifies, but it is irrefutable that the images constituted a unique type of evidence. As Zeb Tortorici has noted for sodomy cases, inquisitors privileged eyewitness evidence, insight encapsulated in the common phrase *lo vido ocularmente* ("I saw it ocularly," or with one's own eyes), a phrase that saturates Inquisition cases.[76] In a crucial sense, the images drawn by Tebanillo were unmediated proof that heretical productions had been made. Here, inquisitors did not need to reconstruct what a group of witnesses had heard; they could see it with their very own eyes.

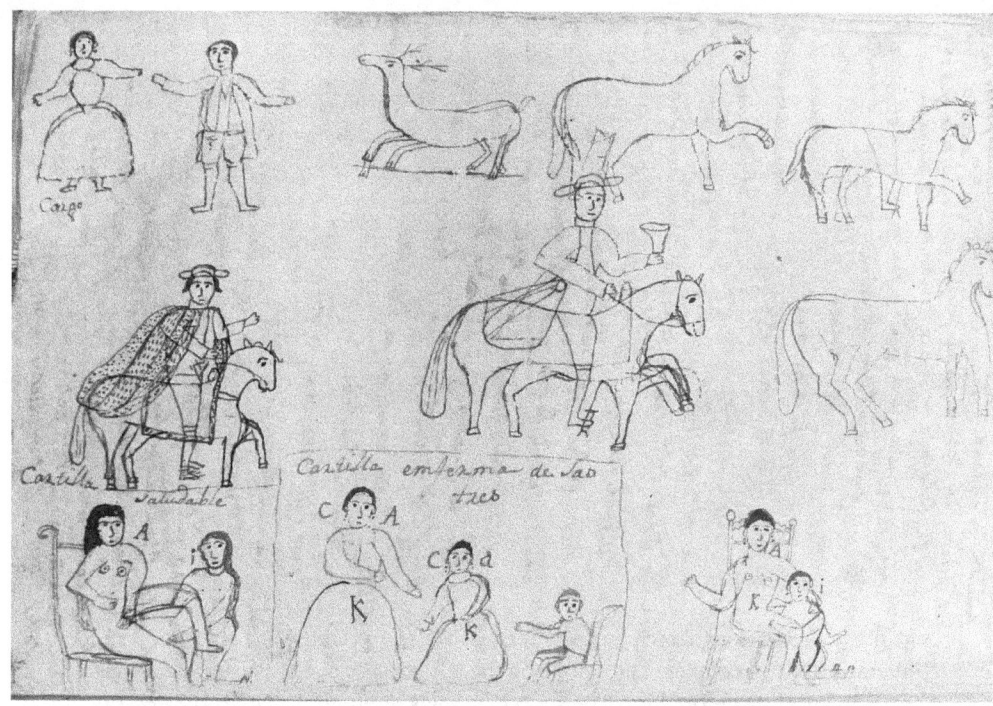

FIGURE 3.3 Salacious sketch by José "Tebanillo" Ventura Gonzalez, ca. 1789. Drawing shows two men on horseback at center and a man and woman in the upper left-hand corner. The lower half of the image shows a man masturbating a woman on each corner, and a woman standing next to a young girl and a little boy at center. Source: AGN, Inquisición, vol. 1505, exp. 3.

And yet like the cases previously analyzed, madness stymied inquisitorial procedure. To the inquisitors, charged with extirpating heresy and enforcing Christian morality in the Americas, the sexually charged and indecent images materialized in a disquieting way the perverse ideas of a troubled mind and the broader problem of managing the crimes of the mentally disturbed within a pastoral religious framework. Under normal circumstances, inquisitors could manage sexual sin and indecency among the laity through confession and penance. But a madman like Tebanillo could not be made to repent, since in theory he had never really violated the faith in the first place because all sin was voluntary. This fact placed Gonzalez's obscene drawings in a moral gray area, much to the inquisitors' discomfort. To be sure, this problem was not specific to Tebanillo's naughty sketches. The madman's incoherent speech and flimsy control over his body turned irreverent utterances and gestures into equally ambiguous affronts. Tebanillo's drawings

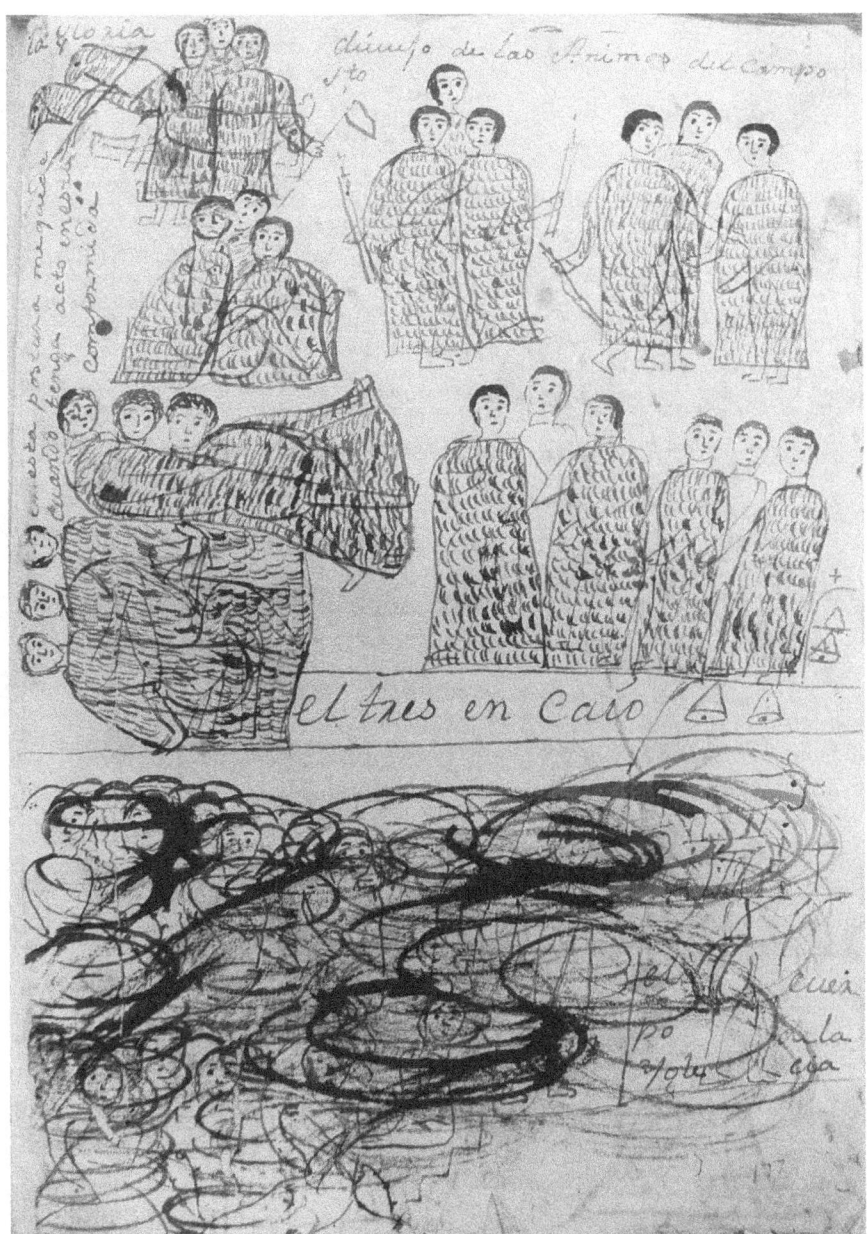

FIGURE 3.4 Salacious sketch by José "Tebanillo" Ventura Gonzalez, ca. 1789. Ostensibly a portrayal of purgatory, drawing illustrates various figures engaged in sexual acts, including bestiality (on the upper left side), beneath their gowns. Source: AGN, Inquisición, vol. 1505, exp. 3.

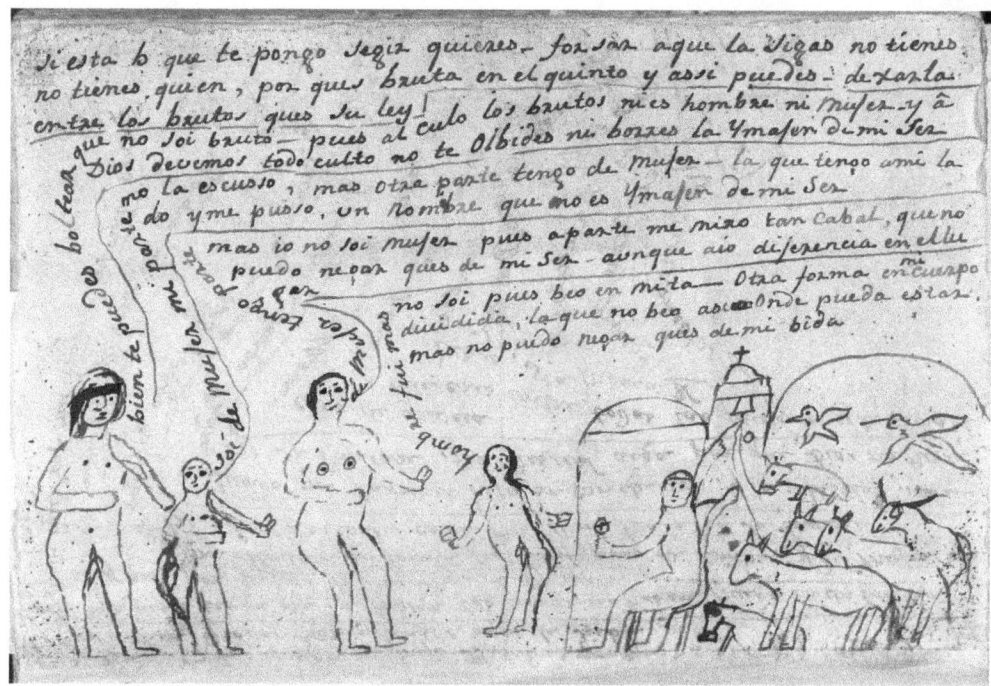

FIGURE 3.5 Salacious sketch by José "Tebanillo" Ventura Gonzalez, ca. 1789. Illustration of naked figures; the captions above make disparaging references to sodomy. Source: AGN, Inquisición, vol. 1505, exp. 3.

only materialized these issues, making them difficult to ignore. Technically, he was innocent by reason of insanity, but his graphic drawings were hard to dismiss as meaningless.

Auto-Denunciation and Female Pathology

Tebanillo's notebook was exceptional in that authorities linked, however vaguely, his troubled mind with his sexuality. For women in colonial Mexico, this was far more common. As Monica Calabritto has observed, "Women's insanity had to do with a more or less explicit deviance from accepted moral behavior, and it often had a sexual connotation."[77] This insight can be extended to the inquisitorial context of New Spain, where due to sexist views of women's intellectual inferiority, female madness was both expressed physically and understood as arising from the body—usually in overtly sexual tones. For the majority of cases involving women, sexuality was the pathology. Nora Jaffary's study of Mexican "false mystics," for in-

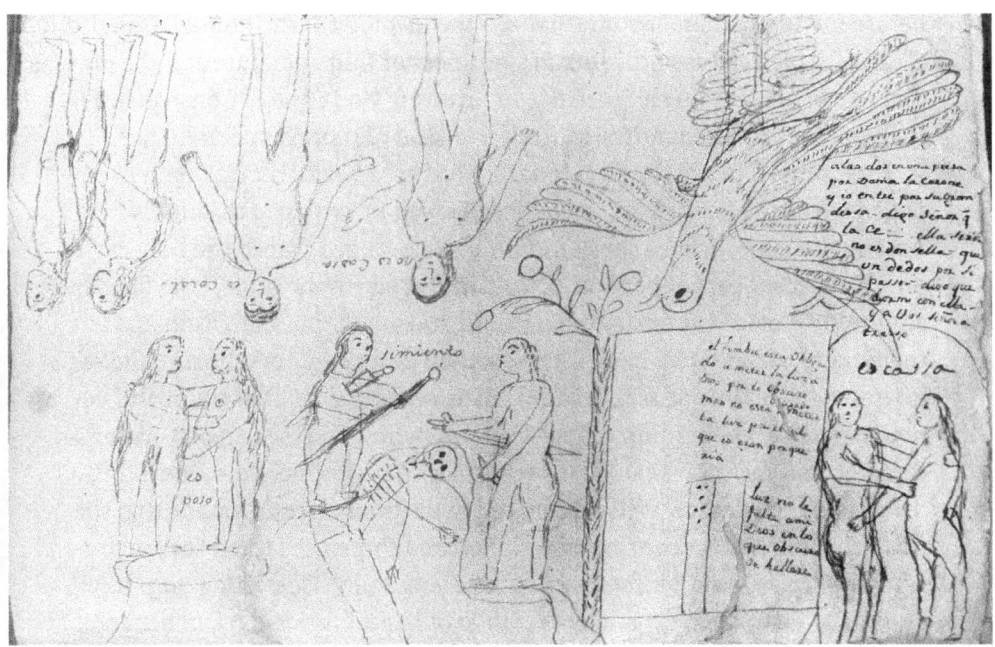

FIGURE 3.6 Salacious sketch by José "Tebanillo" Ventura Gonzalez, ca. 1789. The top half of the image (upside down) includes a bird and two same-sex male couples, one of them possibly engaged in anal sex. The bottom half showcases a violent scene of death depicting a stabbed couple and a skeleton, with an additional couple on either side. The writing states that while men are "obligated" to place their male members in "obscure" places, sodomy is a "great act of indecency" (*gran porquería*). Source: AGN, Inquisición, vol. 1505, exp. 3.

stance, has emphasized how the physical symptoms of mystical rapture experienced by female visionaries—seizures, convulsions, contortions, erotic visions—were often interpreted by inquisitors and physicians as signs of malady, particularly insanity or hysteria.[78] The Inquisition interpreted female madness within a long philosophical tradition in the West that associated women with flesh and carnal appetites.[79]

Evidence from the archives also suggests that mentally afflicted women often approached the Holy Office of their own volition—either out of personal initiative or through the mediation of a male confessor. And although the inquisitors tended to interpret their heightened sense of remorse and emotional distress as pathological, these women often denied, quite vehemently, being ill. Instead, they demanded that the Holy Office acknowledge and pardon their transgressions. In other words, madwomen who appeared

It Is Easy to Mistake a Heretic for a Madman 105

before the Inquisition had internalized the ideology of the Roman Catholic Church, which stressed the innate sinfulness of human nature and the pivotal role of confession and penance in restoring God's grace. Consequently, their madness often manifested itself as a kind of moral hypervigilance.[80]

For example, in 1774 Rafaela Ignacia Alvarez, a novice nun at the Convent of Santa Ines in Mexico City, denounced herself in writing to the Inquisition. Among the many crimes she committed, Rafaela had placed the holy cross on an "indecent part of her body." "And in this very same place," she further admitted, "I placed an image of Our Lord and another of the Virgin and left them there for about an hour." Rafaela then described how she tore the sacred images in a fit of rage (*coraje*), then repeatedly spit at them and renounced God, calling him a "cruel tyrant" who possessed the "heart of a dog." Overcome with shame and remorse, she eventually disclosed these deeds to her confessor, who exonerated her actions on the grounds that she was "impassioned" at the time she sinned and therefore lacked "full understanding" (*pleno conocimiento*) of what she was doing. The young nun, however, rejected this generous interpretation of her transgressions. In her letter to the Inquisition, she emphasized total cognizance of her actions, claiming that although she was overcome with desperation, she knowingly sinned and was now penitent, pleading for mercy and absolution.[81]

Rafaela was subsequently made to appear before the tribunal and interrogated by the inquisitor, Julian Vicente Gonzáles de Andia. Rafaela told Andia that the blaspheming started during Easter three years earlier. While fasting, her head had become dazed (*ataranto la cabeza*) and she found herself "violently tempted by thoughts against [the] faith." Here, too, the nun stressed her sanity and culpability, maintaining that she "always executed [her crimes] with the full understanding that she was gravely sinning" and with a "depraved intention to offend God."[82] Andia then asked Rafaela if there were any witnesses present, but the nun stated that she committed most of her offenses in private.

Rafaela suspected that everyone at the Convent of Santa Ines judged her to be mad. She told Andia that at one point she was locked in a room, medically examined, diagnosed as a hysteric, and subjected to "infinite" amounts of medication.[83] The inquisitors immediately solicited one of Rafaela's physicians, José Toribio, for questioning. Toribio had treated Rafaela since before she entered the convent and had cured her of dysentery when she was younger. At her parents' behest, he would make routine visits to Santa Ines to attend to her health, and in his testimony, the doctor reported that on one particular visit a nurse informed him that Rafaela was stricken with madness (*demencia*), "completely lost in delirium," and undergoing bouts of "furor." The nurses believed the onset of menstruation had provoked Rafaela's affliction, and they summoned another physician, Segura, who administered medicine but was unable to restore Rafaela's health. Because she did not respond to his treatment, Segura suspected Rafaela's illness was feigned, possibly staged on account of her discontent with the cloistered life, but Toribio believed otherwise: Rafaela's appearance, symptoms, and behavior all suggested she was *verdaderamente loca* (completely insane).[84]

The inquisitors accepted Toribio's assessment of Rafaela's mental health and abruptly suspended the charges. The nun was mentally ill and therefore not accountable for her crimes. In their closing remarks on the case, they ordered a confessor to absolve Rafaela of her sins *ad cautelam* and administer the "penitential medicines" necessary to assuage her conscience.[85]

As a nun, Rafaela came from the colonial elite, but similar behavior and understandings of madness arose in all classes of women in colonial Mexico. Between 1768 and 1784, Mauricia Josefa de Apelo, a *mestiza* servant and *doncella* (unmarried woman) residing in Mexico City, denounced herself to the Inquisition on multiple occasions. The first denunciation reached the Holy Office via a letter drafted by Mauricia's confessor, Joseph Gonzalez. The letter detailed how Mauricia, overwhelmed with *aborrecimiento*, or loathing toward God, had crushed a crucifix while shouting "furious words." On another occasion, she tore an image of the Holy Trinity, placing the pieces on the "most shameful parts of her body." Mauricia was also guilty of renouncing the faith and sacraments and worshipping the devil.[86]

In her interrogation before the inquisitor, Francisco Larrea, Mauricia disclosed additional details about her *amistad*, or friendship with the devil. Just fifteen days earlier, she informed Larrea, she had removed her rosary and scapular, throwing these to the ground, and proceeded to invoke the devil "with the desire to see him and the intention to worship him." Mauricia confessed she had surrendered her soul to the devil and that she would have sexual relations (*comercio carnal*) with him. Her devotion to the devil prompted her to increasingly reject God and the tenets and rituals of the faith, such that when she took communion she was often overcome by the urge to spit out the host and toss it into the latrine. Mauricia further revealed that her illicit relationship with the devil had developed at a young age, around six or seven, when she began to feel the early stirrings of lust (*movimientos fuertes de la carne*) and summoned the devil to satiate her sexual appetite. From then on, Mauricia reported that she frequently engaged in "carnal acts" with the devil, who sometimes appeared to her in the shape of a man, other times in the form of a dog.[87]

Such lurid stories about worshipping and cavorting with the devil were not unfamiliar to inquisitors. They were the stuff of European demonological treatises like the *Malleus Maleficarum*, which expounded at length about witches who had love affairs with Satan. These ideas reflected views of women as more vulnerable to the influences of demonic powers and as sexually voracious. Mauricia's claim to have fornicated with the devil, who appeared to her in both human and animal form, fit not only with existing European traditions but also with the Mesoamerican belief in the shape-shifting phenomenon known as *nahualism*, which was often associated with the devil's machinations.[88] However, by the time Mauricia subjected herself to the Inquisition, these notions had little traction among skeptical inquisitors, and Larrea seems to have entirely dismissed them in favor of impaired reasoning. In a side note made during her *audiencia* on December 1, 1768, he remarked that the suspect's imagination seemed "preoccupied" and that her *potencias* were clearly "obfuscated."[89] Unlike Rafaela's case, however, Mauricia's raised concerns about her *casta* (race). Although she claimed to be *mestiza* (of "mixed" blood), the tribunal suspected she was possibly Indian and therefore even more deserving of leniency, since it was the Inquisition's policy not to prosecute natives.[90]

Although Mauricia was ultimately granted absolution following her first denunciation, her mind and soul remained ill at ease, and she reappeared before the Holy Office three additional times, in 1769, 1773, and 1784. With each ensuing auto-denunciation, Mauricia's race, which appears to have been a mitigating factor in securing her a pardon initially, became less and less of an issue, and the Inquisition took much more seriously whether she was, in fact, mentally ill.

The process began after her second auto-denunciation in 1769, when Larrea retracted his initial impression of Mauricia's mental abilities, determining her to be competent to stand trial for heresy. Although he noted that her capacity was dull (*capacidad es corta*), Larrea declared her judgment intact (*entero juicio*).[91] Mauricia was subsequently examined by friar Pedro de Arrieta, who listened carefully to the suspect's testimony, searching for inconsistencies in her statements and the outward signs of mental instability. Mauricia now claimed she had an actual written pact with the devil, but when Arrieta requested to see it, she told him it was lost. The first session of questioning ended early because the defendant was scared (she was crying) and reluctant to speak. During the second meeting, she mustered the confidence to declare that not only had she fornicated with the devil countless times—in the form of a man, a brute, a dog, and a cat—but "were God to place Himself [before her] in human form, she would sin carnally" with him as well. Her shocking confession did not stop there; she admitted to violating the host and to placing an image of Christ in her "venereal parts." She went on to say that this last deed had caused the earth to shake, which she took as a sign of God's omnipotence and, since then, was a true believer of the faith.[92] Like Larrea, Arrieta believed the suspect sane, but his reasoning was odd. According to Arrieta, Mauricia's story about the missing devil's pact was dubious, but her willingness to divulge her crimes was inconsistent with the hesitance she had displayed earlier.[93]

In spite of this conclusion, the Holy Office was reluctant to take action and prosecute the suspect for heresy. Instead, she was shipped to the Hospital del Divino Salvador for a period of three months. The Inquisition eventually suspended the case when it received confirmation from the hospital that, contrary to Larrea's and Arrieta's assumption, Mauricia was indeed *demente*.[94] The insanity verdict was issued once more in 1773, following her third auto-denunciation, when friar Juan Gregorio de Campos, Mauricia's spiritual adviser during her stay at the Divino Salvador, informed the tribunal that Mauricia suffered from a "lesion of the imagination," the source of which was "uterine fury."[95]

Following each dismissed denunciation, the Inquisition had Mauricia placed under the care of a parish priest who absolved her of her crimes. This, in essence, was "spiritual physic," a form of mental health care practiced by the clergy that "aimed at restoring equilibrium in the souls of troubled individuals."[96] According to Stephen Haliczer, one of the central aspects of post-Tridentine Spanish Catholicism was the "greatly enhanced role for the priest/confessor as the 'doctor of souls.'"[97] As a physician of the soul, the confessor possessed the power to appease the tortured consciences of penitents like Mauricia. Furthermore, so went the thinking, through his familiarity with the penitent's thoughts and intentions, as well as her personal history, he had privileged insight into her psyche and could proffer a diagnosis that would assist the inquisitors in their negotiations. In this way, the confessor served as both spiritual doctor and judge.

The role of confessor was particularly important in Mauricia's fourth and final auto-denunciation in 1784. Like her first denunciation, this one was mediated by a confessor, in this case Antonio Pichardo, who had received Mauricia's confession but was unwilling to absolve the penitent, fearing she had committed a form of "mixed heresy." Instead, he urged her to seek out the Inquisition. By 1784, Mauricia was an infirm and destitute older woman residing in the capital's Hospicio de Pobres (poorhouse). In his letter to the Holy Office, Pichardo underscored the pathos of Mauricia's situation and requested that the tribunal use discretion in their proceedings against the suspect so that she would not suffer ridicule or alienation from the other poorhouse inmates.[98]

The Inquisition's response was to fully enlist the help of Mauricia's previous confessors. They first summoned Cristobal de Folger, who had confessed Mauricia on many occasions at the Hospicio and once when she was gravely ill at the Hospital of San Juan de Dios. According to Folger, Mauricia suffered from an asthmatic condition known as a "suffocated chest" and, based on his personal observations, displayed a "species of furor" and *frenesi*. The priest recalled how on one occasion she appeared for confession crying for her lost kitten and later began to hallucinate, pointing to a cat that did not exist.[99] Another priest, friar Pasqual Equiía, held a vastly different opinion: Mauricia was "excessively dumb" (*demasiadamente tonta*) and "simple"—not mad.[100]

The most persuasive testimony came from Pichardo himself, who visited the Hospicio to question the attendants, physicians, and fellow inmates about Mauricia's conduct and mental health. The tribunal had particularly requested to know if Mauricia was a good Christian who attended mass regularly and observed the sacraments. In his letter, Pichardo offered a balanced and painstakingly nuanced testimony. He reported that many people at the Hospicio considered Mauricia to be a dedicated Christian and an honest woman, and in the words of one of the nurses, Mauricia was a "saintly soul."[101] Many witnesses commented that although she was virtuous, her moods were highly unpredictable. According to Francisca Alanis, another nurse, Mauricia's "mood was very variable, and sometimes she would speak with much warmth, and friendliness," while on other occasions she was taciturn and depressed.[102] Other witnesses noted that Mauricia was overly zealous about confessing. For example, Doña Josepha Vasquez, an honorable matron who held a position of authority at the Hospicio, characterized Mauricia as someone who was "scrupulous" and "timid," "always [to be found] behind the confession booth, praying, or confessing herself."[103]

Pichardo's letter also included medical testimony. According to the physician attending to Mauricia, she was not mad but rather suffering from a suffocated chest. Whatever the cause, her situation merited compassion, Pichardo emphasized. Mauricia's body was severely damaged and wounded (*lastimado y rasgado*) from the bloodletting and other "cruel medicines" that the physician had applied.[104] He also noted that her age and ill health rendered her excessively weak to fulfill any punishment that the Holy Office might wish to administer. "She is also worthy of mercy," he went on, "for wanting to present herself [to the Inquisition] so many times."[105] Swayed by Pichardo's letter, the Inquisition acted leniently. As in previous occasions, Mauricia was once again absolved of her sins—no matter how she might have felt about them. The Inquisition would act as the rational conscious they deemed she lacked.

In comparing the two cases, it is worth noting Rafaela's enclosure in the Convent of Santa Ines and Mauricia's forced internment at the Hospital del Divino Salvador for poor madwomen and later at the Hospicio de Pobres. At a time when the hospital had yet to become the primary custodial institution for managing madness, individuals suffering from its affliction, if not cared for at home by relatives, might find themselves confined in a variety of institutions, whether medical or otherwise. This was especially the case for women in a colonial patriarchal society that sanctioned enclosure as a means of protecting women's bodies and enforcing gender norms. Surplus elite women like Rafaela often found themselves funneled into convents, where the conditions of enclosure and religious life, especially if imposed involuntarily, could provoke despair, suicidal ideation, and other forms of psychological distress.[106] Poor and marginal women like Mauricia faced grimmer options, and in many ways their plight mirrored that of fallen women placed into *casas de recogimiento* for their correction. Nancy van Deusen has documented the widespread practice of *recogimiento* in the Spanish Americas, a practice that involved the depositing of girls and women into institutions such as convents, pious houses, schools, and hospitals. Although originally intended to educate and Hispanicize the mestizo daughters of conquistadores and young women of the Indigenous nobility, by this period *casas de recogimiento* were more concerned with regulating the behavior of socially and sexually deviant women such as prostitutes, adulteresses, single mothers, and *divorciadas* (women seeking divorce litigation). Colonial officials variously labeled these problematic women as "repentant" (*arrepentidas*), "evil" (*mujeres de mal vivir*), or "lost" (*perdidas*).[107] Poor madwomen like Mauricia were subsumed into this broader category of marginal, vulnerable, and dishonored women, and the main institution designed to contain them—the Divino Salvador—assumed many of the characteristics of houses for wayward women. In fact, in 1722 the Mexican periodical *Gaceta de*

Mexico revealingly described the Divino Salvador not as a hospital but as a "*recogimiento.*"[108]

THERE WAS A TIME when historians praised Pinel's late eighteenth-century intervention in French hospitals—encapsulated in the unchaining of the mad at the Bicêtre and Salpêtrière—as the moment that ushered in a period of humane treatment toward the mentally disturbed, when "moral treatment" replaced chains and brute force, and madness became managed through humane medical techniques, including the "talking cure" and the inculcation of moral self-discipline. Whether praised or, as in the case of Foucault, attacked, the moment has stood as a convenient touchstone of the Enlightenment and a decided shift from the barbarism that came before it. Yet while recent regional histories have shown that the pre-Enlightenment period was anything but barbaric—indeed, the history of San Hipólito fits well into this growing field—histories of madness have failed to fully account for the role of the Inquisition as an engine of medicalization and a proponent of a humane and rational approach to madness.

Why? The Holy Office itself is partly to blame. In the late eighteenth century, the institution became a reactionary force against Francophile influences, including French Protestantism and the revolutionary ideas of the philosophes. On this matter, they treaded on delicate ground. Before the French Revolution, the French leanings of Charles III, who drew inspiration from the enlightened despotism of French monarchs, created an atmosphere that promoted French literature for its utilitarian knowledge. After the Revolution, however, elite fears that the more subversive elements of Enlightenment thought would infiltrate New Spain and set it on a similar path prompted the Inquisition to embark on what Richard Greenleaf has characterized as a "resurgence of inquisitorial activity."[109] Its index of prohibited books—essentially a compilation of the Enlightenment canon from Voltaire to Pope—only reinforced its image, then and now, of a backward institution mired in intolerance and staunchly opposed to the forces of progressive social change.[110]

Yet though the Inquisition never set out to be a radical bastion of social change, its commitment to what it saw as a divine mandate to uncover and adjudicate on sin made it into one of the most humane, and in this sense even modern, institutions in the Hispanic world—certainly so in New Spain. Differentiating sin from mere error or mistake demanded entering into a suspect's interiority thoughtfully, and in many cases empathetically, to deduce the conscience of the actor and the reasoning for his or her choices, and it is clear that by the mid-eighteenth century, the Inquisition was willing to do this. A powerful, influential institution, the Inquisition not only had embraced the principle of insanity in matters of religious orthodoxy but was actively working to discern where individual responsibility ended and insanity began. To do this, it would lean on the insights and opinions of medical experts, unleashing a process that lent greater legitimacy to physicians in matters of madness—albeit slowly, hesitantly, and not without contestation.

CHAPTER FOUR

Medicalization and Its Discontents

On March 18, 1770, José de Silva, a Creole tailor from Puebla and a prisoner of the Inquisition, was escorted from the secret cells to the Church of Santo Domingo in the center of Mexico City to attend mass and receive his sentence.[1] The infamous staging of judgment known as the auto-da-fé (act of faith) required Silva to wear a number of penitential trappings, including a gag fastened to his mouth (*mordaza*), a rope around his neck, and a cone-shaped hat (*coroza*) bearing the insignias of a blasphemous heretic. He also carried in his palms a lit wax candle, which he humbly offered to the priest once the mass had concluded. Then the sentence was read. For his numerous crimes, which involved heretical propositions and various other scandalous acts against the Catholic Church, including publicly slandering and physically threatening an ecclesiastic, Silva was condemned to ten years of exile, four of which would consist of forced labor on the presidio in Havana. Following the sentencing, the disgraced tailor was shamefully paraded through the crowded streets of the capital in his penitential attire while the town crier announced his crime and punishment to spectators—a stark but customary example of the Holy Office's resolve to use shame as much as corporal punishment to discipline those who stepped outside Church orthodoxy. Two days later he performed his penance, abjuring his sins *de levi*, for "minor offenses," and was subsequently carted off to the royal prison to await his transfer to Havana.[2]

But Silva never made it to Havana—he never even boarded the ship—because in the weeks that followed, he lost his wits. On April 4, the priest Juan de Dios Loreto Bestan descended into the cold and murky royal cells to hear the prisoners's confession, but he was unable to confess Silva, who was taciturn and resistant and whose *juicio* appeared to be, in Bestan's words, "perturbed." The other prisoners quickly affirmed the priest's suspicions that the condemned Creole tailor had gone utterly mad.[3] Upon learning of Silva's questionable mental state, the Holy Office summoned its physician, Juan Joseph de la Peña y Brizuela, who, over a course of a week, examined the prisoner on multiple occasions and, after careful deliberations, delivered a concise medical report. By his careful estimation, Silva displayed a "morbid melancholy," a "strange sadness with much peevishness," and an "inclination towards solitude." He further noted that the prisoner "would not allow his pulse to be taken, nor his body to be touched, [as he was] fearful of everyone," and that he would often indulge in "ridiculous conversations." These were the classic symptoms, the physician concluded, of a "melancholic delirium, an accident or illness" that stemmed from the "cooling and drying of the brain." He explained how humoral imbalance and putrefaction had produced "melancholic vapors" in Silva's body, which had "risen to the brain," distorting his mental faculties—particularly his imagination. Disequilibrium of vital humors and spirits explained why some men were prone to outlandish hallucinations and "imagined [that] they were kings . . . or made of glass . . . or gods."[4] Confident in his diagnosis, the physician proceeded to caution the Holy Office against prolonging Silva's confinement within the royal prison. Such conditions, he stated, "originate from sadness, or what one calls discord of soul and body," and would likely intensify within inhospitable environments. He then went on to cite examples—largely from natural philosophical texts—in which extended imprisonment had prompted sudden death as evidence of the heavy toll emotions took on both mind and body.[5]

As shown in previous cases, *any* manifestation of madness among the accused put the Holy Office in any uneasy conundrum, but Silva's situation was especially challenging. As a medically diagnosed melancholic, he was clearly incapable of serving the terms of his sentence, nor could he continue to remain imprisoned within the royal cells on the brink of sudden and calamitous death—a devastating outcome indeed for a tribunal whose primary obligation was to salvage rather than imperil misguided souls. Further complicating the situation, Silva *was* a convicted heretic who could hardly be allowed to go free. Technically, the insanity defense applied only to those subjects who had offended the faith during moments of compromised intellect, but Silva had been sane when he committed his crimes and became mad only *after*; did that entitle him to the leniency of the insanity defense? Unable to forge a consensus or render a firm determination about whether or not *when* madness manifests in the accused matters in granting leniency, Julian Vicente González de Andia dodged the issue and had the tailor committed to San Hipólito indefinitely. Thus, on May 12, 1770, more than a year after his unfortunate run-in with the Holy Office and less than two months following his sentencing and public shaming, the heretical and now mad tailor was admitted to the hospital with a warning from the Holy Office to the prior general that he should keep a close watch on the patient-prisoner to ensure that he did not flee.[6]

While not all patients made their way to San Hipólito in such dramatic fashion, Silva's case underscores a number of critical developments. First, it exposes the Holy Office's growing dependency on the mental hospital for the purposes of managing *locura* and the challenges it introduced to inquisitorial procedure. Second, it highlights the centrality of medical opinion not only for prompting hospital confinement but for addressing questions of human cognition that were at the root of inquisitorial investigation in a rational, scientific way. As chapter 3 argued, the Inquisition's obsession with the intricacies of human interiority and the nuances of volition generated some of the most sophisticated uses of the insanity defense in late colonial Mexico and fostered an unexpectedly conducive environment for the medicalization of madness. This chapter builds on these insights, paying closer attention to the role of medical expertise and medical discourse within the inquisitorial courts. While university-trained physicians had long counted among the Inquisition's salaried personnel and attended to the health of prisoners, it was in the eighteenth century that they began to serve as key witnesses in matters in which a suspect's sanity was in doubt. In so doing, they equipped inquisitors with a more refined set of tools for gauging interiority, such as empiricism and a rational theoretical framework for understanding mental disorder. Nevertheless, this chapter argues that in spite of their expanded role and prestige as diagnostic experts, these physicians were but secondary actors in a process of medicalization that was ultimately propelled by the Inquisition and its religious imperatives.

As the individuals charged with determining and characterizing a suspect's interiority, inquisitors faced a challenging task, but they could expect to rely on other witnesses—including local spectators, friends and neighbors, fellow prison inmates, lawyers, and parish priests—to chime in and provide insight. In fact, in the sixteenth and seventeenth centuries, these were the main witnesses on which the Inquisition relied in their deliberations.[7] However, beginning in the 1730s and particularly from 1760 on, these figures declined in importance as inquisitors came to privilege medical testimony as the highest form of evidentiary proof. They thus served as key agents of medicalization, lending legitimacy to rationalist models of illness and of *locura* in particular. Seen in this light, confinement at San Hipólito was not necessarily punitive. Rather, it was the practical, imperfect, and at times creative outcome of the Holy Office's willingness to insist on madness's physiological underpinnings.

Returning to the case of José de Silva, it is worth expounding on one of the paradoxes his situation and others so consistently reveal: the contrast between the Holy Office's unbridled commitment to its time-tested procedures and traditions—in this instance, its continued reliance on the outdated auto-da-fé for enacting what Toby Green has called its "reign of fear"—and its eager embrace of medical theory and medical forms of discernment as a heuristic device to complement its already hefty arsenal for gauging interiority.[8] It is precisely this juxtaposition of tradition and innovation that speaks to the central theme of the Hispanic Enlightenment when approached from the vantage point of one of the empire's most maligned and stereotyped institutions. While Enlightenment intellectuals excoriated against the Holy Office, casting it as a symbol of Old Regime decadence, backwardness, and religious intolerance, in practice it was not as hostile to the forces of rationalism as its critics opined.[9] Certainly, in many ways eighteenth-century inquisitors remained tethered to the medieval worldview from which the Holy Office originated and understood their work in terms of a cosmic battle between God and Satan for the bodies and souls of mortals.[10] But when faced with instances of suspected madness in their courts, they turned to medicine as a valuable epistemological tool, generating the kinds of questions and seeking the kinds of solutions that facilitated madness's medicalization.

Witnesses of the Mind and Body

Chapter 3 introduced the figure of Felipe Antonio Alvarez, the spiritually lapsed Franciscan friar whose heretical articulations sent inquisitors on a legal merry-go-around as they tried to figure out whether the friar was a heretic or a madman. Confounded by the evidence and circumstances of his case, and worried that their deliberations would plummet into endless speculation, the inquisitors reached out to whatever expertise was available. In addition to consulting three medical professionals, who filed extensive reports on the friar's mental state, they eagerly thumbed through the writings of seventeenth-century Roman physician and jurist Paolo Zacchia. "Zacchia," they announced, quoting the opinion of the enlightened cleric Benito Feijoo, "has more authority than twenty gullible authors who write whatever they want without any reflection."[11] In his *Quaestiones medico-legales*, the text under the inquisitors' scrutiny, Zacchia had called attention to the utility of medical knowledge within legal settings.[12] It was a ponderous work that transformed the body into legal evidence whose physical manifestations were best left to the physician's erudite interpretation. On the subject of madness—a disease with somatic origins—Zacchia had plenty to say, stressing that there was "scarcely another disease more easily and more frequently feigned than insanity (*insania*) and no disease more difficult to discern."[13]

The *calificadores* who deliberated ad nauseam in the case of the recalcitrant friar found Zacchia's work compelling, as it applied principles of medicine to the law through cases studies and offered an exhaustive treatment of madness's manifold causes and physical symptoms. In discerning madness in legal subjects, Zacchia advocated for a comprehensive approach that took into account a wide range of criteria, including the individual's words and actions, his or her emotional state, physical symptoms as observed by a competent physician, and "exterior causes," such as the environment or lifestyle.[14]

With Zacchia as their guide, the *calificadores* navigated Alvarez's complicated case, emphasizing first and foremost that the "most certain and infallible signs of madness" resided in what they called the *passiones de animo* (emotions). By inspecting the suspect's emotional state and sentiments, a careful observer might discern his or her mental facilities. Based on their careful reading of Zacchia, they concluded that a defective emotional state consisted of "despising what was worthy of praise, praising the despicable; not fearing what was fearsome and horrendous; desiring the adverse," and exhibiting "courage and audacity" in the presence of people or situations that should inspire "shame and confusion."[15] Alvarez, the heretical friar, satisfied all these criteria, particularly in his shocking contempt for religious authority, casual dismissal of scripture, and brazen confidence—even in the face of stern punishment from the Holy Office. The inquisitors found that even Alvarez's eyes possessed the dull obscure look that Zacchia reported characterized madness. As if it were not enough that the accused both acted and looked insane in the present moment, the inquisitors employed Zacchia's insight that overstimulated senses could corrupt a person's faculties of reason to explain the friar's checkered past and, in particular, his predilection for what they characterized as "various species of lust" and "effusions of semen."[16]

The *calificadores*' use of Zacchia's text as a valuable diagnostic aid signaled important changes in how medicine was to be deployed within the inquisitorial courts. As scholars have shown, the dissemination of Zacchia's work in the courts of continental Europe in the seventeenth and eighteenth centuries went hand in hand with the elevated status of physicians and surgeons as authoritative witnesses. From canonization proceedings to support or refute claims of bodily incorruption or miraculous healing to criminal trials involving murder or infanticide, medical professionals appeared as increasingly prominent fixtures in legal disputes.[17] They differentiated themselves from other witnesses on account of their specialized knowledge of the body, both its internal processes and its outward manifestations, and became, in Silvia de Renzi's words, "witnesses of the body"—that is, expert evaluators who were uniquely and adeptly skilled at interpreting the body and its physical symptoms as a novel form of legal evidence.[18]

In New Spain, a perpetual dearth of university-trained practitioners meant that the "medical turn" within the courts consolidated much later, in the mid- to late eighteenth century, precisely around the time the Enlightenment had made itself felt within the mature Spanish colony.[19] It was during this period that New Spain witnessed recurring examples of medical experts testifying in Inquisition cases, especially on questions of madness. From the late seventeenth century on, physical evidence in the form of bodily examination by a medical expert or midwife played an important role in resolving cases involving *esturpo* (rape) and sodomy, crimes with muddled jurisdiction that entangled both the secular and the episcopal courts, and with respect to sodomy, even the inquisitorial courts.[20] For trials on *alumbradismo* (illuminism), a form of mysticism prosecuted as a Lutheran heresy, inquisitors had to evaluate ecstatic fits, visions, trances, convulsions, and contortions in order to determine whether divine or demonic powers were at play. Here, too, by the eighteenth century, medical categories worked to discredit alleged visionaries by attributing their symptoms to malady, especially insanity, epilepsy, and, for women, hysteria.[21]

The penetration of medical discourse and medical expertise into the courts occurred in tandem with the nascent consolidation of the medical profession. Throughout the colonial period, university-trained physicians remained an elite minority, eclipsed in daily practice by a diverse landscape of unorthodox healers whom the crown failed to fully regulate. Nevertheless, in this period, they began to differentiate themselves from irregular healers, wrap themselves in a mantle of greater legitimacy, and more closely align their profession with the emerging reformist policies of the state. In the late eighteenth century, physicians revamped the university medical curriculum to incorporate formal training in the more empirical sciences of surgery and botany and would go on to enforce stipulations for mandatory clinical training.[22] The theoretical foundation of medicine also shifted to accommodate a proliferating set of texts written by more contemporary authors. Whereas medical training had long centered on humoral theory as expounded in the canonical works of Galen, Hippocrates, and Avicenna, following the second half of the eighteenth century physicians enjoyed access to a diverse authorship that included physicians and scientists like Herman Boerhaave,

Andres Piquer, Johannes de Gorter, and Lorenzo Bellini, as well as a growing body of homegrown authors.[23]

While the eighteenth century saw little medical professionalization within the halls of San Hipólito, physicians were beginning to carve a niche for themselves within the spaces of the Holy Office as experts in diagnosing *locura*. On this front, medical professionals brought a unique skill set to the table. First, they came armed with theoretical training and were able to draw on rationalist models of illness to explain nonsensical thought and behavior. While ordinary colonial people spoke of *demencia* or *locura* in the generic sense, learned physicians employed more technical terminology and conveyed a firm grasp of the internal mechanisms underlying aberrant or inferior mental states.

By the late eighteenth century, medical understandings of *locura* had undergone significant transformation, although they remained indebted to terminology derived from humoral medicine and its fixation on physiological equilibrium and correlations between illness and larger environmental and lifestyle factors. In his *Compendio de la medicina practica*, published in 1788, the Creole physician Juan Manuel Venegas defined madness as "that illness in which the afflicted . . . think, act, [or] speak . . . [in a manner] that is not in agreement with his or her reasoning." He then proceeded to enumerate a series of causes, with the most immediate being "pressure or dryness of the sensory vessels" and "thickness of the cerebral liquids." Other factors included hereditary disposition; injury or contusions to the brain; irritations to the cerebral membranes caused by fevers; hysterical or convulsive "accidents"; poisons or toxins in the body; excessive "sadness, care, fright, pride, avarice, lust, ire"; hypochondriacal excesses or extreme fixation on a particular object; "the movement of acrid or ichorous humors into the head"; and "grave debility of the body."[24] This blanket but highly technical definition, which reflected mechanical models of the body, encompassed a broad spectrum of disordered thought and action, with the most extreme and violent manifestation being mania. The maniacal individual was essentially a *loco furioso* with a fancy diagnosis—that is, a person who exhibited unwarranted bouts of intense anger and violence, labored incessantly, all the while withstanding long durations without food or sleep. Venega explained that this most severe and episodic form of *locura* originated in the "irritation of the membranes of the brain" due to an excess of corrupt material or fluid.[25] If mania was one end of the spectrum of madness, its opposite was the condition widely known as *melancolía* (melancholy), which, in keeping with contemporary thought, Venegas defined as a form of hypochondria arising from corrupt matter passing from the liver to the blood and whose symptoms comprised anxiety, sadness, constant fear, predilection to solitude, and delirium.[26]

In addition to specialized knowledge of the body—its internal machinations and effects on the faculties of reason—medical professionals summoned in Inquisition cases arrived with something even more valuable: empirical evidence. Physicians and surgeons derived their expertise not only from the thorough digestion of erudite tomes but through firsthand interaction with patients and careful scrutiny of their symptoms. As chapter 3 emphasized, the inquisitor's favored route to "fact-finding" or arriving at guilt or innocence—the accumulation of testimony from lay witnesses and interrogation of the accused—was notoriously unreliable and inconclusive at best in cases of suspected *locura*. Medical testimony of the kind offered by skilled professionals not only promised an attractive alternative but carried the hallmark of objective truth: rooted scientific theory backed by empirical observation. It certainly was not the case that heresy disappeared in the second half of the eighteenth century, but in this period, incriminating actions could easily become something categorically different: symptoms. In the same way, sin could become illness.

Familiar Bedfellows

To be sure, the Inquisition had long embraced medicine in its proceedings and, since the mid-sixteenth century, had maintained its own permanently staffed physician and surgeon among its ranks. As salaried employees complicit in the inquisitorial apparatus, medical practitioners had long performed two basic but vital functions. First, they attended to the health of prisoners confined within the secret cells. This task was usually reserved for the surgeon, who made routine visits to the prison cells and operated in consultation with the supervising physician. Only in specific cases, such as when a prisoner had died or fallen gravely ill, or in situations complicated by pregnancy, did the physician deliver personal examinations. Second, medical practitioners had long furnished the inquisitorial court with a specific type of expert evaluation: whether a suspect was physically fit to undergo torture and, in the case of convicted heretics, whether they could withstand the typical punishment of public whippings or forced labor. Throughout the sixteenth and seventeenth centuries, the Inquisition's physicians, at least for New Spain, had little concern for—and consequently little to say about—a suspect's mental state.[27]

For the licensed practitioner, employment within the Holy Office bestowed numerous benefits. Although physicians and surgeons generally received less salary than other officials, they reaped surplus income from medical costs and services, usually paid for out of funds generated from the prisoner's confiscated property. Moreover, staff practitioners could count on the Holy Office's sizable body of court officials—inquisitors as well as *familiares*, or low-level functionaries—as steady and prestigious clientele. In addition to the comforts of financial security, affiliation with the Inquisition brought legal protection and enhanced one's reputation and social status, no small perk in a colonial society structured according to the ideals of honor, inherited privilege, and racial purity. Worth emphasizing is that membership within this exclusive community of *letrados* testified irrefutably to one's *limpieza de sangre* (purity of blood), a prerequisite both for joining the ranks of the Inquisition and for obtaining a university education.[28]

The Holy Office and the medical profession thus enjoyed a mutually beneficial relationship. In a crucial sense, both bodies were conjoined in an effort to uphold a colonial status quo rooted in Catholic orthodoxy and racial and class hierarchy. By affixing themselves to the Inquisition not only as salaried employees and expert witnesses but also by taking up posts as local functionaries (the so-called *familiares*), university-trained medical practitioners lent legitimacy to their aspiring profession. Moreover, they stood to profit from the tribunal's agenda to prosecute popular or irregular healers whose beliefs and practices smacked of superstition or witchcraft.[29] In short, the Holy Office played a critical role in buttressing the ascendancy of the medical profession in the late colonial period, while the latter furnished the former with new models of evidence, rooted in scientific theory and empiricism, for addressing the long-standing mysteries of human reasoning and intent.

Diagnosing *Locura*, or The Inquisitor's Quandary Revisited

In spite of the physician's claim to specialized expertise and authoritative knowledge of the mind and body, how medicalization unfolded in actual practice was a complex, contested, and untidy process. For starters, *locura* proved notoriously difficult to unequivocally identify, even for the most expert and trained eyes. While medical theory had parsed madness into several distinct varieties—mania, melancholy, furor, or frenzy—diagnosing a particular disorder was never straightforward and unambiguous. Indeed, madness possessed many faces, and its symptoms were seemingly infinite.

On one extreme, it could manifest itself on the fringes of human behavior: in bouts of intense wrath, perpetual motion, and senseless, incoherent babble. On the opposite end of the spectrum, madness might only present itself through subtle shifts in mood or behavior, or through heightened attention on a particular subject or object. Any of these symptoms, exaggerated or barely perceptible, could easily be mistaken for other conditions, such as stupidity, inebriation, or simply altered states of emotion that did not impinge on the powers of reasoning sufficiently to warrant a diagnosis of insanity. Further complicating this already messy picture, doctors had known for centuries that madness could be episodic, with states of impaired judgment punctuated by lucid intervals (*intervales*), making it that much harder to link deviant thought and action to defective cognition.

In addition, medical professionals did not enjoy unchecked authority in deciding who was mad and who was sane. Diagnosing *locura* was very often a collective effort, and the power to issue a verdict ultimately resided with the inquisitor, who found medical evidence both useful and compelling but did not necessarily regard it as hegemonic knowledge. While doctors had begun to stake their territory in claiming to know the mechanisms by which physiological processes ensnared the mind, in the era before psychiatry they had yet to fully colonize matters of thought and emotion, which resided very much still in the hands of the religious.

Chapter 3 discussed the "inquisitor's quandary"—that is, the moral, legal, and epistemological predicament the inquisitor found himself in when grappling with cases of alleged madness. The mad individual's presumed innocence before the law meant that the inquisitor needed to tread cautiously, even err on the side of lenience, in situations in which the suspect's sanity was in doubt. At the same time, the Holy Office had to guard against the devious and cunning who might act insane to avoid punishment. In the end, the Inquisition's purpose rested in assuring that Church doctrine remained secure, and if it opened an enormous loophole for the heretical to pass through, it would be violating its own mission. Medicine promised a way out of this predicament, furnishing inquisitors with rationalist models of madness that bypassed many of the uncertainties that came from relying on witness testimony, or the endless and inconclusive questioning that resulted from interrogation of the accused. However, the introduction of medical expertise was hardly a magic bullet. Quite to the contrary, it often served to amplify uncertainty and confusion. Inquisitors indeed became agents of medicalization, but they often did so hesitantly and only through a process, at times clumsy, of trial and error.

When the Holy Office called in medical experts to delve into the mental state of Felipe Zarate in 1790, it discovered how much—and how little—help physicians had to offer. In particular, Zarate's case demonstrates that while medical expertise helped inquisitors navigate the nebulous terrain demarcating madness from inebriation, it did not entirely eradicate fears of simulated illness, which perpetually loomed large. A year earlier, in the summer of 1789, Zarate caused a scandal when he ran amok down the streets of Texcoco hurling blasphemies in what appeared to be a drunken stupor. According to witnesses, he had cried, "Me cago en Dios, y en la María Santissima" (I shit on God and the Virgin Mary!), "Es un carajo Dios" (God be damned!), and "Maldito sea el que me crio" (Damn the one who created me!). Eventually, he was subdued by a group of angry neighbors and deposited in the local jail. While incarcerated, Zarate persisted to blaspheme well into the night, much to the irritation of the other inmates, who beat him in a vain effort to silence him. When the priest of Texcoco, friar Manuel de Arpide, learned of Zarate's verbal assaults on the faith, he immediately denounced him to the Holy Office.[30]

As with many cases that came before the Inquisition, testimony from witnesses—from local spectators to prison deputies and inmates—produced unsatisfactory results. In particular, there was much confusion as to whether Zarate's offensive utterances stemmed from mental illness or inordinate drinking. Most people who knew him simply dismissed Zarate as a drunkard. Zarate's employer, Joaquín de Campos, had many times heard him renounce the faith and issue other *disparates* (foolish remarks) but attributed them to his fondness for *pulque* (an alcoholic beverage made from fermented cactus).[31] Josef de Ariza, a weaver who had known Zarate for nearly eighteen years, cited his drinking habit in a long list of vices that included gambling, living in concubinage, and not confessing regularly.[32] Another witness reported that Zarate was "inclined to drink, and when he drank something, he would begin to laugh" and talk to himself.[33] Zarate's drinking was an added problem for the doctors called to diagnosis him, for they had been trained to believe that alcohol could cause mental disorder by producing hot vapors, which would rise up toward the brain, resulting in muddled judgment and delirium. In his treatise on practical medicine, Venegas included *embriaguez*, or inebriation, as a form of mental illness, describing excessive drinking as a "species of *frenesi*" (frenzy) in which the imbiber became "heated" and "infuriated"; was prone to "shout," "tremble," and "do petulant things"; and experience "anxiety, violent vomiting, fluxes in the blood, and palpitations of the heart."[34]

To add another dimension to the unfolding saga, Zarate himself offered an alternative explanation for his unruly conduct: he was under the sway of the devil. According to one of the prison deputies, Zarate had stated than an ominous "wind" had whispered in his ear, urging him to utter blasphemies and the following scandalous chant in particular: "Ave María, tu barriga con la mía" (Ave Maria, your belly against mine). Zarate also told the deputy that

> on some occasions when he was weaving he saw on the fabric an image of our lady of Ocotlán who appeared dancing with a crucifix, and because the fabric was moving, he could no longer continue to weave. . . . That one night he went to sleep in a barn, and the next day while he was shaking off the hay that was stuck to his sleeve, a voice spoke into his ear and it told him not to shake off [the hay]. . . . That on another night as he was about to go to bed he saw a worm crawling around the end of the candlestick, and the same voice said that it was the worm of [his] conscience.

When questioned before the tribunal, Zarate confirmed to have experienced this vision. He was not a drunkard, he adamantly told the inquisitors, but a victim of the devil's malice.

Similar to the case of Mauricia Josefa de Apelo—who also claimed to cavort with the devil—Zarate's appeal to malicious demonic influences carried little traction among skeptical inquisitors. While the devil remained a powerful figure in popular religion, embodying the convergence of native concepts and Christian beliefs, by the late colonial period, belief in the devil's existence appears to have waned, "demoted to mere 'superstition'" in the eyes of educated Spanish officials and ecclesiastics.[35] Thus, while Zarate tethered his criminal actions to demonic forces, his defense held little sway over the inquisitors, who proved to be increasingly wedded to "rationalist standards of evidence."[36]

Ultimately, they sided with the testimony provided by the tribunal's appointed physician, Francisco Rada—but not without significant reservations. In a concise report dated April 22, 1790, Rada confirmed that while Zarate did not display the symptoms of "melancholy delirium, furor, or mania," his judgment was most certainly impaired by a "form of fatuity" that indicated that his "mind was not perfect."[37] However, in medical terms, this diagnosis was vague; unlike melancholy or mania, *fatuidad* did not correspond to a concrete set of symptoms rooted in an underlying physiological imbalance, leaving room for uncertainty. In effect, Rada announced to the court that

Medicalization and Its Discontents   125

while he was certain Zarate was in fact mad, he could not specify *why* he was mad. And while the inquisitors valued the physician's input, they did not accept it blindly. Rather, they considered it alongside their own observations of the suspect's conduct and responsiveness during his interrogation. Thus, the prosecuting judge, or *fiscal*, noted that Zarate "responded with understanding [*acuerdo*] and reflection" to questions pertaining to his "genealogy, provenance, occupation, and [knowledge of] doctrine." However, when pressured to discuss the circumstances of his imprisonment, he became reticent and reserved. To the *fiscal*, these inconsistencies pointed to the fact that Zarate was more inclined to "malice rather than fatuousness."[38]

Yet even he could not come to a firm conclusion. If Zarate was not unambiguously mad, he was still bizarre enough to clearly not be sane in any ordinary sense, and the *fiscal* sent him to San Hipólito for a period of twelve to fifteen days so that his condition could be closely monitored. After even closer observation, the brothers at the hospital could do no better than the court's physicians, and in the end, they declared Zarate to be "medio demente" (somewhat mad).[39]

Of course, not all of this ambiguity can be laid at the feet of doctors. Madness, like sanity, was a slippery spectrum, its liminality stumbling physicians as much as inquisitors and lay audiences. Inquisitors, however, could not afford to truck in liminality. Suspects were guilty or innocent—deserving of punishment, penance, or release. The Holy Office needed more from physicians than ambiguity and highly qualified judgments; they needed conviction and struggled to get it from a profession not fully confident in its authority.

The Melancholy Bigamist and the Enlightened Melancholic

If identifying fatuity could be tricky, proving melancholy could be vexing. A disease recognized since classical antiquity, melancholy had long been associated with the preponderance of the melancholic humor, or black bile; when corrupted or present in excess proportions, this bile produced toxic vapors that migrated to different parts of the body, including the brain, wreaking havoc and impairing proper physiological and mental function. In his *Florilegio medicinal* (1712), Juan Esteyneffer explained how the protean symptoms of *melancolía* reflected the inner movement of noxious vapors and their effects on different body parts. If the vapors stayed still, then the individual was "content and joyful, as if he or she had never suffered from any ailment." However, if they reached the head, then the sufferer experienced headaches, buzzing in ears, and blurry vision, and if the vapors dispersed throughout the brain, the disorder expressed itself in more intense ways: delirium or disordered thoughts, fantasies, poor sleep, nightmares, and an aversion to people. If they engulfed the heart, the patient might expect palpitations, anxiety, fainting, and fright to ensue; in the stomach, they generated flatulence, belching, and vomiting.[40]

From the fifteenth century on, melancholy proved an alluring and malleable metaphor for mental and emotional suffering that captivated the attention of artists, writers, philosophers, and theologians.[41] In the courts of the Holy Office, however, it surfaced as an unglamorous condition whose unwieldy symptoms confounded inquisitors and medical professionals alike. Two cases from the eighteenth century, sixty years apart—one involving a humble mulatto accused of bigamy, the other a literate military lieutenant under fire for subversive statements—capture the climate of confusion and ambiguity that reigned in efforts to diagnose melancholy. They also demonstrate that while medical knowledge imposed a semblance of transparency on what was a messy state of affairs, it often did so while exacerbating the very states of quandary it was intended to resolve.

The first case begins in 1737, when the *alcalde mayor* of Taxco arrested Antonio de la Cruz for the "bad treatment" of his wife, Polonía Rosales. In addition to the charge of abuse, authorities suspected that Cruz had committed bigamy in marrying Polonía when his first wife was still alive.[42] Detained in the Taxco prison for nearly a year, he was eventually transferred to the cells of the Holy Office and, on April 21, 1738, summoned for interrogation by the inquisitor, Pedro Navarro de Isla. In his testimony, Cruz identified himself as a free mulatto, a native of Periban, forty years of age, and a former slave to Don Domingo de Revollar.[43] He emphatically denied the charges of bigamy, insisting that his first wife, María de Mendoza, was long since dead. In his defense, Cruz crafted a captivating story that detailed how he and his first wife were married and then forcefully separated during the course of an acrimonious suit against Revollar for María's freedom. It was during this period of hardship, while undertaking a six-year stint to work in the Amilpas, that a group of mule drivers from Zamora informed him that his wife had died.[44] However, the Inquisition uncovered a different version of events: Cruz had indeed been formerly married, but according to witnesses he had abandoned his first wife following a series of domestic disputes. He then proceeded to falsely conduct himself as a bachelor in the pueblo of Mazatepec, where he illicitly married Polonía, a free mulatta, blatantly lying to the priest about his marital history.[45]

Although the *fiscal*, Diego Arangado y Chavez, fully intended to prosecute the humble mulatto for the crime of bigamy, his plan fell through when Cruz began to exhibit odd behavior, for by the time of the third *audiencia*, Cruz began to speak "impertinent and foolish things."[46] In came the medical experts. Cruz was subsequently examined by the physician Juan José de Zuniga and the surgeon Francisco Dorantes, both of whom could not initially deliver a definitive diagnosis. On their first visit, they "found him to be agreeable [*acorde*] and by looks of it sane," exhibiting a sound memory and a sensible grasp of the present. Yet while his demeanor betrayed no evidence of *demencia*, they did identify in him a state of altered emotion—what they labeled a *passión de animo*—which, while it stifled the heart, left his powers of reasoning "free."[47] He was, for the purposes of his trial, sane.

On their second visit, however, Dorantes and Zuniga expressed uncertainty. Although Cruz's disposition had improved thanks to the "frequency of medicines," they hesitated to diagnosis him this time around as sane. Instead, they believed his symptoms suggested the "beginnings of melancholia," which, if left untreated, could escalate into full-blown mania.[48] Examined for a third time by Dorantes alone, Cruz not only continued to display *passión de animo* but reported hearing voices. The surgeon hoped a transfer to a different cell might both improve Cruz's condition and allow experts to better study the suspect's symptoms.[49]

The examinations continued, and throughout the month of November Cruz was repeatedly visited by Zuniga. Although his condition appeared to worsen—Cruz continued to hear voices and claimed to see his first wife in an apparition—Zuniga ultimately concluded that Cruz only suffered a *passión de animo* that had not yet descended into madness. In addition, his skepticism compelled him to wonder if some of Cruz's symptoms were perhaps staged to avoid trial. The physician formed this opinion largely by engaging the humble mulatto in a lengthy dialogue. During the course of their conversation, Cruz made a series of revealing statements, including that his "legitimate wife" (Polonía) was pregnant—but presumably not by Cruz, who by now had been imprisoned for close to two years—and that he "would lose his mind to see her [his first wife, María] alive." Based on his reasoned responses to the physician's questions and the "jealous passion" he displayed at having been cuckolded by his second wife, Zuniga became convinced that Cruz was in his *juicio natural* (natural judgment), "without injury" to his powers of reasoning. He proceeded to question Cruz about his children and personal history, to which Cruz responded in a coarse (*bronco*) but logical fashion, illustrating a *sano juicio* (sane judgment).

Zuniga brought to bear every weapon in his medical arsenal. He and Dorantes had applied medicines, taken note of Cruz's appearance, changed his environment, and scrutinized his speech; all that was left was to study how the heavenly bodies affected the patient's behavior. Zuniga began by observing how the "mutation of the moon"—that is, during the new and full moons—affected Cruz's behavior. He observed that during the former Cruz exhibited much *llanto* (weeping), while during the latter he displayed a "tolerable inedia," refusing some of his meals. While Cruz's weeping indicated "fear" and a "recognizable sadness," the physician contended that fear and sadness—like "love, jealously, [and] anger"—were classic symptoms of a *passión de animo*, which was the true source of Cruz's mental and emotional malaise.[50] Zuniga followed his lunar observations by comparing Cruz's symptoms and his response to certain medications against these larger astrological mutations.

As with his earlier visit, the physician's arsenal featured the diagnostic power of dialogue, documenting medicine's early encroachment into domains long dominated by the religious.[51] In engaging the humble mulatto in conversation, Zuniga could observe whether Cruz could string together coherent, cogent statements, which would provide clear evidence of sound reasoning. More importantly, it would help him deduce whether Cruz had experienced any significant life events that aroused the emotions, which could adversely affect the faculties of cognition. As the conversation revealed, Cruz had indeed suffered trauma in learning of his wife's infidelity, which incited feelings of jealous rage and inconsolable sorrow. However, in colonial Mexico's patriarchal society, where masculine honor was tied to the control of female sexuality, the physician concluded that Cruz's reaction was that of a normal jealous husband, not a madman.

In addition, the case of Antonio de la Cruz points to the ways in which medical models could be strategically employed by defendants—specifically lawyers—to claim the insanity defense. If medical expertise had finally granted the inquisitors clearance to pursue charges, Cruz's defense lawyer (*defensor*), Joseph Mendez, would undermine consensus. Mendez mounted an equally sophisticated, if prejudicial, defense of the humble mulatto that rested on two points. The first was that Cruz, sincerely believing that his first wife was dead, did not *knowingly* commit bigamy. The second argument, which elaborated a kind of racial pathology, emphasized a "defect" in the defendant's mental faculties. Having examined Cruz on repeated occasions, Mendez found Cruz to be "manifestly stupid [*leso*] and empty of judgment" (*bacio de entendimiento*). He further argued that Cruz's simplemindedness was not only due to his "rusticity" and lack of education but the product of an underlying medical condition: Cruz suffered, according to his attorney, from a "species of *demencia* . . . where judgment and intelligence in the internal faculties [*potencias internas*] are lacking." He added, "While these species of madness [*enajenación*] are almost innumerable and difficult to diagnose," since Cruz's condition did not manifest itself as *furor*, his chief symptom was "fatuity, stupidity, and what is called idiocy [*mentecas*]." Mendez further cited Cruz's propensity to "sudden tears" whenever he was questioned about the "bad treatment" of his second wife as further evidence of "invisible interior afflictions" whose source was not only guilt but humoral imbalance. The lawyer went on to give Cruz's condition a proper if broad diagnosis: *insania*. This *insania*, he observed, was known to "harm whichever melancholy humor possessed the brain, or imagination, or cognitive or discursive faculty." In Cruz's case, the illness had injured his faculties of imagination and discourse, such as there was "no argument or truth" that could convince the *defensor* that Cruz was "penetrated by reason."[52]

Cruz's case had reached a stalemate: while the *defensor* argued that Cruz should be diagnosed as insane and his trial suspended, the medical experts believed that Cruz's *passión de animo* had not fully shifted into melancholy. This convoluted debate exposes, among many things, the malleability of medical models, which enabled learned men on opposite fronts to arrive at staggeringly different conclusions. While ordinary people spoke of *demencia* or *locura* in a generic sense, learned physicians used technical terminology to explain the relationship between life events, bodily processes, and their effects (or lack thereof) on cognition. Yet their limited authority was made clear in the lawyer's ability to latch on to similar language to muddy the waters and craft a competing interpretation. Such narratives represented highly intricate readings of human interiority offered to quench the inquisitor's appetite for evidence that was both rational and objective. However, and for a variety of reasons ranging from the inquisitor's skepticism to the physician's own diagnostic limitations in the face of an intractable disorder, this testimony rarely resulted in the expediency of procedure.

The inquisitor's response to the gridlock was to stall the delivery of a verdict until Cruz's condition had deteriorated to the point that his madness was undeniable. On January 24, 1739, the Holy Office excused him from his trial and sent him to San Hipólito to be treated for melancholy. During the interim, Dorantes and Zuniga had issued an additional series of wavering assessments regarding Cruz's condition. By this point, the humble mulatto had endured over two years of incarceration and bullying, which had clearly taken their toll. His behavior was more extreme than ever. On January 5, the *alcalde* who visited his cell noted that while he took his breakfast quietly, he "began to scream" and thrust "furious blows" against the doors once they had shut.[53] In his final medical report, Zuniga diagnosed Cruz with a "profound melancholy" that was complemented by a "species of *furor*" and the nascent beginnings of "mania."[54] It would appear that in wavering and prolonging the case, the Inquisition had in fact taken some action and come down harshly on the humble mulatto. Here, the very process of coming before the Inquisition and attempting to prove insanity actually drove the accused further insane.

Over half a century later, melancholy was still a common condition brought before the Inquisition, and though it remained a knotty dilemma, as the case of José María Calderón will show, much had changed in the interval. In the world of eighteenth-century Mexico, Calderón was everything Cruz was not. He was a military officer of European descent enraptured with that bane of religious conservatives on both sides of the Atlantic, Voltaire. Most notably, his case went before the Inquisition nearly two generations after Cruz, in 1795, during a period of intense revolutionary thought and activity, whose currents had reached Calderón's pueblo of Xequelchacan in the bishopric of Yucatán. Unlike Cruz, who affronted the sanctity of marriage and colonial morality, Calderón, according to the Inquisition, had unleashed "scandalous and heretical propositions" against the very bedrocks of New Spain's society. According to various witnesses, Calderón had made slanderous attacks on the Catholic faith, claiming that religion was merely a tool of the elite to subjugate the lower classes, that fornication was not a sin, that hell was not eternal but temporary, that purgatory did not exist, and that the Inquisition was "tiempo perdido" (a waste of time).[55] As if launching a fusillade against the Church, its teachings, and its institutions was not daring enough, Calderón had made a number of politically subversive statements that challenged the authority of the crown. For instance, he was widely known in Xequelchacan for having "applauded" the success of the French Revolution, exalting the superiority of the French government, and forecasting that New Spain would soon follow in its footsteps. His admiration for Voltaire was also no secret.

The *comisario* of Xequelchacan, investigating rumors of Calderón's madness, had questioned witnesses but failed to produce compelling evidence. Although most Xequelchacan residents dismissed his heretical and revolutionary pronouncements as the meaningless babble of a delusional madman, the inquisitors interpreted their testimonies with skepticism. As the *fiscal* explained, "He may have a reputation as a madman because of his scandalous actions without being [mad] in reality."⁵⁶ Because Calderón was stationed in Campeche at the time of the accusation, the *comisario* there had the first opportunity to interview him directly, but he found that Calderón's long-winded answers only raised more questions. At key points, Calderón himself blamed his questionable behavior on "delirium" and "disordered judgment [*juicio trastornado*]." Cryptically, he explained his crimes thus: "Just as the mad have their moments of sanity, [so too do] the sane have their moments of madness."⁵⁷

Calderón was subsequently examined by three military surgeons—Fernando Guerrero, Gabriel Barrero, and José Ruíz Triano—all of whom diagnosed him with melancholy, although some more confidently than others. The strongest conviction—and, notably, the most technical explanation—came from Guerrero, a retired surgeon of the Royal Navy. Basing his assessment on contemporary mechanical explanations of the body, he claimed that Calderón's melancholy originated from an interruption in the movement of blood that "disrupted the course of the spirits to their [corresponding] organs."⁵⁸ From this, the mind would become fixed on a particular thing or idea, resulting in the "perverted imagination" that often compelled men to entertain the most ludicrous of fantasies. It was for this reason, he explained, that some melancholics believed themselves to be "dogs, wolves, or lions"; others "pontificated," thinking they were "kings" or "emperors"; and still others imagined themselves as "angels, demons, [or] gods." In Calderón's case, his compromised intellect was easily swayed by the teachings of anti-Catholic books—which were deliberately designed to "flatter the passions" and "disseminate with malicious sweetness the poison of their pernicious doctrine"—and the "fanaticism" of the French Revolution, which captivated even sane but "ignorant" people. Searching for a cause for Calderón's unfortunate condition, something to make sense of why a respectable officer might utter such revolting ideas, Guerrero found it in a tragedy: the death of his mother had, in the surgeon's judgment, "touched his brain."⁵⁹ Thus, in Guerrero's estimation, Calderón was no dangerous insurgent; his heterodox utterances, he assured inquisitors, had no grounded basis in rational belief because he was a suffering melancholic.

In far simpler terms, the other two surgeons agreed but expressed more doubt. Barrero only affirmed a "tightness or affliction on the left lateral part of his [Calderón's] chest near the heart, the result of having been injured, or possessed of the melancholy humor."⁶⁰ Triano, perhaps in language designed to not contradict his colleagues, bluntly admitted that even both classical and modern authors "confused the true signs" of diseases of the mind and spirit.[61]

Compared to the case of Cruz, the surgeons who examined Calderón arrived at a more compelling diagnosis. Nevertheless, the inquisitors mulled over these reports, never abandoning the possibility that the lieutenant could be feigning illness. They waited a stunning three years until ordering that Calderón be transferred from Campeche to the secret cells in Mexico City so that he could be examined by the tribunal's appointed physician, Francisco Rada—the same expert who had diagnosed Zarate. Rada observed in Calderón the classic symptoms of melancholy: "much taciturnity," the "obscure color" of his face, "the opacity and sadness of his eyes," and conversation that was "not one bit intelligible"—and diagnosed him accordingly.[62] After almost four years of deliberation, the court finally agreed, confident that it was not being duped, and allowed the melancholy lieutenant to enter San Hipólito, where he remained for nearly three years until he suffered a delirium that claimed his life. The inquisitors no doubt took some satisfaction in the hospital's report that Calderón had achieved a lucid "interval" during which he received the last rites.[63]

Send Them to San Hipólito! The Problem of Custody and the Uses of the Mental Hospital

It was not the mere presence of physicians in Inquisition cases that pointed to the medicalization of *locura* in eighteenth-century Mexico but how much they contributed, the shifting language and models they employed, and, even more, how much inquisitors mulled and debated their findings. Yet as the cases discussed here prove, the authority of medical experts had its limits. Time and again, the court expressed doubts as to how well medical expertise could truly reveal the interior of the suspects before them. Terrified that it might be duped by an accused feigning illness, the Holy Office not only required more proof but needed a custodial solution, a place to send cases for observation, treatment, and potentially even cure.

Prior to the eighteenth century, the hospital played only a limited role in the Inquisition's deliberations. Madness was a collective affair best managed at the level of family and household, and on the rare occasions they found it, inquisitors quickly returned suspects back to their communities.[64] There were, however, some noteworthy exceptions, such as in the case of Luis de Zarate, who was tried for *alumbradismo* in 1598. Convicted as a heretic and poised to be burned at the stake, he lost his sanity while awaiting execution in the Holy Office's secret prisons and was duly shipped to San Hipólito.⁶⁵ Luis de Carvajal the Younger—the famous sixteenth-century crypto-Jew, martyr, and memoirist—likewise spent time in San Hipólito's facilities following his first inquisitorial trial for Judaism. To be sure, the Inquisition sent Carvajal to San Hipólito not as a confirmed madman but as a penitent ordered to "occupy himself in constructive duties and services as determined by the administrator."⁶⁶ Indeed, it was not uncommon during this period for colonial authorities to punish criminals by ordering them to serve the sick poor inside hospitals for designated stretches of time. Such sentences brought with them dishonor, imposed both moral and physical discipline, and reflected a long history in which penal servitude was the norm, trumping public executions.⁶⁷

By contrast, after 1700, and especially between 1760 and 1821, roughly a third of the cases involving *locura* entailed hospital confinement as an outcome.⁶⁸ This included suspects the Inquisition had deemed clearly insane as well as indeterminate cases that had stymied judicial process. The indeterminate cases posed an especially serious problem. The Inquisition could not, in good conscience, return potential frauds back to their communities and risk sending the signal that heresy would be tolerated, nor could these suspects be left to languish in prison, a solution that was not only inhumane but ineffectual. As illustrated in the case of José de Silva, whose trials in prison opened this chapter, confinement within the secret cells of the Holy Office was an insalubrious experience that by any standards imposed a heavy emotional burden on even the most composed of individuals. Not only were prison cells dark, dank, inhospitable places, but the Inquisition upheld a "pedagogy of fear" through the techniques of secrecy, torture (or its implied use), and the threat of infamy.⁶⁹ Suspects were usually detained without knowing the charges against them, kept in a state of bewilderment, and isolated from the outside world in trials that could drag on for years. That the occasional prisoner lost his or her wits while enduring these hardships hardly startles. Indeed, the spaces and techniques of the Holy Office had been deliberately designed to get suspects to mentally and emotionally crack.

The archival record bears witness to these grim realities. Like Silva, the inquisitorial process took its toll on the rebellious friar Felipe Alvarez, who divulged desires to hang himself upon experiencing the "gravest sadness" due to lengthy imprisonment and the dread of impending punishment.⁷⁰ Juan Pablo Echegoyen, a Basque royal naval pilot imprisoned on charges of heretical propositions and Freemasonry in 1762, likewise lost his sanity while in custody and proceeded to experience visions, pace frantically throughout his room, and tear his mattress to shreds. One afternoon, as he was being taken back to his cell following yet another hearing, he began to bash himself against the stairs as if "wanting to harm his head," much to the horror of the prison guards escorting him.[71] Medical opinion accounted for these experiences by explaining that prolonged incarceration agitated the emotions, which in turn affected mental function.[72] It was because of this that physicians and inquisitors alike often advocated for hospitalization; maintaining prisoners in such states of extended duress was deleterious to mind, body, and soul.

Hospitalization, however, did not necessarily solve the problem of *locura* within the Inquisition's courts. In one of the paradoxes this book sheds light on, medicalization occurred at the very same time that confinement remained an ad hoc arrangement—a last-ditch solution or even an experiment—that reproduced some of the very same obstacles and uncertainties inquisitors encountered in their courtroom deliberations. Put differently, many of the same issues that informed inquisitors' quandary extended to the mental hospital, shaping how it was used and why. At center stage were concerns about feigned madness and the ambiguities of diagnosis that plagued so many cases. In the cases of Antonio de la Cruz and José María Calderón, inquisitors only decided to have the prisoners hospitalized once they had exhausted all possible alternatives and the health of both men had worsened to the point that their lives were in peril. In other instances, inquisitors turned to San Hipólito as a means of practicing caution and managing skepticism. Although the hospital delivered care and appropriate facilities to those genuinely in need, it could also provide a space for deducing whether the illness was authentic or fraudulent. Because of this, the terms of committal were not necessarily indefinite; quite often, they were temporary, contingent on recovery or further evidence the hospital could produce regarding the precise nature of symptoms. It will be recalled that Felipe Zarate, the mestizo weaver, was sent to San Hipólito for only twelve to fifteen days, long enough for the Holy Office to ascertain whether his fatuity was genuine or feigned. Likewise, Diego Mendoza, the mad pauper discussed in chapter 3, faced a limited two-month committal following his run-in with the Holy Office for spewing offensive remarks.

In sending deserving suspects to San Hipólito, the Inquisition intended to be humane, but the conditions there could be as miserable as those in the Inquisition's prison. Indeed, they could be so wretched that the Holy Office may have unnecessarily fretted over the danger of frauds. In one revealing case, a prurient priest from Puebla, Joseph Ruíz Cañete, pretended to be mad rather than face trial for making untoward advances on at least four female confessants and was soon after committed to San Hipólito. However, once there, confined to his cell and haunted by the shrilling screams and curses of the *locos furiosos*, he found it unbearable, indeed far worse than any punishment the Holy Office could inflict. On January 24, 1772, Cañete issued an apology to the Inquisition, in which he confessed, and sincerely regretted, his scheme to fake mental illness and went on to not only insist on his sanity but to beseech the Holy Office for mercy:

> I also declare before the Holy Tribunal, that I am in my full judgment, and reasoning, that I feigned madness, and later suffered a [fit of] passion, but I am recovered. . . . I also declare that it is my desire to flee this madhouse [*casa de los locos*], and since it is possible that I may be caught during my flight, and therefore imprisoned like a *furioso*, it is my wish that this Holy Tribunal understand, that it is my desire to leave on my own [*por mi propio pie*] and deliver myself like a prisoner of this Holy Office to request clemency, and [demonstrate] that I am not by any means mad.[73]

Cañete's ploy to simulate madness provides an example of the ways in which colonial subjects used an institution like San Hipólito to undermine the imperatives of the Inquisition. However, that his plan ultimately backfired simultaneously testifies to the utility of the mental hospital as an outlet for suspect madmen. Only the testimony of a professed sane man could fully demonstrate how wretched life inside San Hipólito could be and why it suited the Inquisition so well. If a suspect was truly insane, then the court was right to send him or her there, but if not, there was nothing about residing in a madhouse that was pleasant. Unless a prisoner successfully fled—which they sometimes did—choosing between hospital confinement or punishment from the Holy Office was very often a contest between the lesser of two evils. In the case of Cañete, confinement worked successfully to expose an impostor and buttress the Inquisition's desire to resume trial and execute punishment.

The Inquisitor's Laboratory

Because San Hipólito so adequately served the institutional needs of the Inquisition—a proper place for the insane, a form of punishment for those faking—it is tempting to see the latter's reliance on the former as a mere convenience. However, the facts do not support this. While hospitalized suspects could, and often were, lost in the piles of cases that cluttered inquisitors' desks, Inquisition documents attest to lengthy correspondence with the hospital over the status of certain patients. As noted in chapter 3 regarding the cases of Juan de la Vega and José Ventura Gonzalez, by the eighteenth century the Inquisition had come to rely on testimony from the hospital's nurses for suspects who had been previously interned to arrive at expeditious dismissals. They had come, in other words, to not only privilege expert testimony over that of lay witnesses but to recognize San Hipólito as a legitimate site for the production of medical knowledge concerning madness and its elusive diagnosis. They continued to do this for patients held in duress, their trials stalled due to the onset of madness, and demanded of the brothers of San Hipólito close observation and routine reporting of suspects' symptoms and their progression and even sent their own physician(s) to check up on them when circumstances warranted. If medical models and theory alone were of marginal aid in resolving their "quandary," inquisitors came to insist on the evidence of closely monitored observation—and, in this way, San Hipólito served for them a kind of colonial laboratory.[74] This is, of course, not to conflate San Hipólito with the modern laboratories that appeared in the late nineteenth century, which have distinct genealogies in the artisanal and especially alchemical workshops of the late middle ages and their seventeenth-century transformation into sites for the practice of the experimental "new science."[75] Rather, it is to suggest that the hospital was being put to new and creative uses that emphasized firsthand observation and the production of experiential knowledge and proof.

In the case of Juan Pablo Echegoyen, the colonial laboratory aided to resolve an indeterminate case and have the accused stand trial for crimes that were, by the Inquisition's standards, grossly egregious. In 1762, the Basque royal naval pilot had been arrested on charges of alleged Protestant leanings and ties to Freemasonry. In addition to ample witness testimony corroborating the charges, Inquisitors had unearthed compelling physical evidence: an illicit religious text published in English and an embroidered insignia testifying to membership in a lodge of Scottish Freemasons. Echegoyen languished in prison for eight months while enduring grueling rounds of questioning before his mind finally snapped and he began to experience visions, declare himself bewitched, and pace frantically around his cell.[76]

When Echegoyen was hospitalized in 1763, expert opinion regarding the authenticity of his symptoms was highly tentative. Indeed, the medical report emphasized the "ease and frequency" with which someone could "simulate madness." The inquisitors nevertheless had Echegoyen institutionalized as a precaution against his wild delusions and untamed behavior.[77] Nearly two months later, the hospital's head nurse, friar Felipe Ruíz, notified inquisitors of Echegoyen's condition. In accordance with inquisitorial orders, Echegoyen had been kept isolated from the other inmates and forbidden from conversing with the visitors who came to see the *pobres dementes*. His delusions and sense of being persecuted persisted. As he had done within the inquisitorial cells, he shunned food, claiming it was "bewitched," and undid his mattress for the same reason. He continued to experience vivid dreams, one of them involving two ships bound for New Spain to wreak destruction on the capital city.[78] Nevertheless, because Echegoyen spoke cogently on some matters, the head nurse attributed his antics and occasional verbal tantrums not to madness but to a "fever in the head."[79] Likewise, the prior general, who also issued a report to the Holy Office, claimed to have not discerned any signs of mania in Echegoyen, only a "hardness of temperament, or stubbornness born out of an oppressed spirit and lack of freedom."[80] Elaborating on these assessments, the Holy Office's appointed medical adviser, the physician Fierro, asserted that Echegoyen's symptoms "could perhaps be artificial or feigned"; at the very least, he stated, they were manifestations of his "headstrong and impatient character that should not stand as an obstacle to prosecution and punishment."[81] Echegoyen remained in San Hipólito for a little over six months before the *fiscal* ordered him transferred back to the secret prisons to stand trial.

No case more clearly illustrates the hospital's role as a laboratory for studying mental disorder than that of José de Silva, whose auto-da-fé and descent into madness opened this chapter. At a time when hospital confinement remained an ad hoc solution for cases in which madness surfaced in the colonial courts, in this particular instance inquisitors appear to have stumbled across its diagnostic promise accidentally. Following his committal in 1770, the Inquisition ignored Silva's pending case for an astounding thirteen years. When it revisited the case, it was at the instigation of the tribunal of the Acordada, New Spain's law enforcement agency, which requested to know Silva's status, as he also had criminal charges pending with them. Following this request, the Holy Office sent the physician Rada to the hospital to apprise them of Silva's health. In a letter dated September 14, 1783, Rada concluded that Silva's mind was still "perturbed" and that he should remain hospitalized. This assessment is initially puzzling, given that Rada reported that Silva's condition had remarkably improved and that the tailor could engage in "agreeable conversation, without giving the slightest indication of *demencia*." Nevertheless, he hesitated to unequivocally declare Silva as sane, since "experience" had taught him that madmen tended to exhibit moments of "perfect sanity" only to later decline in mental health.[82]

If Rada could offer only a tentative diagnosis, the hospital's nurses who had attended to Silva for over a decade could provide much more detailed and persuasive evidence. It was friar Pedro Granados who convinced the Inquisition that Silva remained unwell. Drawing on his experience treating the countless other patients who frequented San Hipólito's wards, Granados explained to the Holy Office that Silva exhibited a mania that was "very contrary" to anything he had ever observed. When he first arrived at San Hipólito, Silva was quiet and reclusive, willingly isolating himself from everyone. Then, as time passed, he began to lead a "life that was almost religious." He became a model inmate: he prayed, sometimes in accompaniment of the *pobres dementes*; he spent his money on mass and candles; he exhibited "almost rational conversation."[83] But such admirable conduct did not last long. Abruptly, Silva would succumb to an "interval of passion or delirium"; he would "burst out" against religion, sometimes in tears, and refuse to confess because, he stated, "the evil spirits [*hechiceros*] were speaking inside his body."[84] To Granados, these shifting moods amply illustrated that Silva had not reached "perfect sanity."[85]

Thus, the Holy Office consented that Silva should remain in confinement, with the stipulation that "under no circumstance" should he be permitted to leave the hospital grounds.[86] This was not, however, a definitive sentence. Having reopened the case, the inquisitors took renewed interest in monitoring the prisoner's health, with a plan to eventually transport him to Havana to fulfill his sentence. In the year that followed, they ordered that the physician Vicente de la Peña y Brizuela and the surgeon Matheo de la Fuente, in addition to Rada, make repeated visits to the hospital to examine the patient-prisoner. The inquisitors specifically wanted to know if Silva would be able to withstand the harsh conditions of exiled labor on the Havana presidio.[87] Ultimately, the Holy Office would not achieve its goal to punish Silva. De la Peña y Brizuela and de la Fuente concurred that while Silva displayed "intermissions" of sanity, in which his characteristic "fury" and "audaciousness" were absent, he was most certainly possessed by a "refined mania, or madness."[88] Rada, in an extensive evaluation written following routine visits to the hospital and consultation with a colleague, likewise concluded that Silva was a "maniacal madman" (*demente maniaco*).[89] Silva's case thus remained suspended and he stayed in San Hipólito.

There may have been a certain degree of distinction for San Hipólito in having an institution as important as the Inquisition call on it for aid, but serving as the court's laboratory may have been more trouble than it was worth. Even with all the changes the hospital underwent in the eighteenth century, detailed, comprehensive reports took precious time, and a complete redesign of the building did not make it any easier to keep those suspected of feigning madness from escaping, which required extra surveillance. Moreover, although the prisoners paid for their hospitalization—just as they were expected to fund their incarceration in the secret prisons of the Holy Office—these prisoner-patients nevertheless occupied precious space, while their reputation as alleged blasphemers and heretics tainted the hospital's charitable mission. This last point was not merely a symbolic violation, as the prior general, Joseph de la Peña, explained to the Holy Office in a letter dated 1785. Written in response to a request by the Inquisition to intern an additional prisoner, Peña's letter cautioned against the "grave harm" of housing two Inquisition prisoners in such close proximity. He went on to request that the Holy Office transfer Silva to "another destination." Having been hospitalized for fifteen years, the heretical mad tailor had outworn his welcome: his madness was "very malicious," the prior general stated, for Silva had "discovered the vice of drinking, together with that of gambling," and he had "perverted" at least two of the brothers "with these vices."[90] Keeping the brothers moral and virtuous was challenging enough without having patients compounding the problem. However, the records provide no indication that the prior general's request was ever granted. In the Inquisition's view, the colonial laboratory had exposed Silva as a confirmed madman with heretical proclivities, and the most viable solution was to extend his confinement at San Hipólito.

In addition to highlighting the Inquisition's use of the hospital's diagnostic potential, these cases disclose nascent tensions between physicians bent on expanding their authority on matters of mental interiority and the brothers of San Hipólito, who had long been entrusted with the care of the mad—tensions that would only intensify in the following century. Professional and vocational conflicts between secular and religious healers often worked to obfuscate the hospital's laboratory-like capabilities, accentuating the quandary inquisitors had hoped to bypass. This was especially apparent in the case of Francisco Ferris, a resident of Pachuca and a former officer of the royal treasury, whom the Inquisition investigated for heretical propositions in 1794. According to various witnesses, Ferris had made a series of ghastly claims, such that "children, even if they were baptized . . . did not go to heaven but to limbo," and that "Christians live in error, and they are deceived by their own faith."[91] Inquisitors soon learned that Ferris had been committed to San Hipólito just two months earlier by his father, whom he lived with and who, according to multiple witnesses, had been alarmed to discover that his son owned an illicit copy of "Wolter" (Voltaire).[92]

Although Ferris's father had failed to secure the necessary medical certification to intern his son, San Hipólito took him in nonetheless and housed him as a "distinguished" client on account of a prestigious recommendation. In Pachuca, rumors widely circulated that Ferris had been released because he was not ill, a suspicion confirmed by the hospital's prior general, friar José Martínez, who told inquisitors that he had "not observed any delirium more than a grave seriousness, and very little speech."[93] Confirmed sane, the trial continued, unearthing additional scandals, including claims that Ferris welcomed French invasion, inviting the foreigners to unleash their revolutionary ire on the Inquisition itself and employ the dreaded guillotine on every cleric in the colony.[94] No doubt shocked by these threats, inquisitors nevertheless worried that the mounting evidence amounted to hearsay and decided to return Ferris to San Hipólito for additional observation.

Dating to 1796, the second round of medical reports emanating from the hospital disclosed conflicts and much confusion, as both the nurses and the physicians debated the etiology of Ferris's heretical and seditious actions. Significantly, one report came from José Castillo, who identified himself as the *medico* (doctor) of the General Hospital for Dementes. Notably, this comprises the earliest and most concrete evidence that San Hipólito had succeeded in financing the services of a physician (although how long Castillo remained there is unclear). Contradicting the prior general's earlier report, the physician confirmed that Ferris had indeed entered San Hipólito two years earlier in a state of *demencia* and took credit for restoring him to sanity and securing his release. However, during this second internment, he conceded that not only had Ferris undeniably relapsed, but he was now fully resisting the doctor's measures to cure him. "He is mad," Castillo affirmed, and suffering from madness that was "almost incurable."[95] Six months later, the Inquisition received a new report from the prior general, not Castillo, reiterating Ferris's sanity, noting only emotional agitation at being forcefully admitted to the hospital "without considering himself mad." He appended the written testimony of friar Eucebio Figueroa, a member of the order and a licensed surgeon, who had examined the suspect during his initial stay, closely monitoring him for one month. Contrary to Martínez, Figueroa had identified in the suspect the early beginnings of *demencia*, the product of "maniacal passion and affect." To this conflicting assessment, Martínez could only reaffirm his initial opinion that Ferris was sane while admitting that

Ferris's condition was "undeniably confusing."[96] Although the Inquisition would ultimately send its own experts, Francisco Rada and Mariano Armarero, to San Hipólito, their reports also produced conflicting assessments and augmented the state of quandary, confusion, and chaos surrounding this determination of madness. In this particular case, the colonial laboratory failed—and failed stupendously. Ferris's intractable condition proved too complicated to discern, rendered all the more elusive by emerging jurisdictional battles between religious and medical authorities. In the end, Ferris exploited this situation and took flight.

From the halls of the Inquisition, inquisitors wrestled to understand behavior and emotional and mental states that defied the boundaries of what was considered reasonable. While in the previous century it might have been easier to attribute unusual phenomena—from bizarre antics to hallucinations—to supernatural forces, by the eighteenth century inquisitors had come to accept a more secular-minded worldview and embrace the notion that certain mental and emotional states had an underlying physiological basis that could be understood, diagnosed, and managed in a more rational and scientific way. However, this process of medicalization was unequivocally messy and contested, with physicians ultimately playing an important if subsidiary role, informing the verdicts of inquisitors but only capable of penetrating the hospital's spaces from the margins. By the close of the eighteenth century, jurisdictional fights between medical and religious healers over the power to diagnose *locura* had come to penetrate San Hipólito itself, setting the stage for struggles that would come to characterize the nineteenth century and shape psychiatry's rise.

CHAPTER FIVE

Crime and Punishment

When in 1804 the governor of Veracruz petitioned Viceroy Iturrigaray for permission to transfer Pedro José Zetina to San Hipólito, he crudely referred to the hospital as a *casa de los locos* (madhouse). Absent from his appeal were the charitable connotations of San Hipólito as a *hospital para pobres dementes* (hospital for mad paupers). Instead, the governor referenced Mexico City's oldest public institution for the mad as a place where insane and dangerous criminals like Zetina could be "incarcerated." Little is known of Zetina—who was admitted to San Hipólito on September 24 of that year—beyond his criminal history: in 1800 he was sentenced to ten years of hard labor on the presidio in Isla del Carmen for murdering one man and wounding another in the village of Tenasco, located in modern day Jalisco. Four years into his sentence, he lost all sanity and self-control, overcome by what the governor described as a "mania for wanting to kill people." Troubled by these violent and erratic outbursts and worried that Zetina would commit another deadly crime, the governor had him locked up "in a room with the greatest security possible." When it became apparent that the prisoner's fits would not abate, he pleaded to the viceroy for assistance; shortly after, the governor had Zetina shipped out to San Hipólito.[1]

The Inquisition, with its deeply rooted interest in the interiority of accused suspects, was not the only institution in New Spain that saw value in San Hipólito. Others, far less interested in the motivations for condemnable—even criminal—actions, simply needed someplace to house murderers and criminals with violent predilections like Pedro José Zetina. If the Inquisition looked to San Hipólito as a place that might finally bear practical witness to the problem of liminal insanity, secular authorities—viceroys, local governors, law enforcement deputies, and magistrates—were far more inclined to treat San Hipólito as a custodial space to hold those they could not manage. For them, the *why* mattered far less than the *how* of managing those afflicted.[2]

Of course, the confinement of recalcitrant *locos furiosos* who disrupted the public peace and endangered society had always formed a valuable if understated part of San Hipólito's institutional mission. However, it was only in the late eighteenth and early nineteenth centuries that colonial authorities operating outside ecclesiastical jurisdictions began to exploit its resources with recurring frequency. While this pattern forms part of the larger history of medicalization this book documents, it was also tightly linked to Enlightenment notions of utility, rational order, and the public good. In the 1770s, as described in chapter 2, San Hipólito was physically renovated and its mission reimagined in terms of a utilitarian service to the state and wider public, a transformation that materialized only through the financial and symbolic muscle of the crown and city council. In exchange for a higher profile, the hospital found itself obligated to receive those peace- and lawbreakers authorities identified as fit for confinement. While this hardly amounted to a colonial "great confinement," the rising presence of criminal inmates within San Hipólito's wards certainly yields the impression that the hospital's penal character had intensified on the eve of social and political revolution.[3]

In the closing decades of the eighteenth century, lawlessness and disorder became a growing concern for colonial authorities, and as part of the Bourbon reforms, leaders introduced more aggressive state measures to enforce law and order to combat escalating levels of crime, especially in urban areas. In the eyes of state authorities and the colonial elite, crime and immorality had scaled to epidemic heights, and the principle culprits were the racially mixed poorer and marginal classes: the *gente baja* (underclass), whose size in the capital had considerably swelled as the city's population more than doubled between 1742 and 1810.[4] In 1785, the lawyer Hipólito Villaroel captured official sentiment when he described the viceregal capital as a seedbed for vice, mendacity, and crime—in his words, "a receptacle for vagabonds, the depraved and the wickedly preoccupied, a refuge for evil-doers, a brothel of infamy and dissolution, [and] a cradle of thieves [*picaros*]."[5]

In this climate, it was inevitable that San Hipólito, a flagship institution of its kind, would be called on to do its part to combat the problems that authorities saw swirling around them. But it was far from the front lines of change. Indeed, it stood on the fringes of larger efforts to fortify the police force, expand the judiciary, and transform the capital city into a rationally ordered space. The history of modern policing in New Spain began in 1719 with the establishment of the Tribunal of the Acordada, an agency intended to police rural banditry. By 1756, the crown had extended the tribunal's jurisdiction to include crime within the city and its neighboring districts, along with the criminal courts (*sala del crimen*) and, in later decades, urban military patrols.[6] In 1782, a second major development in law enforcement occurred when the viceroy, Martín de Mayorga, divided the city into eight major administrative and police districts (*cuarteles mayores*), each of which contained four smaller subdistricts (*cuarteles menores*). Modeled on similar systems in Spanish cities, the *cuartel* system was designed to make law enforcement more rational and efficient, permitting "a greater degree of coordination between the *sala del crimen*, the municipal authorities, and their respective law enforcement agencies."[7] These reforms were soon followed by the addition of a ninth municipal court in 1790 by Viceroy Revillagidedo, who also furnished the capital with its first street lighting system, fully equipped with its own force of watchmen (*guardafaroles*) to expose and police devious nighttime activity.[8] Taken together, as Michael Scardaville has observed, "this proactive approach to law enforcement in Mexico City resulted in a tenfold increase in the number of arrests and trials, the vast majority involving the urban poor, between the early 1780s and the late 1790s."[9]

These more stringent efforts at *policía* provide critical context for why San Hipólito was solicited with requests by law enforcement officials to house and treat insane criminals with a frequency unparalleled in earlier periods. By this point, the hospital had widely promoted its new utilitarian mission, which powerfully resonated with the Bourbon state's embrace of Enlightenment notions of the public good and public happiness. Describing the Bourbon reforms, particularly those that targeted crime and public morality, as nothing short of a "radical social engineering [project] to produce a more rational and productive citizen," Pamela Voekel observes that the "Bourbon state justified its unprecedented interventions into daily life by claiming to act in the interest of the 'public,' a concept foreign to previous regimes."[10] To some extent, this language seeped into the highly contested arena of the criminal courts, where deviant and criminal actions were not simply construed by local justices as attacks on the king but began to be seen more generally as "sinning against the public."[11] Likewise, in cases involving madness, colonial magistrates often followed a similar "utilitarian rationale," justifying decisions to commit perpetrators to mental hospitals on the basis of the danger—usually physical rather than moral—they posed not just to themselves but to the wider public.[12]

The utilitarian logic at the heart of these transformations also echoed the opinions of Enlightenment intellectuals who argued for the more rational treatment of criminals. Eighteenth-century reformers such as Manuel de la Roda, Juan Meléndez Valdéz, Gaspar Melchor de Jovellanos, and Manuel de Lardizábal y Uribe urged an overhaul of the penal system, including the elimination of torture, maintaining that punishment should be "rehabilitative" and rational rather than vindictive.[13] Commissioned by the Spanish king to analyze criminal jurisprudence, the Mexican-born jurist Lardizábal y Uribe confidently asserted that a reformed and rationalized criminal justice system—where punishment was "public, prompt, proportionate to the crime, impartial, and certain"—would eliminate crime entirely by deterring future lawlessness.[14] Lardizábal y Uribe and his contemporaries were influenced by the work of the Italian criminologist Cesare Beccaria, whose essay *On Crime and Punishment*, a foundational text of modern penology, was translated into Spanish in 1774.[15] With respect to the mentally disturbed, Lardizábal y Uribe quoted Beccaria, who contended that the insane merited different treatment from that of the average criminal because, as he wrote, "the madman caused less injury to society than the sane man, being that the [latter] taught others to commit crimes, and [the former] gives no example but of his furious madness."[16] Thus, in arguing that the gravity of a crime should be judged according to the harm it inflicted on society, it stood to reason that "[the sane] should be punished more severely than [the madman]."[17]

The criminal courts were slower than their ecclesiastical counterparts to embrace the medicalization of madness, but when they finally did, they did it with gusto. If San Hipólito was a "laboratory" of practical observation for the Inquisition, a site for observing the authenticity and progression of symptoms in order to mete out the appropriate sentence, for the secular courts the hospital would ideally be an essential component of a more calculated, rational, and enlightened form of criminal justice in the colony—with all the contradictions, failures, and incoherence that accompanied it. Despite the ambitious visions of enlightened reformers like Lardizábal y Uribe, the reform of the penal system would not occur until the late nineteenth century, when a liberal government was fully installed. Until then, criminal trials—especially those involving madness—comprised an eclectic blend of Enlightenment rationalism, colonial paternalism, and jurisprudence, as well as more practical local concerns about containing violent and dangerous individuals. At times they became circuses, where no one—not lawyers, not judges, and certainly not defendants—had any idea what to expect. The only certainty in these cases was that San Hipólito was the most viable solution to the problem of insane violent criminals. But the hospital was, in many respects, an eclectic mix. It was repressive and unwelcoming enough to meet older notions of punishment yet ostensibly committed to caring for and, ideally, healing the ill. And like the reform impulse in the years before independence, even the hospital's greatest successes were never absolute and could only be measured by degrees of effectiveness. Its failures, however, could be utter and obvious, for it took little effort for resourceful criminals to escape and expose the impotence of the colonial state.

Colonial Order and Mental Disorder

The ambiguous successes of the Bourbon effort to eradicate crime and enforce public order began in its legal foundations, which, as Michael Scardaville has emphasized, "did not fully displace traditional Habsburg notions of justice." Indeed, he contends that while tightening its grip on crime with renewed rigor fueled by Enlightenment rationalism, the state continued to assume the traditional role of the "paternalistic and benevolent" government, a ruling entity that would, in his words, "preserve stability and order through guidance, not merely through coercion or open force."[18] In other words, during the late colonial period, the wheels of justice were propelled by the alchemy of Bourbon and Habsburg philosophies. Outwardly, the colonial courts and police force "operated in accordance with Bourbon notions, most notably the imperative to attack the vices of the populace not simply on moral grounds, but primarily for economic and utilitarian reasons."[19] Inwardly, however, the local magistrates continued to issue verdicts in keeping with traditional Habsburg legal "principles and processes," which cast the king as the compassionate and just mediator of social conflict.[20]

Thus, in spite of Enlightenment appeals for penal reform by jurists like Beccaria and Lardizábal y Uribe, criminal law and court procedures, both in Spain and in its overseas possessions, were deeply entrenched in age-old Roman and medieval traditions.[21] Colonial law (*derecho indiano*) consisted of a diverse series of *leyes* (legal codes) compiled in the kingdom of Castille, local Spanish customs developed around these written doctrines (*derecho vulgar*), and another body of edicts formulated exclusively for the Indies.[22] The *Recopilación de leyes de los reinos de las Indias*—the main compendium of Spanish law produced for the colonies—contained only marginal references to criminal law.[23] Thus, when issuing sentences in criminal trials, colonial legal officials generally relied on the ranked body of corpora that made up *derecho Castellano* (Castilian law), while also thumbing through learned legal commentaries and supplemental manuals of court procedure.

In addition, judges had at their disposal the power of judicial discretion or free will, a concept known as *arbitrio judicial*. Rooted in medieval jurisprudence, the doctrine of *arbitrio judicial* entrusted judges with the whim and authority to deviate from the prescribed punishment for the crime in question and customize a sentence according to his own conviction and sense of *equidad* (equity).²⁴ The law not only allowed but encouraged colonial magistrates to calibrate their verdicts according to the nuances of each particular case, weighing such factors as motive, conscious intent, the gravity of the crime committed, and even the social ranking and race of the suspect in question.²⁵ It was a potent if subjective power judges wielded, and one that cut through the often Byzantine legal codes of New Spain.

Drawing on Roman civil and criminal jurisprudence, Spanish law awarded the mad—along with those deemed worthy of the crown's paternal guardianship, such as minors—certain legal protections when charged with crimes.²⁶ For example, *Las Siete Partidas*, the medieval compendium of Spanish law mentioned in chapter 3, exempted the insane and children under the age of ten from punishment for murder "for the reason that he does not understand or appreciate the offense which he committed."²⁷ Like perpetual children, the insane lacked the capacity to be held accountable for the severity of their crimes, and also like children, they deserved the crown's paternalistic care. Lest there be any confusion on the matter, elsewhere *Las Siete Partidas* explicitly exculpated the mad from criminal liability for "offenses" vaguely and broadly defined.²⁸

Such doctrines left ample room for interpretation and exegesis, and Spanish jurists writing on both sides of the Atlantic elaborated on the idea of reduced culpability and the range of individuals and circumstances that could lay claim to it. For example, Juan de Hevia Bolaños's *Curia Philipica*, a widely used manual of legal procedure, emphasized *entendimiento* ("reasoning" or "understanding") as the deciding factor in determining criminal responsibility. Thus, he argued, a deaf or mute person who lacked *entendimiento* and was unable to communicate through *señales* (signs) was "incapable of committing a crime, being accused, or being punished." However, he continued, even when judgment was intact, and the deaf or mute person was able to express him or herself through gestures, they could not be condemned, as it would be impossible to extract a clear and unmediated confession.²⁹ By contrast, the old and decrepit were liable to punishment, he stated, "because even though they lacked natural strength, they did not lack *entendimiento*." (Although here he conceded that their fragility and maturity could occasionally warrant lighter punishment than what would normally be inflicted on the "robust.")³⁰

Bolaños's argument about the need for *entendimiento* to be present in order to prosecute criminal action and his emphasis on the importance of obtaining a coherent and rational confession from the accused had clear implications for judicial leniency toward insane individuals who came before the court. The "*furioso*, or the *loco*," he declared, "cannot be punished for the crime he committed meanwhile the madness or fury persists, since he lacks judgment."[31] Of course, if the accused lacked judgment, no ability to communicate could ever deliver the clear, rational confession necessary for a guilty verdict. Interestingly, his position, while reaffirming the necessity of full rational judgment to be present in order to pursue a conviction, nonetheless left open the possibility that punishment could be inflicted if the criminal ever recovered his senses. Recognizing that certain forms of *locura* were episodic rather than chronic, Bolaños went on to say that mad individuals who committed crimes during intervals (*intervalos*) of sanity could indeed be punished, but only during moments of restored lucidity.[32] Thus, Bolaños emphasized less the innocence of the insane due to a lack of judgment and an absence of criminal intent than the illegitimacy of punishing irrational individuals, regardless of intentions when they perpetrated the crime.

But Bolaños's legal prescriptions, like that of so many of his contemporaries, remained frustratingly devoid of nuance and subject to wide interpretation, and thus fell glaringly short when it came to resolving the complicated problems legal officials encountered when they tried to mete out justice in trials involving the allegedly insane. While they established a legal foundation for issuing an insanity defense (and likewise for imposing punishment on the recovered if the justice so wished it), they did not provide a blueprint for how to determine the presence or absence of *entendimiento*. And as was illustrated in the struggles of inquisitors to wade through the "quandary" madness produced, diagnosing *locura* in all its subtle and extreme manifestations was no simple task, even though secular magistrates showed less concern with the intricacies of human reasoning and motive than did their religious counterparts. More troubling for the agents of the criminal courts who faced mentally compromised individuals who had perpetrated violent crimes was that Spanish law did not dictate how to provide for the care and detention of insane offenders who were potentially prone to inflict harm. Given this state of affairs, the agents of the criminal courts acted on a case-by-case basis, their decisions generally lenient and heavily mediated by the prerogative of *arbitrio judicial*. Judicial discretion allowed for a great deal of experimentation and negotiation, especially with regard to the use of hospitals as custodial solutions for the criminally insane.[33] But the courts' growing reliance on hospitals was double edged. True, they could both confine and—ideally—heal, but relying on hospitals opened new avenues for abuse, on the part of resourceful and cunning criminals as well as the justices assigned to correct them.

Before proceeding to the individual cases, it is useful to chronicle the procedural norms of the criminal trial. In colonial Mexico, when a crime occurred, the first notified was the nearest local official (governor, *alcalde*, *alguacil*, *regidor*). After a preliminary investigation, or sometimes immediately upon notification, the suspect was apprehended and taken to either a public jail or the royal prison. While the suspect was in custody, a magistrate and his assistants would undertake the *sumaria* (the investigatory phase of the legal process), questioning the aggrieved party, witnesses, and the accused (called a *confesión*). In cases involving homicide or physical injury, a medical practitioner, usually a surgeon, would issue a *fé de heridas*, providing a graphic description of the wound and its severity. During the *plenario* segment of the trial, the magistrate would formally charge the defendant and appoint a defense attorney (*defensor*). At this point, the magistrate would once again interrogate the suspect, who could speak on their own behalf or through their legal representative. In the final phase of the judicial proceeding—the sentencing—the magistrate would exercise the power of *arbitrio judicial* to arrive at an appropriate punishment for the offense, if indeed the suspect was judged to be guilty.[34]

Indian Rebellion and the Mad Count of Moctezuma

In all the cases discussed in the following pages, the law allowed legal authorities to act like fathers, who would reason and judge for those who, like children, could not advocate for themselves. These dynamics, and their contradictory combination of benevolence and discipline, were especially cast into bold relief in cases involving Indians. Since the sixteenth century, Spaniards had expounded at length on the weak mental capabilities of the Indigenous population, regarding them as *gente sin razón* (people without reason) and granting them the legal status of minors. While in many ways exceptional, the case of Manuel Antonio Chimalpopoca—a self-styled "noble" Indian from the southern isthmus of Tehuantepec, admitted to San Hipólito in 1781—shows how discourses regarding the protected legal status of the mad and Indians combined to persuade judicial officials to issue a lenient verdict that entailed institutional confinement. It also illustrates the way in which mandated committals could sometimes serve state interests to effectively silence a rebel who questioned the crown's legitimacy. While we have no way of knowing if Chimalpopoca was truly mad or not, the circumstances surrounding his confinement in San Hipólito hint of a more sinister motive to delegitimize a political adversary and squelch a potential Indian uprising on the eve of the empire's decline.[35]

The case opens in the summer of 1781, when the *fiscal del crimen*—the chief prosecuting attorney of the high criminal court—requested permission from the viceroy, Martín de Mayorga, to transfer Chimalpopoca from the royal cells to the Hospital de San Hipólito. The motives for Chimalpopoca's imprisonment were initially unclear, as the prisoner's name did not appear in the entry books nor could the *fiscal* locate Chimalpopoca's criminal file. The only established facts were hidden in coded language: that the prisoner committed certain "excesses" and possessed "immunity."[36]

Months later, the *fiscal* found the appropriate documents pertaining to Chimalpopoca's incarceration buried among paperwork. The file reported that the prisoner had been arrested in 1773 by the *teniente* of Tehuantepec, and the aforementioned "excesses" for which he was charged consisted of pretenses to grandeur and agitating for possession of royal land. Titling himself as the Count of Moctezuma—although in other instances he raised himself to the status of marquis—Chimalpopoca claimed to be an Indian of noble ancestry and dared to refer to the viceroy of New Spain as his "cousin." On the day of his arrest, he had appeared "with a demonstration only used by decorated people" before the church of the village of Guadalcázar and, proclaiming himself the descendant of Don Juan de Velasco Zuniga de Guzmán Moctezuma y Austria, he demanded the "enjoyment of status and privilege."[37]

Chimalpopoca's bold claims to noble blood and property were not entirely preposterous.[38] The Spanish crown had long recognized pre-Hispanic lineages and, as part of its program to segregate Indigenous communities into a *república de indios* (Indian republic), had made a concerted effort to preserve internal Indigenous hierarchies, in addition to granting native communities certain rights to land and political semi-autonomy. Moreover, as María Elena Martínez has discussed, the creation of a separate but subordinate Indian polity in New Spain resulted in the gradual restructuring of Indigenous concepts of genealogy. In particular, it imposed the Spanish concept of the "purity of blood" (*limpieza de sangre*) onto Indigenous notions of lineage, inheritance, and property, producing a "discourse of Indian purity" that Indians like Chimalpopoca readily appealed to when voicing their rights as citizens.[39] In fact, upon his arrest, there was no mention that Chimalpopoca was *demente*; his crime resided less in his outlandish delusions than in violating the "colonial relationship of vassalage," in which Indians enjoyed special citizenship in exchange for subservience, loyalty, and tribute to the Spanish monarch.[40]

Only in 1781, after eight years of being held in the cells of the Real Audiencia without trial, Spanish authorities began to see delusion in Chimalpopoca's actions and claims—or, what had previously been viewed as a political act had now become the product of compromised mental function. That year, the *fiscal* argued that his conduct "should not be judged as criminal, but as the effects of mental fatuity [*fatuidad*] and a weak comprehension," not to mention "a vivid imagination" and "foolishness." He therefore advocated for leniency in the prosecution, emphasizing, in addition to Chimalpopoca's poor faculties of reasoning, the fact that he had not "manifested an inclination towards uprising or disobedience." On the contrary, he had exhibited the appropriate deference to colonial rule. Apparently two years after his arrest, Chimalpopoca had rescinded his contentious claims to land and entitlement, making the voyage across the Atlantic to kiss the hand of the Spanish king and beseech clemency.[41] Taking these factors into consideration, plus the fact that he had patiently endured nearly a decade of imprisonment, the *fiscal* maintained that Chimalpopoca was more worthy of "pity than punishment."[42]

Though he did not intend it, the *fiscal*'s appeal touched on the heart of Chimalpopoca's case. On the surface, it was a call for the insanity defense, but on a deeper level it harked back to the very foundations of Spanish subjugation of Indigenous people and their protected and inferior legal and cultural status as *miserables* (wretched people). The idea that certain people—because of their misfortune and helplessness—merited compassion and assistance has a long history, but the Spanish reinvigorated and reinvented this concept in the Americas when they applied it to the Indigenous population in its totality to account for the fact that the natives, in their view, were rationally weak and incapable of governing themselves. These ideas had legal ramifications for Indians charged with crimes: they were to be treated as legal minors, and their responsibility for criminal actions was often viewed as limited.[43] Thus, the seventeenth-century jurist Juan de Solórzano Pereira claimed that Indians, on account of their "ignorance" and inferior "natural intellect," should be "less [severely] punished for their crimes" than non-Indians.[44]

However, closer inspection reveals that Chimalpopoca's committal to San Hipólito was only on the surface a gesture of lenience and benign paternalism. For one, he was not accorded certain privileges on account of his ethnic status as *indio*, namely the right to a speedy trial and legal counsel.[45]

Moreover, because of his "immunity"—though it is not clear where it originated from—he should have been granted liberty, a fact that was not lost on the *fiscal*.[46] Nevertheless, the *fiscal* advocated for Chimalpopoca's internment in San Hipólito out of fear that his ideas might incite rebellion among the Indigenous masses of Tehuantepec. Although the prosecuting judge had earlier noted that the Count of Moctezuma was not personally disposed to "uprising and disobedience," this did not mean that he could not, like a contagious scourge, "infect" (*contagiar*) the rest of the Indians with his madness, "giving them a bad example" and "imprinting" on their "docile" minds "ridiculous and pernicious" ideas.[47] The underlying assumption here was that while sophisticated and mentally keen Spaniards could recognize the differences, nuanced or obvious, between reason and unreason, the simple-minded Indians could not and thus could easily be misled to revolt against the king by the fanciful convictions of the delusional Indian "count."

These apprehensions, though racially biased, were not entirely unfounded. While the viceregal capital remained relatively free of open riot (though clearly not devoid of crime), rural areas in New Spain witnessed countless revolts against Spanish rule throughout the late colonial period. The isthmus of Tehuantepec, marked by its massive Indigenous population, was the scene of a large-scale rebellion in the 1660s, followed by two smaller revolts in the early 1700s.[48] Moreover, fresh on the *fiscal*'s mind, no doubt, was the insurgency led by the mestizo *kuraka* (local lord), Tupac Amaru II, and similar rebellions throughout the Andean highlands, which threatened to overturn the entire colonial system.[49] Colonial officials were thus especially anxious and eager to stifle any and all signs of local discontent and uprising, and it was for this particular reason—a utilitarian desire to preserve law and order—that Chimalpopoca was denied liberty and instead transferred to San Hipólito, where the *fiscal*, in his capacity as a spokesperson of royal benevolence, ordered that he be treated "with the greatest piety."[50]

To be sure, the intention here was not to keep Chimalpopoca imprisoned in San Hipólito indefinitely but to release him once his health recovered, his delusions vanished, and the image of an audacious Indian who considered himself entitled to property and status—implicitly exposing the injustices of colonial rule—was rendered nonthreatening. Six months following his admission to the hospital, the prospect of discharging Chimalpopoca became a reality when the physician, Francisco Rada, who had examined countless mad suspects from the Inquisition, reported to the Real Audiencia that he "could not observe [in Chimalpopoca] insanity or fatuity, ire, sadness or any other passion"; he was indeed "perfectly recovered."[51] It was then that the *fiscal* entertained in earnest the possibility of freeing Chimalpopoca. But he issued one important caveat: Chimalpopoca "must abstain from falling into similar delusions and pernicious kinds [of thoughts]," and he must be warned that should he continue to "impress upon those of his class, or another *casta*, he would not be treated with benignity, but rather be punished with the utmost rigor."[52]

Chimalpopoca did indeed leave San Hipólito, but not on court orders. On the morning of September 13, 1782, as the head nurse was making his routine rounds through the hospital's halls to deliver breakfast to the patients, he noticed that cell number 82, belonging to Chimalpopoca, was empty.[53] Like many before and after him, the Count of Moctezuma had fled forced internment and, according to the ensuing investigation, was hiding in the cemetery of the parish of Santa Catarina with the intention of proceeding to the nearby church, where he might acquire *derecho de asilo eclesiastico* (ecclesiastical asylum). It was a shrewd maneuver for a man authorities had once identified as mad and simpleminded. Having no idea about his impending release and believing that the secular authorities would do him no favors, Chimalpopoca had decided to try his luck with the church rather than remain imprisoned in San Hipólito.

Chimalpopoca never received ecclesiastical asylum. A deputy, pretending to be his nephew, lured him out from his religious sanctuary. Once captured, the Count of Moctezuma was promptly returned, but not to the mental hospital from which he had so stealthily fled; rather, he was taken back to the royal prison and chastised by officials for his "desperate illusions" and "malicious plots."[54] Whether worn down by despondency or crushed by his tribulations, Chimalpopoca died in custody soon after, but we should not throw aside the importance of his case. While it is exceptional in many regards, it clearly illustrates how the crown's paternalism toward the *pobres dementes* resonated in the Americas with colonial discourses and practices surrounding the inferior intellectual abilities of the natives and their protected legal and social status. It also highlights the fact that for these two types of *miserables*, protection and coercion were not necessarily on opposite ends of the spectrum but often two sides of the same coin. While couched in the language of royal benevolence, Chimalpopoca's confinement in San Hipólito was a way for colonial officials to temporarily do away with, if not necessarily punish, a vulnerable but threatening individual whose demands, whether grounded in reason or fantasy, exposed the injustices of Spanish colonialism.

Murder, Madness, and the Prison of Last Resort

The case of Chimalpopoca illustrates a recurring feature of criminal cases involving madness: namely, that the secular magistrates, unlike their inquisitorial counterparts, were far less invested in tethering their verdicts to the nuances and accuracies of medical diagnosis. Their chief concern was what to do with insane offenders who exhibited violent proclivities but whose madness impeded formal punishment. It must be recalled that punishment during the colonial period did not amount to a prison sentence but consisted of public whippings or executions and, far more common in the Spanish Empire, temporary or permanent exile and forced labor.[55] To inflict such harsh sentences on the mentally incapacitated was considered inhumane and an abuse of power. What, then, to do with a violent homicidal madman? The *furiosos* could not be left to suffer or run amok in the colony's public jails, which were intended only for temporary custody. But neither could the magistrates in good conscience allow them to go free, risking the danger that they might perpetrate a second, potentially fatal crime. San Hipólito, then, was the most obvious and convenient answer to this practical and moral dilemma, and we can see the colonial justices arriving at this solution in two criminal cases involving homicide in Teotihuacan, a small village located about thirty miles northeast of the viceregal capital.

Atanasio Guadalupe Delgadillo, a humble Creole *arriero* (muleteer) of *pulque*, did not murder Ignacio Cruz on a December evening in 1798 in a state of *locura*. He was definitely angry, but not mad. According to Delgadillo's testimony, the two *arrieros* quarreled after Cruz trampled up against his cargo as both made their way into Mexico City. Following a heated exchange of insults and threats, Cruz pulled out his whip and lashed out at Delgadillo, who responded by hurling rocks back. The two men then ended up brawling in the road, during which Delgadillo—although he claimed he could not recall the act—fatally stabbed Cruz twice. Witnesses immediately pulled Delgadillo off, subdued him, and delivered him to the custody of the chief deputy of Teotihuacan. Four months into his incarceration at a local jail, while the deputy was in the thick of his investigation, Delgadillo and four other prisoners managed to escape.[56]

The issue of Delgadillo's insanity would arise five years later, when he was discovered and rearrested in Teotihuacan. For the next two years, Delgadillo languished in the local prison while officials investigated both his first crime and his escape. While the process dragged on for what seemed like an interminable amount of time, he lost his wits and began to act out in vicious, furious bouts of violence. According to the new *subdelegado* of Teotihuacan, Manuel Joseph Gutiérrez, Delgadillo was "very *furioso*" and regularly harassed his fellow prisoners. His repeated blows against the walls were so fierce that they forced the jail door to open, inviting one inmate to flee. The officers then placed the raging muleteer into a prison stock, but that experiment failed, since he eventually broke it to "pieces." They then took Delgadillo to a cell in the basement, but much to their frustration and horror, he began removing bricks from the walls and hurling them at both prisoners and guards. Finding his resources and options exhausted, the *subdelegado* finally ordered that Delgadillo be placed into shackles (*grillos*) to "restrain his furor" and, as a last ditch solution, had the other prisoners transferred to an older and less secure jail nearby, leaving the raving muleteer to self-destruct in isolation.[57]

Clearly, Delgadillo could not remain in the provincial jail, but where could he go? It appeared the *subdelegado* had a destination clearly in mind. He summoned the surgeon, Felipe Herrera, to observe the deranged prisoner. If Delgadillo was destined for San Hipólito, he would require an official diagnosis. But while the *subdelegado* had attributed Delgadillo's deranged antics to a *demencia furiosa* (furious madness), Herrera claimed that the muleteer was not suffering from "total madness" but from a "grave hysterical passion" (*passión histerica*), which he could easily overcome "if he was taken out of the jail" and his heart allowed to recover.[58] Either diagnosis worked for the *subdelegado*, confirming that Delgadillo could not remain confined in prison. He immediately sent him to San Hipólito, instructing the prior general to notify the Real Audiencia once the prisoner's health was restored.[59]

There was no simple, one-size-fits-all description for which criminals ended up interned at San Hipólito; the only thing they shared was a propensity to violence and the authorities' desire to shield the public from it. Whereas Delgadillo had murdered in an act of rage and only later became mad, another criminal from Teotihuacan, José Mariano García, was a madman who murdered and, like Delgadillo, wound up inside the halls of San Hipólito. The case concerns the familiar scene of tavern spat gone ugly. On the evening of April 22, 1819, Francisco Bargas, also known as Pancho Peseta, stumbled through the doors of the local *pulquería*, or drinking tavern for *pulque*, while crying out in pain, "García has killed me!" Bargas bore a knife wound to his chest; he was faint and bleeding. According to witnesses, he and the culprit had earlier been drinking at the tavern when a game over a pint of *pulque* quickly escalated into threats, fighting, and stabbing.[60]

After authorities were notified of the crime and the murder suspect apprehended, the *subdelegado* of Teotihuacan, Francisco Lomarriba, collected witness testimony. Given the crime scene, investigators began with the assumption that alcohol had played a factor in the fatal altercation. Despite the crown's perpetual efforts to regulate the countless *pulquerías, vinaterías, tepacherías*, and other formal and informal drinking houses dispersed throughout the capital city and countryside, and to issue prohibitions against public inebriation, taverns and heavy alcohol consumption remained a central facet of plebeian culture.[61] Not just sites of merriment, recreation, and socializing, taverns were often places where intoxication, violence, and normative codes of masculine honor combined into a volatile, deadly mix. In eighteenth-century central Mexico, the majority of homicides were linked in some way to alcohol and often precipitated by a *riña*—that is, a superficial fight over a perceived affront or disagreement.[62] Teasing, jibes, and insults—an important part of plebeian masculine culture—forged bonds but also easily deteriorated into violence under the sway of heavy drinking in a society where manhood was vulnerable and easily challenged.[63]

Witnesses' testimony supported the centrality of alcohol to Bargas's killing. One man, who had visited the tavern earlier on the day of the assault, informed authorities that the "killer was fully loaded with *pulque* and *aguardiente*."[64] The tavern owner, a widow named Doña Margarita Oveido, also testified on García's obvious intoxication. However, she attributed the violent crime not just to inordinate drinking alone but to its lethal coupling with *locura*, recalling the suspect's rumored history with madness. Her suggestion that García's violent actions were not purely the result of inebriation but possibly driven by some underlying mental defect was quickly confirmed during his interrogation.[65] When prompted by Lomarriba to identify himself, García retorted the following nonsense: "I am the captain of the Divine Troop, which is part of the Celestial Fatherland." The *subdelgado* then observed that the suspect stood "in silence for a long time without being able to say anything but look about all places, cover his mouth, gaze foolishly at those around him, and, with a stuttering tongue, announce that he wished to die."[66] Lomarriba subsequently had García examined by a surgeon, who, after closely scrutinizing the suspect's "appearance and character," found García to be "completely insane" (*enteramente fatuo*) and with much "furious madness" (*demencia furiosa*).[67]

All evidence and testimony in the case guided the magistrates toward issuing the insanity verdict. Even the victim's wife urged the justices to act with clemency, stating that the "wretched" García should be treated with the "piety and compassion befitting his fatuity and drunkenness."[68] García's *defensor* (defense lawyer) built on this, stressing that it was "public" knowledge throughout the pueblo of Teotihuacan that his client struggled with madness, and that it was his condition, exacerbated "by the accident of becoming drunk," that instigated the victim's death.[69] Indeed, he emphasized, if García "was previously *demente* he became even *more* [mad] through inebriation," and given this state of double impairment, his crime should be judged as less severe.[70] Turning to legal doctrine, the *defensor* went on to remind the justices that the laws "dictate" that a mad person—whether identified as *furioso*, *demente*, or *fatuo*—"is not deserving of punishment," and because of this, he demanded that García be released and allowed to return home, giving some "comfort to his unhappy wife," who was "eager to apply some medicines at his side."[71]

Along with madness, Spanish law had long considered drunkenness a mitigating factor in a suspect's culpability. García's defense essentially argued that he was doubly impaired. Referencing *Las Siete Partidas*, Bolaños's *Curia Philipica* had instructed the justices to deliver mitigated sentences to those who were *borracho* (drunk), since they lacked full *entendimiento*.[72] Thus, by combining evidence of madness with intoxication, García's *defensor* mounted a persuasive defense that ultimately compelled the justices to declare the suspect "free of all punishment." That said, they would not consent to returning him home, even though his wife seemed willing to care for him. The legal consultant summoned in the case, the *licenciado* (lawyer) José Antonio Robles, had advised the magistrates to exonerate the culprit in keeping with the dictates of the law, but he urged caution in considering the best method to "contain him." Placing García in back in society, he argued, would be an egregious mistake, since it would present "new occasions" for the madman to commit "similar acts and many other excesses."[73] Thus, as they had done with Delgadillo years earlier, the colonial magistrates ordered that a man with no legal conviction against him be removed from a local jail and confined in San Hipólito. But unlike Delgadillo, in García's case the court offered no hint that he might someday be released.[74]

Colonial magistrates interned Atanasio Guadalupe Delgadillo and José Mariano García in San Hipólito not as retribution for their violent crimes but because, quite simply, they did not know where else to put them. At first glance, the magistrates' exercise of the legal principle of *arbitrio judicial* reads like a nearly unchecked power, but as both cases demonstrate, the administration of justice in late colonial Mexico was very much a collective enterprise.[75] The opinions of physicians or surgeons, lawyers, legal consultants, and lay witnesses, including the aggrieved party, all weighed in on the judge's verdict and sentence. Faced with a strong sentiment for humane leniency but also desirous of serving the more abstract notion of the "public"—particularly public safety—both judges leaned on San Hipólito as a solution. However, unlike their counterparts in the Inquisition, secular courts showed no interest in scrutinizing the behavior of those interned. Rather, the hospital was merely convenient, and if a convict regained mental health, then they would respond. But otherwise, once in the halls of San Hipólito, the criminal became a patient and no longer the court's responsibility.

Dangerous Passion: The Criminal Fantasies of María Getrudis Torres

One pattern that emerges from the archival records of the secular courts is that there were far more insane and violent men than women. Even more than in the case of the Inquisition, where instances of madness among male suspects outnumbered those of women, criminal cases of insanity among women were so rare as to make them almost negligible. But when they did arise, they revealed plenty about the social structure of life in New Spain. The case of María Getrudis Torres lays bare the gendered nature of status and hierarchy in New Spain, how women were expected to help ensure social stability by reproducing social castes and classes, and how cultural expectations ultimately infused legal institutions to make sure a woman dared not set her ambitions too high. Indeed, the case of María Getrudis is a lesson that for women in the early nineteenth century—supposedly an age of revolution and freedom—stepping out of one's social place was, by definition, insane.

The case begins on the morning of April 6, 1806, in Mexico City, when María Getrudis committed a dreadful act of violence. Her victim was the thirteen-year-old *criolla* María Manuela Moreno y Jove, the daughter of Rosalía Jove, María Getrudis's former employer. One shocked witness, Petra Ilachea—the servant who was accompanying María Manuela as she attended mass at the Church of San Francisco—reported to have seen the *castiza* seamstress attack the *niña* (young girl) as they were leaving the church. "So it is you who says you will kill me!" María Getrudis had shouted before proceeding to stab María Manuela in the back with a sharp instrument. Petra was horrified but reacted immediately. In her testimony, she described how she attempted to restrain María Getrudis while María Manuela, wounded and bleeding, ran away toward the nearby cemetery. Struggling to free herself

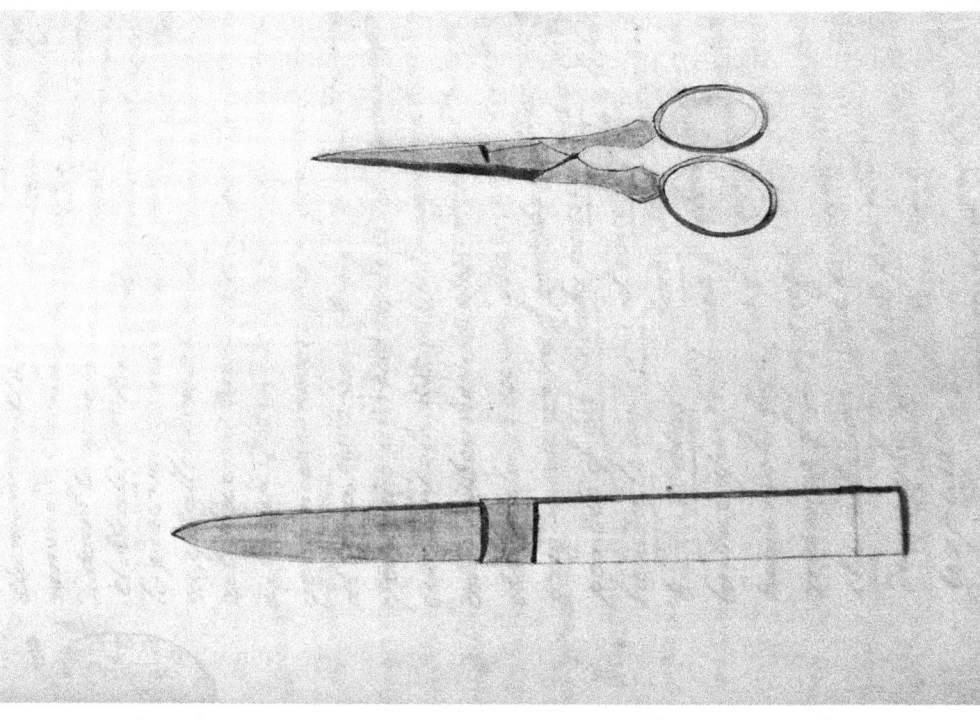

FIGURE 5.1 Illustration of a small knife and pair of scissors belonging to the *castiza* seamstress María Getrudis Torres, the knife being the assault weapon used to wound her thirteen-year-old victim, 1806. Source: AGN, Criminal, vol. 712, exp. 3.

from Petra's grip, María Getrudis repeatedly struck the older woman in the shoulder with what appeared to be a dark and pointed knife. She then fled the scene of the crime.[76]

While Petra received only some minor scrapes, the young María Manuela fared much worse. Following the attack, she was medically treated by a surgeon who went on to inform authorities that a "sharp and pointed instrument" had pierced through her chest, possibly damaging the left lung and resulting in "great hemorrhaging" and heavy, labored breathing. Although María Manuela survived, she had come frighteningly close to death.[77] The weapon in question, it was later revealed, was a small knife that María Getrudis kept tucked away near her bosom, next to a pair of sharp scissors. Upon her arrest the following evening, she produced both of these and handed them over to the *alguacil* (constable), who had them illustrated and deposited as evidence (see figure 5.1). When asked by the *alguacil* why she carried the scissors in addition to the blade, she responded that both were intended for her own protection and that should she lose the knife, she could "make use of the scissors."[78]

What compelled the *castiza* seamstress to violently stab an innocent girl in cold blood? Searching for motive, the magistrates constructed a narrative that cast María Getrudis as a vindictive and delusional woman incited to violent acts by her own jealous fantasies and unchecked passions. Although María Getrudis had worked as a seamstress for the Jove family without incident, when she ended her employment, her conduct showed signs of mental instability. In particular, the entire Jove household, both servants and family, recalled an ominous series of letters the seamstress had delivered to her former employer, Doña Rosalía, in which she accused Doña Rosalía of attempting to thwart her marriage to Don Rafael Sagaz, a physician well acquainted with the Jove family, by enticing him to marry María Manuela instead.[79] It is not clear whether Doña Rosalía truly intended to marry her adolescent daughter to the prominent physician, but María Getrudis's belief that Sagaz pined after her was, according to witnesses—Sagaz included—ludicrous. In his testimony, Sagaz revealed that María Getrudis had earlier sent him a doting letter, which he readily tore to pieces, dismissing her advances and deeming the whole affair a source of amusement and "laughter."[80]

Although witnesses mocked her intention to marry at her mature age—she was thirty-six—and outside her social station, María Getrudis remained fixed in her beliefs.[81] In her testimony, she described how Sagaz "viewed her with affection" and told others he desired to marry her, going so far as to obtain a marriage license. If the marriage had failed to materialize, María Getrudis believed it was because Doña Rosalía had intervened by defaming her character, calling her a "pig who was lazy and did not know how to sew," and persuading Sagaz to engage himself to María Manuela instead, who was youthful, vibrant, and wealthy.[82] María Getrudis told the judges that when she learned of Doña Rosalía's plot to thwart her marriage, she was overcome with a violent surge of "choler" that, she later elaborated, caused her to "feel a disturbance in her head" and a "shakiness" throughout her body. Only then did she write the letters to Doña Rosalía—although she could not recall their contents—and on the morning of April 6, upon encountering her imagined nemesis, María Manuela, at mass, she angrily launched at her.[83]

María Getrudis's madness expressed itself in strikingly gendered ways. Cases before the Inquisition often focused on a woman's illicit carnal desires and imagined copulation with the devil, pointing to colonial Mexico's sexual double standards and the frustration that it inevitably stirred within women. María Getrudis's case, by contrast, was hardly as sexually titillating but far more revealing of the stakes women faced when confronting marriage. In colonial Spanish America's patriarchal society, an honorable marriage represented the highest and most dignified state to which women could aspire. But not all women in the viceregal capital were capable of contracting an advantageous marriage; indeed, many never married at all.[84] Overwhelmingly, it was the colonial Spanish elite (and those with material means for upward mobility) who contracted legal and endogamous marriages, driven by their concerns with legitimacy and status.[85] María Getrudis's obsession with her imagined betrothal to the physician thus reflected a longing to participate in a normative institution that perpetuated social and racial hierarchies, buttressed male authority, and protected women's bodies from dishonor. Moreover, the *castiza* seamstress's conviction that her former employer had purposefully besmirched her character and convinced the physician to break off the intended engagement was a perceived assault on her sexual honor and reputation. The only valid reason for a suitor to call off an engagement—if, in María Getrudis's imagination, she was indeed engaged—was the discovery that the bride-to-be was not sexually virtuous.[86] And as Sonya Lipsett-Rivera has demonstrated, ordinary plebeian women like María Getrudis were just as concerned about their honor as were their male counterparts, and willing to engage in direct confrontations, often violent, with other women to defend it.[87]

Regardless of María Getrudis's reasoning, she had committed a grave crime and, worse yet, against someone who was socially superior. As a self-identified *castiza*, María Getrudis benefited from being on the lighter end of the color-coded racial ladder, but she was clearly poor and forced to work for a living. By contrast, her victim's mother, Doña Rosalía, came from a respectable Creole family with strong ties to the medical establishment, being the daughter of the president of the Protomedicato and widow to the former director of the Royal Amphitheatre of Anatomy. As a widow of social standing, Doña Rosalía was both appalled that her daughter's safety had been violated and indignant that the crime transgressed racial and class boundaries. Her contempt for her former seamstress burned bright, as she described María Getrudis as a woman "of little Christian sentiment and honor."[88] No doubt, the notion that María Getrudis presumed to imagine herself as a genuine competitor with her daughter was like gasoline poured on her anger.

Readily diagnosed by physicians as a "true maniac," the *alcalde ordinario* of Mexico City's *cabildo* (municipal council) proved willing to grant her the insanity defense. However, he faced active resistance from the aggrieved party. Doña Rosalía's brother, Don Pedro José García Jove, a lawyer for the Real Audiencia, deftly maneuvered to ensure sterner punishment for the assailant. A few months after the assault, Doña Rosalía and her attorney-brother crafted a letter on behalf of the family to the municipal justices that emphatically argued against treating the *castiza* seamstress with leniency. The letter undermined the idea that María Getrudis was insane, instead casting her as a volatile woman who, prompted by "unregulated amorous passion," had committed the violent deed of wounding María Manuela "with premeditated cruelty" (*con crueldad alevosamente*). "There is no doubt," Doña Rosalía and her brother wrote, "that [the crime] was premeditated with the measures and precautions of someone who is not *demente*, but very sane." The fact that María Getrudis had fled the scene of the crime, clearly "fearful" that she would be apprehended, betrayed thoughts and actions "little consistent with the disturbed brain of a madwoman." Moreover, they argued that her intention was not just to injure María Manuela but to kill her, a point they drove home by underscoring that she "invaded [the victim] from behind" with a weapon "deliberately designed to cause death." Her brother's legal skill shone in the letter, pointing to the "direction" of the stabbing, perilously close to a vital organ, and the fact that she carried not one weapon on her person but two on that fateful day. Given what they believed was ample evidence of malicious intent, the victim's family urged the local justices to condemn the jealous seamstress to a life sentence at the Casa de Recogidas, a punishment they considered both just and mitigated.[89]

Perhaps knowing that they had an uphill fight against popular opinion that María Getrudris was insane, Doña Rosalía and her attorney-brother faced the issue head-on. The last scenario they wanted was for her to enjoy her freedom. While it was true, they stated, that the genuinely mad could not be punished, this protection did not apply to those whose madness stemmed from amorous passion (*locos de amores*). To grant the lovesick seamstress the insanity defense, they reasoned, would be tantamount to issuing impunity to the countless crimes committed by men overcome by a "fanatic love" or "jealously" that also "to some extent distorts judgment."[90] However, even if María Getrudis was indeed determined to be an authentic maniac rather than, as they believed, a jealous woman suffering from unrequited love, the Joves implored the justices to consider the "threat" she posed both to their safety and security and to the "public" at large.[91] The *castiza* seamstress clearly did not lack the "temerity" to harm an "innocent victim" like María Manuela, and they warned she was therefore likely to lash out again if her distorted and obsessive mind ever re-entertained the notion of marrying someone well

Crime and Punishment 163

beyond her grasp. Whether sane or not, the Joves demanded María Getrudis's "perpetual reclusion"—if not at the Casa de Recogidas, as they desired, then at the very least at the Hospital del Divino Salvador. Only with the seamstress confined for perpetuity, they insisted, could their family feel "secure and tranquil"; only then could they be truly "liberated" of "this woman, our cruel enemy."[92]

The municipal justices disagreed that the crime was maliciously premeditated, concurring with the physicians—Juan José Bermudez and José Vásquez—that the seamstress was mentally unstable, showing signs of suffering from a mania that rendered her sane in all matters except that which touched on the subject of her imagined marriage to Sagaz.[93] But they concurred that María Getrudis was a dangerous and unstable woman, liable to act on her delusions in a violent manner once again, and so on August 4, 1806, by court order, she entered the Divino Salvador.

The active involvement of Doña Rosalía and her attorney-brother in the prosecution against the *castiza* seamstress exposes the role of local interests in shaping not just verdicts but the terms of confinement in a mental hospital and its duration. Although the Jove family had desired a life sentence for the culprit at the Casa de Recogidas, once the *alcalde ordinario* granted María Getrudis the insanity defense and the more lenient sentence of committal to the Divino Salvador, they went to great lengths to ensure that she did not leave, challenging her repeated petitions to the *cabildo* for her release on the grounds that she remained mentally unsound and continued to pose a threat to their family.

The first request to leave the Divino Salvador came three months after the sentencing, when the hospital's director, Joseph Antonio Martín de los Ríos, informed the court that María Getrudis was fully "restored," submitting with his report an official certificate of health issued by the surgeon, José Colima.[94] Immediately, the Joves voiced their objections. In his response, Pedro José García Jove attacked Colima's credibility, arguing that his training as a surgeon did not render him qualified to assess states of disordered reasoning and demanded that María Getrudis be reexamined by the two physicians who had originally diagnosed her as a maniac. Having cast doubt on the surgeon's diagnosis, Doña Rosalía's brother proceeded to remind the magistrates of the seamstress's "fierce character" and her deviation from modes of proper feminine conduct in a society where women were ideally expected to be demure, passive, and quiet. María Getrudis's conduct at the Divino Salvador had been reprehensible, Pedro José Garcia Jove reported, providing "more signs that she is mad rather than sane." Aside from what he described as her characteristic "obscenity and foul words," María Getrudis had reportedly unleashed her "ire" on the other female inmates on a number of occasions. "If she behaves this way with the innocent [patients] who are incapable of malice," he implored the magistrates to consider, "what will she do with those of my house whom she supposes criminal, those of us who have taken her freedom?"[95]

The Joves ultimately succeeded in keeping María Getrudis confined at the Divino Salvador. At their behest, the municipal justices sent Juan José Bermudez to the hospital, who concluded that the *castiza* seamstress was indeed still mad. Although she had responded "perfectly" to all his questions, Bermudez observed that her imagination was still stubbornly "fixed" on the notion of marrying Sagaz and that she remained convinced she was an innocent victim of Doña Rosalía's machinations. By his estimation, her mind could not accept the reality of her age, race, and class, and preferred to latch on to wild, imagined scenarios. Her refusal to come to harmony with her standing in colonial society, the physician believed, rendered her a continued danger.[96]

Bermudez's opinion was enough to keep María Getrudis quiet for the next four years, but in 1811 she submitted a second petition for release. By this point, the seamstress's health had improved to the point that she was no longer even treated in the hospital as a patient. According to the hospital's director, she was now holding steady work inside the institution, caring for the other female inmates, for which she earned a modest salary. She loathed her situation, repeatedly clamoring for her liberty, insisting that she would "rather go to jail than remain [there]."[97] The court consented, sending her to the city jail while it considered her release. The Joves responded once again, emphasizing her violent impulses, devious character, and the vengeance she would inevitably wreak upon them for keeping her confined. Maniacs, they reminded the court, behaved normally on most occasions but easily relapsed into madness when stirred by their obsession. As an unmarried women fixated on a man she could never hope to have, María Getrudis was sure to suffer in the future.[98]

Once again the Joves' plea moved the magistrates to action, and the seamstress was reexamined by a new physician, Francisco Xavier Tello de Meneses. He reported that María Getrudis appeared perfectly normal and even adorned herself with the trappings of respectable femininity: "ribbons of diverse colors, earrings, fake beauty marks (*chiqueadores*), a choker, and a headband." Nonetheless, like Bermudez four years earlier, Tello de Meneses concluded that she was "truly maniacal." All he had to do was broach the delicate subject of her relationship with Sagaz and her insanity reappeared—

although now she claimed Sagaz "jealously obsessed" over her "during all hours of the night because he believed she was sleeping with various men." The physician pressed her on this irrational conviction, urging her to "reflect" on the differences in status between herself and her fictitious suitor. She then "responded infuriatedly" that "nothing mattered" because she was no longer inclined to marry either Sagaz or Doña Rosalía's attorney-brother, whom, in a new twist, the seamstress now claimed had also "courted" her. Such fanciful beliefs—clearly detached from reality, the physician informed the *cabildo*—were undeniable symptoms of mania, a disease he admitted was difficult to detect and diagnose, even for the most discerning of "medical eyes" (*ojos realmente medicos*).[99] Convinced, the local magistrates overseeing the case sent the maniacal seamstress back to Divino Salvador against her will.

In María Getrudis's case, confinement was never described as a retribution for attempted murder but as a humane and utilitarian measure: it protected her—and others—from herself. Yet it had, in practice, become an intolerable punishment, and in an appeal written prior to her mandated return to the hospital, she objected vehemently to being treated as a "legitimate delinquent," bemoaning having had to endure the "very severe" punishment of being forced "to serve madwomen [*fatuas*] for five years."[100]

It took her five more years, but in 1816 María Getrudis's pleas were finally heard. What had changed in the interval? First, a new municipal magistrate, one sympathetic to her plight, took over her case. Second, that year she penned a letter to the court that voiced contrition and represented herself as a rehabilitated woman. She acknowledged that she had committed a violent and criminal act while "incited by my fantasies," which had caused a "disturbance of the brain." However, she told the justice, the long "reclusion" at the Divino Salvador has had the effect of "excessively cooling my blood, extinguishing my passion, and giving me a place" in which to "reflect." She tethered her prolonged imprisonment to the cruelty of her victim's mother, Doña Rosalía, whose "vehemence" and desire for "vengeance" would not be abated until "she succeeded . . . in exhausting my spirit in this enclosure of sadness and horror." Finally, she shrewdly anticipated potential challenges from medical experts, whom she suspected to be in cahoots with Doña Rosalía (who was, after all, daughter to the president of the Protomedicato). The reformed seamstress informed Calderón that a "virtuous priest" who "directed [her] conscience" had "certified" to her "full and sensible judgment" and went on to assert that claims to sanity were "not limited to physicians"; rather, "it is an illness that is recognized by [any]one who has reason." For good measure, she added a final jab at the experts who had kept her institutionalized: "I wish that in a case similar to mine, these men were sent to San Hipólito, and that they stayed there and experienced what I did," speculating that they too would become partially mad.[101]

The new municipal magistrate saw merit in María Getrudis's petition and had her examined by two physicians, including Tello de Meneses, but notably did not inform Doña Rosalía. Both physicians attested to her recovered mental health, and Tello de Meneses remarked with satisfaction that the seamstress now recognized the delusion in thinking she could ever be engaged to Sagaz. The second physician, Don Miguel María Jiménez, echoed these sentiments while also emphasizing the patient's sense of remorse and her promises to refrain from contacting her former victim and their family should she be granted liberty. She had finally reconciled herself to the "great difference" that existed between the educated and eminent physician and her "humble state."[102] Not only had María Getrudis recuperated her sanity, but she was now a rehabilitated and subdued woman able to accept her inferior status in colonial Mexico's rigidly stratified society and demonstrate due respect to her social superiors. In September 1816, nearly eleven years after she had stabbed a helpless young girl in a fit of jealous rage, she stepped out from the Divino Salvador a free woman, but she was still poor, now nearing fifty, and with even less hope of ever marrying.

The role of medical expertise in defining the terms of madness—in medicalizing María Getrudis's thoughts and actions—also looms large in this case. If tensions over diagnosis ensued, it was because the victim's family generated skepticism and called on additional experts. Less invested in matters of interiority, the secular magistrates were far more inclined to accept medical testimony without question. While inquisitors acted as agents of medicalization in the age of Enlightenment, in the following century it would be the secular criminal courts that would increasingly sanction the medical expert's diagnosis.

The Criminal's Sanctuary: Tales of Suspicious Madness and Escape

Unlike the *castiza* seamstress, not all criminals who pleaded insanity regarded the colonial mental hospital as punishment, or if they did, they fled its confines. If colonial authorities had come to rely increasingly on hospitals, particularly San Hipólito, to store criminals whose insanity rendered them unfit to stand trial or fulfill the terms of a mandated sentence, then a by-product of this trend was that these institutions were also sometimes used by the crafty and resourceful for the purposes of evading the law. Chapter 2 alluded to the striking frequency with which the patients of San Hipólito took flight. Significantly, a large portion of the escapees were soldiers possibly seeking to avoid military duty, slaves escaping bondage, and convicted or suspected felons remanded to the hospital by authorities. In fact, by the late eighteenth century, the problem of feigned madness and hospital flight had escalated to the point that the prior general of San Hipólito, friar Joseph Martínez, lamented to the viceroy that the colonial mental hospital, intended for the charitable care and treatment of *pobres dementes*, had become a "sanctuary" (*asilo*) for criminals, some of "malicious" character, bent on eluding punishment for their crimes.[103] If the case of María Getrudis Torres provided colonial authorities with a model for a successful internment, one that served the purposes of subduing and rehabilitating a violent and maniacal madwoman with delusions of upward mobility, then the cases discussed here loomed large as examples of failure that spoke to broader structural weaknesses, the ad hoc implementation of the law, and the general inability of the colonial state to fully govern the lives of its Spanish American subjects.

The prior general's complaint that San Hipólito had descended into a haven for criminals and devious people was issued in response to the escape of two convicts, Felipe Sierra and Francisco Cosio. On a January evening in 1793, unbeknownst to hospital staff and the two *porteros* (doormen) who guarded the doors to the main entrance and infirmary, the two men quietly removed the shackles that constrained their movement, broke free from their cells, and secretly climbed the walls of the hospital, absconding into the countryside. No one detected the breakout until the following morning, upon which the prior general alerted the deputies, who launched a search. Soon, advisories circulated throughout the capital and neighboring municipalities announcing the flight and the physical attributes of the two fugitives.[104]

According to the prior general, the mastermind behind the escape was Felipe Sierra, a man whom he believed possessed the cunning "ability to seduce" his more dull-witted accomplice.[105] Little is known about Sierra except that in the winter of 1791, while awaiting trial in a Havana prison for an undisclosed crime, he lost his sanity and became irrationally violent, "inclined to kill and offend," according to the governor, at the slightest provocation. With no appropriate institution in Havana to address his madness, the governor had the *furioso* transferred to San Hipólito, but a mere two months later, he escaped.[106] Besides a rumor that he fled to the city of Puebla with the intent to return to Havana, Sierra also escaped from the historical record, seeming to have successfully evaded colonial authorities for the remainder of his life.

Whereas Sierra disappeared leaving no paper trail, within days authorities located his allegedly less conniving accomplice in Valladolid and placed him in a royal prison. The Real Sala del Crimen then undertook a lengthy investigation that left behind scores of documents. They discovered that Cosio, a native of Peru, had arrived in Guanajuato in 1791, "short on fortune" and needing employment. He found it at a local mine and worked without incident for nearly eight months before his overseer noticed he had become "distracted" and his reasoning "perturbed." Cosio confirmed his overseer's suspicion that he was mentally troubled when, on one memorable occasion, he spotted him crouched in the middle of the city surrounded by spectators with a small doll of Christ in his hands, screaming. This led to his firing, but he remained in Guanajuato and, despite some disturbing behavior, avoided arrest until he assaulted and injured—"albeit lightly," officials reported—a local man and a woman. Two days later, he escaped on a stolen horse, evading the law for only fifteen days before returning to prison. Since his reputation as a madman was widely known, the *alcalde* of Guanajuato, Manuel Cevallos, immediately called on the services of the prison's physician, who ultimately concluded that Cosio was indeed *verdaderamente loco* (truly mad); following the confirmed diagnosis, Cevallos had him shipped out to San Hipólito.[107]

The initial diagnosis that took Cosio to San Hipólito did little to assuage the suspicion of the *fiscal* investigating the breakout that the criminal had feigned madness. He was not alone. Indeed, the magistrates overseeing the investigation had instructed the *fiscal* to proceed with skepticism and assume the suspect "invented" his antics in order to "frustrate and undermine" his deserved "punishment."[108] Witness testimony only heightened these apprehensions. A *ladino* (Hispanicized Indian) Cosio met during his flight informed the *fiscal* that he was certainly "not mad."[109] Two medical experts who had recently examined the prisoner at Valladolid also voiced their doubts. One examiner, a physician, could only detect in Cosio a "shameless character," but no madness. The surgeon reached a similar conclusion, stating that the suspect was definitely not *demente* but simply "talkative" and of a "wild temperament" (*genio alocado*).[110]

If the *fiscal* hoped that Cosio's testimony might demonstrate and confirm the suspect's sanity, he would be disappointed. Under interrogation, Cosio explained that he had been institutionalized before in Lima at the Hospital de San Andres but only because a "jealous" woman—whose name he could not recall—had given him a strange beverage that "perturbed his head for four years."¹¹¹ Once recovered, he left for New Spain, hounded by death threats from the woman who had given him the mysterious madness-inducing libation. His account of his previous life was bizarre enough to hint at a barely controlled madness, which was further evidenced by his itinerant lifestyle and inability to hold a job or make a living. Yet when questioned, Cosio adamantly maintained his sanity, and when asked why he had fled San Hipólito, he emphatically stated that it was "to prove that he was not mad."¹¹²

Deeply suspicious that Cosio was faking insanity but clearly troubled by his curious life story, the *fiscal* wavered, but ever so slightly. Could a man who had demonstrable bouts of insanity but who stubbornly insisted on his mental soundness be legally labeled insane? The testimony of José de Villaseca, the physician who had treated Cosio while he was living in Guanajuato and diagnosed him as a hypochondriac with the "beginnings of *demencia*," largely swayed his decision to suspend the case.¹¹³ But what to do with Cosio? The itinerant troublemaker had proven himself to be an annoying thorn in the *fiscal*'s side. The prosecuting attorney reasoned that it was not "convenient to shut him up in a hospice or hospital to the detriment of others" who needed such spaces; and, more pressingly, Cosio had a history of escape. As a reasonable alternative, the *fiscal* turned to what he called the "bonds of blood" and the "compassion of kinship," ordering that Cosio be placed in the custody of his brother, Fernando, who resided in the mining province of Tlalpujahua.¹¹⁴ Cosio's brother had earlier objected to this idea, stressing that his resources were "limited" and that it would be difficult, if not impossible, to keep an eye on his brother, who was "restless" and "not at all tranquil."¹¹⁵ But his pleas fell on deaf ears, and Cosio was soon transferred from his cell in the Valladolid prison to Tlalpujahua, much to his brother's frustration and the relief of colonial authorities.

Francisco Cosio personified all the attributes that Bourbon authorities had come to denounce as sources of the empire's malaise. His peripatetic lifestyle, inability to hold steady employment, and constant troublemaking were precisely the habits and vices Bourbon officials had identified as hindrances to the economic prosperity of what was in fact an empire in a state of rapid decline.¹¹⁶ Indeed, he embodied the social anathema of idleness that centralizing regimes throughout Europe so vehemently condemned and targeted and that historians have linked to the emergence of a heterogeneous range of institutions of confinement and discipline—poorhouses, workhouses, asylums—loosely associated with the "birth of the prison."¹¹⁷ But if Bourbon authorities sought to reform the vices of the local populace in their overseas domains, they rarely used the mental hospital for such purposes. In fact, that the *fiscal* found himself compelled to place the troublesome Cosio in the reluctant custody of his brother shows that colonial authorities were often at a loss when dealing with insane offenders and that the provisioning of their custodial care remained ad hoc.[118] San Hipólito may have loomed large as an attractive solution to the problem of criminal insanity, particularly for cases concerned with violence, but its walls were highly porous.

Another criminal charged with escaping the mental hospital was Rafael Cubo. On the evening of May 14, 1801, in a village adjacent to the capital, Cubo and three accomplices robbed the *tienda* (shop) of Don Manuel Negrete. The men barged in with firearms, assaulted those in the shop, and demanded money before going on to ransack the store and the store owner's adjacent home, stealing linens, jewelry, plates, and various other valuable possessions.[119] Investigating deputies quickly linked the robbery with a similar one that had taken place in the same village months earlier, and the four suspects were eventually identified, apprehended, and subjected to rigorous interrogation, during which their repeated offenses came into full disclosure. Cubo, however, was unable to testify on his own behalf, as he had fallen mad just days after his imprisonment. Not knowing what to do with such a violent—and now insane—prisoner, authorities sent him to San Hipólito on February 4, 1802, "for his recovery."[120] Two months later he fled, and though he evaded arrest for the next six months, he was eventually apprehended and put in a local prison. There, armed with a knife he clandestinely acquired from another inmate, he managed to break free from his cell, but was ultimately spotted by the jail keeper and stabbed in the ensuing altercation. While recovering from a wound to his right shoulder at the Hospital de San Pedro in Puebla, authorities contemplated what to do with him next.[121]

As was the case in any escape from San Hipólito, suspicions immediately emerged that Cubo had feigned his madness all along to flee punishment, so the *teniente provincial* (provincial deputy) of the Acordada had him interrogated. Cubo's testimony exposed a life of lawlessness. He revealed that in 1800, he had been condemned to eight years of hard labor in the Havana presidio for an undisclosed crime. While en route to Havana, he managed to flee on a stolen horse and met the three men who would become his accomplices in his later brutal robberies. But despite his horrible crimes and his penchant for deviousness, Cubo insisted he never lied about his madness. "I was not coaxed to fake madness," he told his investigator, "nor was it my intention to do so." By his estimation, the entire episode had been an "accident." His confinement in jail, he explained, had provoked a surge of "passion" and *frenesí*, during which he was unable to account for or recall his actions. While at San Hipólito, Cubo suddenly and remarkably found himself "restored to his reasoning," and it was only then that he "contemplated escape to liberate himself from the punishment that awaited him." The flight from San Hipólito had been surprisingly effortless: after using a rock to break his shackles, Cubo claimed to have approached the *portero* (doorman) and, "without any violence," requested to leave, to which the doorman curiously conceded.[122]

When prompted by authorities to investigate the incident and corroborate Cubo's version of the escape, the prior general of San Hipólito revealed that the fugitive had not exactly politely asked to leave the hospital. Rather, he had "intimidated" the *portero* guarding the *loquería* (infirmary) using one of the bolts of his broken shackles. However, the prior general's inquiry into the breakout went on to expose San Hipólito's poor and uncoordinated system of surveillance. Not only could the prior general not immediately identify the doorman whom Cubo had violently threatened, since the guards "changed repeatedly," but the second *portero* supervising the doors to the main entrance was apparently not on duty.[123] Understaffed and chaotic, San Hipólito could never hold a clear-minded seasoned criminal who had even the slightest intention of leaving.

Although the authorities remained unconvinced that Cubo had truly fallen ill and was then abruptly restored to his senses, the oppressive and squalid conditions of colonial prisons introduces an element of plausibility to Cubo's rendition of events. Like the secret cells of the Holy Office, public jails were insalubrious places. Prisoners were huddled in tiny cells or in dark, grimy dungeons with no lighting and little to no ventilation. To make matters worse, the jails were usually overcrowded and festered with mice, fleas, lice, and other vermin, and it was often the case that inmates suffered from hunger, malnutrition, and disease.[124] That Cubo might have lost his wits under such wretched conditions, compounded by the stress of his imminent trial, would not be surprising. According to José Manuel Tapía—an inmate who had witnessed Cubo's descent into insanity while in jail—Cubo became "furiously mad" after he was confined in the *bartolina* (dungeon), and then deputies reacted to his maddened fits by beating him and placing him in solitary confinement. Tapía believed these abusive measures were intended "not only to punish the prisoner, but to discover whether he was truly mad."[125] Another inmate stated that Cubo endured the "greatest of miseries" while in prison and that whenever he became *furioso*, he would cease to eat and pace his cell naked.[126]

In the end, whether Cubo feigned his illness or not was a moot point. He was now fully restored to his senses, and authorities had little reason to recruit the opinions of medical experts or delay sentencing in any way. If he had been ill, then the hospital had served its purpose and a mad criminal had now recovered and was capable to stand before the court. If he had been deceiving the court before and been sane all along, he was now going to face the punishment deserving of someone with a long history tarnished by habitual crime and repeated attempts to thwart the law. In January 1804, the justices in Cubo's case decided to make an example out of him for anyone who might want to follow in the footsteps of the resourceful and wily hardened criminal by condemning him to death by hanging.[127]

WHETHER CUBO WOULD HAVE BEEN hanged had he not escaped from San Hipólito and sown doubt as to his sincerity before the court is both unclear and beside the point. San Hipólito had little chance to be what secular courts needed it to be. If its relationship with the Inquisition was a strained, awkward fit, its service to the courts was a farce. The brothers, faced with financial, space, and staff limitations, could never attempt to heal the criminally mad and violent while maintaining their principal mission to serve the *pobres dementes*. Yet by the last decades of the eighteenth century, San Hipólito was too politically and financially indebted to the state to ignore its needs and demands. The state, and more accurately the courts, needed space for those violently inclined but legally exonerated, and the brothers—though the prior general sent off plaintive laments to officials—reluctantly agreed. If San Hipólito's assistance was convenient for the state, the state's support was a necessity for San Hipólito.

Moreover, to a large extent San Hipólito's shortcomings in addressing the problem of criminal insanity did not fully reside within in its walls. Immersed in a colony whose authority over its subjects was weakening, whose coffers were shrinking, whose corruption was growing, and whose infrastructure was crumbling, mental hospitals had little to offer those leaders bent on addressing the disorder, crime, and chaos they saw in the colony. What could San Hipólito offer the secular courts, which, like the Inquisition, broached two worlds: the colonial world of paternalistic leniency, flowing from the crown and enshrined in its laws; and the more modern utilitarian ideas of social improvement, rational order, and public happiness? The strain between the two worlds appeared routinely in the cases of insane criminals—especially violent criminals—and San Hipólito did not have the power, the authority, or the resources to resolve tensions of this magnitude. Frankly, no one did. For all the colonial leaders' pronouncements of reform and improvement throughout the late eighteenth and early nineteenth centuries, legal scholars like Lardizábal y Uribe would never see the penal codes reformed in their lifetimes. Even after Independence, Mexico would have to wait till the late nineteenth century for a systematic reorganization and standardization of its laws.

Conclusion
A Defense of Bedlam

In February 1808, much to the chagrin of a declining global power, the French invader Napoleon and his troops marched toward Madrid, having already sent the Portuguese royal family packing to Rio de Janeiro. What followed signaled the humiliating collapse of the Spanish government, as the king of Spain, Charles IV, and his immediate successor, Ferdinand VII, were placed under house arrest and forced to relinquish the throne to Napoleon's brother, Joseph Bonaparte. The event announced in the Iberian Atlantic the official onset of what has been called the "Age of Revolutions," as Spanish Americans throughout the mainland colonies grappled with questions of local governance and legitimate rule in the absence of the Spanish monarch. By mid-July, news of the monarchy's downfall had reached the viceroyalty of New Spain, heightening brewing tensions between Creoles and Peninsulares.[1] The mature colony, however, did not immediately respond to the imperial crisis by severing ties with the metropolis, nor did it profess obedience to the widely unpopular puppet government of the French emperor. Rather, because of the heavy concentration of royal officials within the colony, and the conservative orientation of the majority of the landed Creole elite, the viceregal government remained loyal to the disgraced Spanish crown and continued to impose local rule in its name.[2] Meanwhile, popular rebellions— most famously, the insurgencies led by the priests Miguel Hidalgo and José María Morelos—began to wreak social and economic havoc, intensifying local discontent and political unrest.

It is difficult to gauge how the whirlwind of events taking place beyond San Hipólito's walls penetrated into the hospital's daily life. Surviving records for this period are sparse, perhaps itself an indication of internal disarray and hardship as the institution weathered the stormy tides of the turbulent decades that preceded independence.[3] To be sure, Hidalgo's army of mostly Indigenous and mestizo peasants—armed with machetes, pitchforks, old guns, and religious symbols, and decrying "death to the *gachupines*"—never sacked the capital city. The Creole priest had mysteriously ordered his troops to retreat to the north and was soon after captured and released to the Inquisition for torture and execution. Were his crimes not so severe, Hidalgo himself might have found himself locked inside San Hipólito, as the priest cited a bout of *frensi* as the source for inciting rebellion.[4] However, one fact remains certain: the popular 1810 uprising and the similar protests it engendered served to aggravate a financial crisis that was sorely felt throughout the capital's charitable establishments.[5] By 1817, the situation was so dire that the viceroy, Juan Ruíz de Apodaca, felt compelled to issue a general fundraising appeal to the city council. As he lamented, "Since that fatal moment in which the atrocious fire of rebellion ignited on this handsome soil, all abundance has disappeared. The corporations, houses, and rich families have been reduced to extreme want, and the asylums of piety, which mostly subsisted on voluntary donations, have been left without funds to support their unhappy inmates."[6]

Local rebellions were not the sole cause of San Hipólito's financial woes. The parsimonious crown, in one of its last-gasp efforts to compete on the global stage, issued in 1793 a controversial decree known as the Consolidación de Vales Reales (Consolidation of Royal Bonds), extending these measures to the Americas in 1804. The decree, a culmination of the Bourbon state's ongoing efforts to wrestle power and wealth from the church, mandated the repayment of all loans whose interest supported pious works, as well as the forced auction of all church property, the proceeds of which would be used to fill the crown's sinking coffers and fund its wars.[7] It is not altogether clear how the Consolidación affected San Hipólito specifically, but the colony's hospitals appear to have experienced a collective pinch in their budgets as a consequence of these harsh measures, which were only compounded by the outbreak of local insurgencies. By 1813, the Royal Indian Hospital had ceased to provide San Hipólito with monthly compensation for the care of Indigenous patients on account of a "lack of funds."[8] Signs of internal turmoil and financial distress were also evident in the fact that it was during this very same year that the number of *pobres dementes* occupying San Hipólito's cells plummeted to a stunning low of just nineteen patients.[9]

San Hipólito was struggling to stay afloat, and in 1816 the new prior general of the hospital, Fray Eusevio Figueroa, filed a complaint with the *fiscal de lo civil* (civil prosecutor) of the Real Audiencia in a desperate effort to retrieve funds. Figueroa began his appeal by noting how even "in times of abundance and prosperity" the hospital had found itself short on resources, juxtaposing that situation to the present day's "calamity and affliction . . . [when] it takes little effort for me to explain . . . the daily tortures I experience finding bread and meat" to feed the *pobres dementes*, or even a "measly linen" to clothe their suffering bodies.[10] The prior general stressed that the hospital's problems did not stem from a "lack of hospitality" but were due to insufficient income, bemoaning the dissolution of the various financial arrangements secured by Viceroy Bucareli during the hospital's illustrious renovation and moment of glory. Figueroa was especially troubled by the failure of many cities in central Mexico to contribute their annual part to the hospital's shrinking coffers, their charitable "spirits," he complained, "deaf to the clamors of humanity."[11] San Hipólito's situation was undeniably pitiful. Although the *fiscal* expressed his sympathy and concern, he reasoned that the "calamities" taking place on home soil would make it difficult, if not impossible, for the designated areas to acquiesce to the prior general's demands.[12] Certainly the city of Guanajuato—which, by Figueroa's accounts, owed San Hipólito 12,000 pesos—was in no position to fulfill payment, having been one of the first places sieged by Hidalgo's band of disgruntled peasants. The *ayuntamiento* eventually granted San Hipólito a "moderate" pension in support of the daily sustenance of the *pobres dementes*, but it is doubtful that this contribution did much to stall the hospital's rapid decline.[13]

Aside from exacerbating conditions of poverty and diminishing quality of care, the fragmentation of the Spanish Empire undermined the central role of the Order of San Hipólito within the hospital's administration. In 1820, the *hipólitos* were dealt a major blow when the Spanish *córtes*—a liberal parliament established in the king's absence that jockeyed for power with Ferdinand VII after the monarchy's restoration in 1814—decreed the suppression of all the hospital orders.[14] Seven years earlier, the *córtes* had likewise decreed the abolishment of the Inquisition, the culmination of decades of disputes over the institution's incompatibility with a modern government rooted in religious tolerance and the separation of church and state.[15]

Soon after the decree, San Hipólito was placed under the direct supervision of the municipal government. Immediately, the *ayuntamiento* appointed a syndicate to oversee the hospital's affairs as well as those of all charitable establishments in Mexico City, led by the *regidor* (governing counselor), Don Manuel Balbotín. In February 1821, just as the royalist-turned-patriot Agustín de Iturbide was entering into an unlikely alliance with Vicente Guerrero and other liberal insurgents in the final push for independence, Balbotín conducted his first inspection of the mental hospital. "In the spacious and beautiful house of San Hipólito," he observed, "there are housed fifty *pobres dementes* under the care of just one religious nurse." Among the patients, he noted, was a "foreign Englishman, or American, for whom it is not known if he is Catholic." Although the patient population had more than doubled from 1813, Balbotín emphasized the hospital's state of "harsh deprivation."

San Hipólito's destitution was so severe that it could not even afford provisions for the patients' regular meals, often relying on leftovers sent from the Colegio de San Fernando.[16] Clothing and bed linens were also in short supply, with Balbotín commenting that the *pobres dementes* were left "almost naked."[17]

Not long after Balbotín's initial inspection and report, San Hipólito's *bienes* (assets) were officially transferred to the municipal government.[18] But this action alone did not necessarily signal the completion of the hospital's shift from religious to secular hands. In spite of the order's suppression, the brothers of San Hipólito remained a visible fixture and continued to assume responsibility for the care of the patients for almost two more decades, its last two members dying in 1843.[19] During that period, they witnessed efforts to restore order to Mexico City's hospitals, including the creation of a public health board, El Consejo Superior de Salubridad (Superior Health Council), to inspect and ensure quality standards of care.[20] When the Scottish travel writer Frances Calderón de la Barca, wife of the Spanish minister to Mexico, toured the hospital's facilities in 1841, its conditions had improved dramatically. As she noted, "The patients were sauntering about, quiet and for the most part sad; some stretched out under the trees, and others gazing on the fountain; all apparently very much under the control of the administrator, who was formerly a monk—this San Hipólito being a dissolved convent of that order."[21] San Hipólito was technically no longer a colonial hospital, but it bore all the vestiges of Mexico's strained ties to Spain.

THE AGE OF SAN HIPÓLITO came to an official halt in 1910 with the establishment of La Castañeda, Mexico's first fully modernized psychiatric facility, located on the peripheries of the capital—far, far away from its predecessor. The asylum's materialization was the culmination of the relentless efforts of a handful of Porfirian psychiatrists, who strategically positioned themselves and their science as a solution to the nation's imperiled future, hindered by uneven industrialization and the perceived degeneration of poor mestizos.[22] This era did not mark the origins of medicalization, however. Rather, it signaled a new phase, whose very beginnings were launched within the wards of San Hipólito, an institution that had once practiced medical care of the mentally ill of a different sort.

In the years after independence, when other colonial institutions gave way to more modern, liberal ones—the famous Palacio of the Inquisition, for instance, ended up in the hands of the Faculty of Medicine in 1853—San Hipólito sputtered along, affected by broader changes occurring beyond its walls. The presidencies of Benito Juarez and the liberal reforms that followed reinvigorated the process of secularization of the capital's welfare system, first unleashed by Bourbon reformers. The creation of a Dirección de Beneficencia Pública in 1861—an agency designed to centralize and nationalize the capital's welfare establishments and make their management more rational and efficient—only artificially signaled the completion of the Enlightenment project to modernize health care. In practice, it was a period of "transitory chaos," marked by continuity and change not unlike that of its late colonial predecessor.[23] The French invasion and the restoration of a Mexican Empire under the Habsburg rule of Austrian monarchs Maximilian and Charlotte followed by a return to liberal governance no doubt stymied dramatic changes. Indeed, the most significant development to have occurred within San Hipólito's wards during this turbulent period was stricter enforcement of the separation of patients based on class and classification of illness, with distinguished patients and epileptics assigned their own wards. Meanwhile, indigents—a remnant of the category of *pobre demente* that had long sustained the hospital's operations—were relegated to the oldest and most deteriorated sections of the building.[24] The requirement of medical diagnosis for admittance was also enforced with greater rigor. This reflected not only legal concerns over the forceful confinement of criminals who were not mad but also the desires of enterprising and encroaching physicians to increasingly police the hospital's spaces on decidedly medical grounds.[25] Taken together, these developments were not wholly remarkable; rather, they were a continuation of practices and ideas well underway during the late colonial period.

Continuities abounded even in the face of significant changes. The secularization of the welfare system in the 1860s had enabled the growing influx of early psychiatrists, both professional and amateur, into San Hipólito and the Divino Salvador, where, within their humid and convent-like confines, protopsychiatrists encountered a concentrated group of patients who suffered from diseases of the mind. There, as Cristina Rivera Garza has remarked, "with little medical equipment and less financial support, physicians concerned with pathologies of the mind slowly but surely developed a branch of medicine, psychiatry, which came to play a fundamental role in identifying, producing knowledge about, and attempting to control behaviors deemed as deviant."[26]

This new stage of medicalization was informed by an eclectic range of approaches to managing mental disorder formulated overseas. From the "moral treatment" devised by Pinel to degeneration theory, new understandings of mental illness—its underpinnings and treatment—began to infiltrate

San Hipólito and its sister institution, enabling psychiatry's precarious rise.[27] While the dawning of a new medical era approached, its debt to older colonial institutions and models was faintly visible. As Jan Goldstein has thoughtfully observed, the moral treatment as a critical paradigm buttressing psychiatry's claim to medical expertise and therapeutic efficacy was not an entirely novel phenomenon: among its "various charlatanistic roots" were forms of religious consolation firmly entrenched in Catholicism and regularly practiced by religious nurses within institutions they had once governed.[28] Although San Hipólito had fully secularized and tried to appeal to a wealthier clientele, poor patients continued to occupy its facilities in overwhelming numbers, demanding access to charitable assistance and enforcing the intersection of poverty and mental illness that had long fueled the hospital's existence. Scientific therapies designed to cure mental illness often failed, physicians and administrators quibbled incessantly, and paltry funds persisted to curb the hospital's ambitions.[29] Indeed, it would appear that Mexico's early psychiatrists grappled with some of the very same dilemmas that daunted their religious forebears.

Yet as was the case for much of the early twentieth century, people applauded La Castañeda by comparing it to what it was not: it was not dank and humid; it was not impotent in the face of suffering; and, in keeping with the social Darwinism that ran rampant throughout the Porfiriato, it was not a place that assumed all castes and races of Mexico were equally plagued by insanity. In short, it was not San Hipólito. Perhaps this was best demonstrated by its location. Whereas San Hipólito sat, and continues to sit, at the center of the capital, anchored by its past and announcing it role as a seminal institution to the creation of colonial Mexico, the nation's emergent psychiatrists built La Castañeda far on the edge of town, away from the bustle and stimulation of the city but also far from the observation of everyday citizens. There would be no public spectacles at La Castañeda. The sick would remain safely removed from the healthy, where professionals could keep in check the polluting effects of their disease and deviancy.

While it is easy to celebrate La Castañeda against the foil of San Hipólito, at least at first, both essentially confronted the same dilemma: how to care for the most vulnerable and marginal in our midst. This question, which haunts psychiatry's past and present, makes it a deeply controversial subject of inquiry. This is doubly so because there are no easy answers. It was no less true that La Castañeda attempted to produce a dreamed-up "modern" world than San Hipólito sought to reproduce the ideal Spanish colonial world. In defining what was "real" and "moral," both institutions essentially defined what was not merely acceptable but even possible. Yet San Hipólito never removed madness from the public. Rather, its model of care—while never celebrating the plight of the insane—kept insanity before the public eye. Madness was part of life, and colonial society allowed for far more voices to weigh in on what should be considered sane or reasonable. While this cacophony of perspectives promoted ambiguity—inquisitors could themselves be driven mad by it—it also made the boundaries of sane and insane less firm and categorical. Definitions of madness could shift according to context and intention.

Most importantly, in the halls of San Hipólito, the brothers did not celebrate clinical detachment but rather a much broader concept of "hospitality." Coming in contact with the mad was not like confronting a disease but rather an opportunity for the sane to improve themselves through mercy, kindness, and generosity. Of course, the actual practice of hospitality depended on the conditions within the hospital and how diligently the brothers administered their duties, but generally speaking, as a custodial solution for the long-term custody of the mentally ill, San Hipólito served Mexico City and its neighboring environs for well over 350 years. In times of war and times of peace, in times of abundance and (far more common) times of scarcity, the brothers provided imperfect care for a predicament that lacked a perfect solution.

APPENDIX

TABLE A.1 Monthly tally of the Indigenous patients at San Hipólito according to the Records of the Royal Indian Hospital (Hospital Real de los Naturales)

1774		1776		1778		1779	
August	17	January	15	January	18	January	18
September	17	February	15	February	18	February	18
October	18	March	15	March	18	March	19
November	16	April	15	April	17	April	19
December	18	May	15	May	17	May	18
		June	15	June	18	June	18
		July	15	July	18	July	18
		August	15	August	18	August	18
		September	15	September	18	September	18
		October	15	October	18	October	18
		November	15	November	18	November	18
		December	15	December	18	December	18

1781		1782		1783		1784	
January	21	January	22	January	22	January	25
February	21	February	22	February	22	February	25
March	21	March	22	March	23	March	25
April	21	April	22	April	23	April	25
May	21	May	23	May	23	May	27
June	21	June	23	June	22	June	27
July	22	July	23	July	22	July	27
August	22	August	23	August	23	August	27
September	22	September	23	September	23	September	27
October	22	October	23	October	23	October	28
November	22	November	22	November	25	November	27
December	22	December	22	December	25	December	27

1785		1786		1790		1791	
January	27	January	26	January	19	January	13
February	27	February	26	February	19	February	13

(*continued*)

TABLE A.1 (continued)

1785		1786		1790		1791	
March	27	March	26	March	19	March	13
April	27	April	26	April	19	April	13
May	27	May	25	May	19	May	13
June	26	June	25	June	19	June	11
July	26	July	25	July	19	July	11
August	26	August	25	August	14	August	11
September	26	September	24	September	13	September	10
October	26	October	24	October	13	October	10
November	26	November	24	November	13	November	10
December	26	December	24	December	13	December	10

1792		1793		1794		1796	
January	10	January	12	January	13	January	14
February	10	February	12	February	13	February	14
March	10	March	13	March	13	March	14
April	9	April	13	April	13	April	15
May	10	May	13	May	13	May	16
June	10	June	13	June	13	June	15
July	11	July	13	July	15	July	15
August	12	August	13	August	15	August	15
September	12	September	13	September	15	September	15
October	12	October	13	October	15	October	15
November	12	November	13	November	15	November	15
December	12	December	13	December	15	December	15

1797		1798	
January	15	January	15
February	15	February	15
March	15	March	15
April	14	April	15
May	14	May	15
June	15	June	15
July	15	July	15
August	15	August	15
September	15	September	15
October	15	October	15
November	15	November	15
December	15	December	15

Source: INAH, Hospital Real de los Naturales, 18:15; 20:5; 24:8; 14:4; 15:9; 17.4; 22:7; 21:9; 23:10; 26:2; 28:12; 29:8; 30:7; 31:6; 32:7; 33:7; 35.1; 36:9; 37:8.

TABLE A.2 San Hipólito's criminal inmates: an overview

Admissions records, 1697–1706

Date of Admission	Name	Personal Details	Source of Admission	Date of Exit, Flight, or Death
March 1698	Francisco Solano	Free Black; married	Real Audiencia	Died April 1698
December 1702	Rafael Antonio	*Mestizo*; 30 years old	Corregidor, sent from jail	
October 1705	Jactinto Ortiz	Indian; widower	Magistrate from Tlaxcala	

Admissions records, 1751–1786

Date of Admission	Name	Personal Details	Source of Admission	Date of Exit, Flight, or Death
August 1751	Antonio Garcia	*Español*, native of Santiago Tianguistengo; married; 48 years old	Real Sala del Crimen	Released September 1751
November 1751	Juan Antonio Reyna	*Castizo*, native of Taneplanta; single	Cárcel de corte	
March 1752	Juan Estevan Perez de Arriola	Free *mulato*; native of Mexico City; married; 23 years old	Real Sala del Crimen	Fled March 1752
December 1752	Manuel Gomez	*Español*; native of Mexico City; single; 37 years old	Viceregal orders	
April 1753	Bonafacio de Vargas	*Español*; native of Acazingo; married; 35 years old	Alcalde del crimen	

(continued)

TABLE A.2 (continued)

Admissions records, 1751–1786

Date of Admission	Name	Personal Details	Source of Admission	Date of Exit, Flight, or Death
May 1753	Juan de Cordova	*Castizo*; native of Orizaba; married	Alcalde mayor	Fled June 1753
July 1754	Gabriel de la Mirada Oveido	*Español*, native of Mexico City; married; 45 years old	Alguacil mayor, señor provisor	
July 1754	Vicente Limon	*Español*; native of Zacatlan; married; 55 years old	Alcalde mayor of Zacatlán	
March 1755	Manuel de Campos	*Español*; native of Mexico City; married; 36 years old	Order of local magistrate; entered for the 4th time	Fled July 1755
April 1755	Francisco (no last name given)	*Gachupine* (peninsular Spaniard)	Viceregal orders	Fled June 1755
April 1755	Juan Baptista Novela	Free *mulato*; native of Colima; married; 40 years old	Magistrate of Colima	Released March 1757
September 1755	Manuel Campos	*Español*; native of Mexico City; married; 36 years old	Court order; entered for the 5th time	
July 1760	Manuel José Velasquez	*Castizo*; native of Mexico City; single; 32 years old	Real Sala del Crimen	Fled March 1762
February 1761	Agustin Pacheco	Indian; native of Oaxaca; single; 38 years old	Real Sala del Crimen	
October 1761	José de Mata	*Español*; native of Alfaiuca; single; 28 years old	Justicia and alcalde mayor of Alfaiuca	

October 1761	Francisco Xavier	*Español*; native of Amacueca; single; 21 years old		Inquisition
March 1763	Don Joaquin Bustillo	Native of Asturias; 38 years old	Corregidor; viceregal orders	Died December 1766
May 1763	Juan Pablo Echegoyen	*Español*; native of San Sebastian de Vizcaia; 39 years old	Inquisition	
July 1763	Marcelino de la Torre	*Español*; native of Guadalajara; single; 60 years old	Real Audiencia de Guadalajara	Fled July 1764
November 1763	José Figueroa y Avila	*Español criollo*; single; 19 years old	Señor provisor, for committing homicide and declaring himself mad	
January 1766	Juan Antonio Infante	*Español*; married	Real Sala del Crimen	Released March 1766
October 1766	Bernabe Garcia	Free *mulato*; native of San Martin Tesmeluca; married	Señor corregidor	
May 1768	Don José Mathias Gamaio	*Español*; native of Pachuca; single; 44 years old	Viceregal orders; transferred from Valladolid	
May 1769	Mariano Ramirez		Local jail	
September 1769	Antonio Trinidad	Married	Alcalde mayor of Otumba	Released January 1770

(*continued*)

TABLE A.2 (continued)

Admissions records, 1751–1786

Date of Admission	Name	Personal Details	Source of Admission	Date of Exit, Flight, or Death
January 1770	Juan de la Luz Cervantes	Single	Corregidor	Fled January 1770 (4 days following admission)
May 1770	Juan de Silva	*Español*	Inquisition	
May 1770	José Montes de Oca	*Español*; 51 years old	Real Sala del Crimen	
August 1770	José Maria Jaime	*Español*; native of San Pedro; 29 years old	Ecclesiastical judge of San Pedro	
September 1770	Antonio Ramirez	*Coyote*; native of Santiago Tecosaucla; married; 40 years old	*Teniente* of Santiago Tecosaucla	
March 1771	Juan de Silva	*Español*; single; native of Madrid	Real Audiencia of Guadalajara	Fled
March 1772	Juan Francisco Mendoza	*Español*; native of Coyoacan; 35 years old	*Teniente* of Coyoacan	
September 1772	Juan Diego Andeaon Roman		Transferred from Oaxaca by order of the alcalde ordinario	Died August 1781
September 1772	Bartolome de Leon, known as "Tabaco"		Transferred from Oaxaca by order of the alcalde ordinario	Fled March 1775; readmitted and died August 1781
March 1773	Diego de Mendoza	Spanish (*Andaluz*)	Inquisition	

December 1773	Phelipe Guillermo Cano	*Español*; widower; 60 years old		Jail
May 1774	*Un pobre demente* (a poor madman)			Courts of Guadalajara
August 1774	Marcos Jacinto	Indian; native of Puebla; married	Orders of the governor of Puebla	Initially sent to Hospital de San Roque (in Puebla), then transferred to San Hipólito
August 1774	Pedro Petarte, "a poor simpleton"		Alcalde	Initially sent to Hospital de San Roque (in Puebla), then transferred to San Hipólito
March 1776	Sebastian Briones	Free *mulato*; native of San Pablo in Cordova; married; 40 years old	Alcalde mayor of Cordova	Died
September 1776	Vicente Berrocal	Married	Inquisition	Died June 1784
January 1777	Diego de Rivera	*Castizo*	Public jail	
June 1777	Vicento Pino	*Español*; native of Veracruz; single; 25 years old	Viceregal orders; came from Cárcel de corte	
July 1777	Don Pedro Portillo	*Español*; native of Fresnillo; married; 41 years old	Alcalde ordinario	Recovered and released, January 1778
November 1777	Jose Joaquin Montezuma	*Español*; native of Sayula in Guadalajara; single; 20 years old	Viceregal orders	Fled December 1778

(*continued*)

TABLE A.2 (continued)

Admissions records, 1751–1786

Date of Admission	Name	Personal Details	Source of Admission	Date of Exit, Flight, or Death
July 1779	Antonio Francisco Rodriguez	*Español*; native of Cosamaluapa; married; 50 years old	Cárcel de corte	Left January 1780
September 1779	Don Manuel Remolina	*Español gachupín*	Cárcel de corte	Died October 1779
January 1781	Bernardo Antonio	*Español*; native of Salvatierra; single; 30 years old	Cárcel de corte	Fled March 1781
November 1781	Antonio Manuel Chimalpopoca	Indian cacique; native of Tlaxcala; married	Real Sala del Crimen	Fled September 1782
December 1781	Don Benito Busta		Viceregal orders	
February 1782	Don Sebastian Posadas	Native of Asturias; single; 29 years old	Viceregal orders	Left recovered, October 1782
February 1782	Jose Ezcorcia	*Español*; native of Real de Monte; married; 36 years old	Cárcel de corte	Fled January 1785; died January 1787
February 1782	Agustin Severino	Black; single; 40 years old	Cárcel de corte "Cárcel de abajo"	
June 1782	Franciso Xavier Manceras	Indian; native of Mexico City; 35 years old		Recovered and released, October 1982
December 1782	Don Nicolas	*Español*; native of Toluca; resident of Mexico City; married; 45 years old	Corregidor	Released May 1783; returned same month; fled August 1783

June 1783	Antonio Aptim	French	Corregidor	Died June 1783
October 1783	Juan Maria de la Pena	*Español*; native of the city of Compostela; married; 48 years old	Real Audiencia of Guadalajara	
1784	Pedro (no last name given)		Acordada	
1784	Cipriano Antonio	Indian; native of Yautepeque	Alcalde mayor	
October 1785	Jose Antonio Tobal	Indian; native of a village near Santuario de Nuestra Señora; married; 26 years old	Real Sala del Crimen	
December 1785	Antonio Reynoso	*Español*; native of Havana; widowed; 58 years old	Inquisition	
March 1786	Tomas Flores	*Mulato*; native of Mexico City; single; 26 years old	Acordada	Entered hospital for the 4th time
March 1786	Jose Ignacio Ledesma	*Español*; native of Zilao; 34 years old	Acordada	
June 1786	Francisco Miguel de Luzes	Native of Guanajuato; single; 34 years old	Inquisition	Fled March 1787
July 1786	Don Melchor Donaique	*Español*; native of Castille; single; 27 years old	Corregidor	
August 1786	Juan Jose Sorribas	Native of Mexico City; married; 30 years old	Provisor	Fled March 1787

Sources: AGN, Indiferente Vireinal, caja 1005, exp. 5; AGN, Indiferente Vireinal, caja 4951, exp. 47.

Notes

Abbreviations

AGI   Archivo General de la Indias, Seville, Spain
AGN   Archivo General de la Nación, Mexico City, Mexico
AHDF Archivo Histórico del Distrito Federal, Mexico City, Mexico
AHSS Archivo Histórico de la Secretaria de Salud, Mexico City, Mexico
INAH Instituto Nacional de Antropología e Historia, Mexico City, Mexico

Introduction

1. AHSS, Fondo Beneficiencia Pública, Sección Establecimientos Hospitalarios, Serie Hospital de San Hipólito, legajo 2, exp. 17, fol. 6r; also quoted in Ballenger, "Modernizing Madness," 32. My analysis echoes Ballenger in reading Labastida's essay as a nostalgic, ahistorical view of San Hipólito's colonial history.

2. AHSS, Fondo Beneficiencia Pública, Sección Establecimientos Hospitalarios, Serie Hospital de San Hipólito, legajo 2, exp. 17, fols. 6r–v.

3. AHSS, Fondo Beneficiencia Pública, Sección Establecimientos Hospitalarios, Serie Hospital de San Hipólito, legajo 2, exp. 17, fols. 6v–7r.

4. Ballenger, "Modernizing Madness," 33–34.

5. See Rivera-Garza, "Dangerous Minds."

6. Ballenger, "Modernizing Madness," 34.

7. Important studies within this vast field include MacDonald, *Mystical Bedlam*; Midelfort, *History of Madness in Sixteenth-Century Germany*; Porter, *Mind-Forg'd Manacles*; Scull, *Most Solitary of Afflictions*; Goldstein, *Console and Classify*; Mellyn, *Mad Tuscans and Their Families*. Published in 2017, Greg Eghigian's *Routledge History of Madness and Mental Health* offers the most updated overview of the field and even includes an excellent chapter on Latin America; however, it makes no mention of San Hipólito.

8. For a revisionist account of Pinel's contributions to "Enlightenment psychiatry," see Weiner, "Madman in the Light of Reason: Part II."

9. Positivist accounts of psychiatry include Alexander and Selesnick, *History of Psychiatry*; Zilboorg, *History of Medical Psychology*. The classic declensionist account is Foucault's *Histoire de la folie à l'âge classique: Folie et déraison*, published in English as *Madness and Civilization*. See also Rothman, *Discovery of the Asylum*; Scull, *Most Solitary of Afflictions*.

10. The most thorough account of Bethlem hospital is Andrews et al., *History of Bethlem*.

11. Allderidge, "Bedlam: Fact or Fantasy?," 18.

12. Important exceptions include Weiner, "Brothers of Charity and the Mentally Ill"; Houston, "Clergy and the Care of the Insane in Eighteenth-Century Britain"; Jones,

The Charitable Imperative. For an important intervention on the dynamic relationship between medicine and religion in Enlightenment Europe see Grell and Cunningham, *Medicine and Religion in Enlightenment Europe*.

13. For an overview of the historiography on medicine and public health in colonial Latin America, see my essay "Beyond the Columbian Exchange."

14. On connections between Goya's art and the Zaragoza hospital, see Kromm, "Archives and Sources."

15. Weiner, "The Madman in the Light of Reason: Part I."

16. For up-to-date overviews of the Hispanic Enlightenment see Meléndez and Stolley, "Enlightenments in Ibero-America," and essays in E. Lewis, et al., *The Routledge Companion to the Hispanic Enlightenment*.

17. Foucault, *Madness and Civilization*. For critiques of Foucault, see Midelfort, "Madness and Civilization in Early Modern Europe; Porter, "Foucault's Great Confinement." Foucault himself offered a more philosophical pondering of the Enlightenment as an "attitude" and way of "thinking and feeling" in his essay "What Is Enlightenment?" For a discussion of this essay in connection to colonial Latin America, see Premo, *Enlightenment on Trial*, 45. For a critique of the Enlightenment as an "age of reason," see Daston, "Afterword: The Ethos of Enlightenment."

18. Philo, "Edinburgh, Enlightenment, and the Geographies of Unreason," 373–74. I thank Mariselle Meléndez for bringing this piece to my attention. For a discussion of Philo's arguments in connection to the medicalization of the female body in eighteenth-century Peru, see Meléndez, *Deviant and Useful Citizens*, chap. 4.

19. Premo, *Enlightenment on Trial*; Stolley, *Domesticating Empire*; Ramirez, *Enlightened Immunity*; Few, *For All of Humanity*; Cañizarez-Esguerra, *How to Write the History of the New World*; Safier, *Measuring the New World*; Bleichmar, *Visible Empire*; Weber, *Bárbaros*; Hesse, "Towards a New Topography of Enlightenment."

20. To be sure, similar claims have recently been made by historians of the European Enlightenment. See, for instance, Bertucci, *Artisanal Enlightenment*.

21. Paquette, *Enlightenment, Governance, and Reform*; Paquette, *Enlightened Reform in Southern Europe*.

22. The scholarship on late colonial church reform is vast. See, for instance, Brading, *Church and State in Bourbon Mexico*; Brading, "Tridentine Catholicism and Enlightened Despotism"; Farriss, *Crown and Clergy in Colonial Mexico*; Zahino Peñafort, *Iglesia y sociedad en Mexico*. On enlightenment piety, see Voekel, *Alone before God*; Larkin, *Very Nature of God*.

23. Gay, *The Enlightenment*, 2:12, 5–6.

24. Gay, 13.

25. A. Warren, *Medicine and Politics in Colonial Peru*; Ramirez, *Enlightened Immunity*; Few, *For All of Humanity*.

26. See, for instance, Bertucci, *Artisanal Enlightenment*; Premo, *Enlightenment on Trial*; Spary, *Eating the Enlightenment*; Takats, *Expert Cook in Enlightenment France*; Jacob, *The Secular Enlightenment*; Sorkin, *Religious Enlightenment*. See also literature on the Catholic Enlightenment cited below.

27. For a discussion of the history and historiography of medicalization, see Nye, "Evolution of the Concept of Medialization."

28. On the "Catholic Enlightenment" and its embrace of science and medicine, see Lehner, *Catholic Enlightenment*; Mazzotti, *World of Maria Gaetana Agnesi*; Ewalt, *Peripheral Wonders*; Messbarger, Johns, and Gavitt, *Benedict XIV and the Enlightenment*.

29. Silverblatt, *Modern Inquisitions*, 5.

30. Peters, *The Inquisition*, 174–88, 231–62.

31. Perez, *The Spanish Inquisition*, 94–98.

32. Greenleaf, "The Inquisition in Eighteenth-Century New Mexico."

33. Peters, *The Inquisition*, 3.

34. Anderson, *Colonial Pathologies*, 111.

35. I borrow this term from Mellyn, *Mad Tuscans and Their Families*, 5.

36. Important revisionist histories include A. Warren, *Medicine and Politics in Colonial Peru*; Ramirez, *Enlightened Immunity*; Milton, *Many Meanings of Poverty*; Arrom, *Containing the Poor*.

37. Stoler and Cooper, "Between Metropole and Colony," 5. See also, Anderson, *Colonial Pathologies*; Tilly, *Africa as a Living Laboratory*.

38. As Stoler and Cooper have remarked, "Europe's colonies were never empty spaces to be made over in Europe's image or fashioned in its interests; nor, indeed, were European states self-contained entities that at one point projected themselves overseas. Europe was made by its imperial projects, as much as colonial encounters were shaped by conflicts within Europe itself." Stoler and Cooper, "Between Metropole and Colony," 1.

39. Butterwick, "Peripheries of the Enlightenment," 6.

40. Dorantes de Carranza, *Suma relación de las cosas de Nueva España*, 113.

41. Gerbi, *Dispute of the New World*, esp. chap. 3; see also Cañizares-Esguerra, "New World, New Stars."

42. Pagden, *Fall of Natural Man*, chap. 4.

43. Fanon, *Wretched of the Earth*.

44. Vaughn, *Curing Their Ills*; Sadowsky, *Imperial Bedlam*; Keller, *Colonial Madness*; Ernst, *Mad Tales from the Raj*; L. Jackson, *Surfacing Up*; Mahone and Vaughn, *Psychiatry and Empire*.

45. Here I follow the lead of Claire Edington, who has called for histories of psychiatry that examine the "dynamics of institutional practice, as opposed to discourse." See Edington, "Going in and Getting out of the Colonial Asylum."

46. Few, *For All of Humanity*, 18. See also Gómez, *The Experiential Caribbean*; Ramirez, *Enlightened Immunity*.

47. Edington, *Beyond the Asylum*, 5.

48. Few, *For All of Humanity*, 21. See also Ramírez, *Enlightened Immunity*; Few, et al., *Baptism through Incision*.

49. The Divino Salvador's records are more intact from the nineteenth century on. See Berkstein Kanarek, "El Hospital del Divino Salvador"; Ballenger, "Modernizing Madness."

50. Tortorici, *Sins against Nature*, 4.

51. On the abolishment of the Inquisition, see Rawlings, *The Spanish Inquisition*, chap. 7; Toribio Medina, *History del Tribunal del Santo Oficio*, capt. 25.

52. Midelfort, *History of Madness in Sixteenth-Century Germany*, 11.

53. For more on this approach, see Rosenberg, "Framing Disease."

54. Mellyn, *Mad Tuscans and Their Families*, 19.
55. Covarrubias Orozco, *Tesoro de la lengua Castellana*, 505.
56. Covarrubias Orozco, 419.
57. This last term implies demonic possession more generally, which could include states of madness. It only surfaces once in the Inquisition cases I consulted as *enagenado demente*.

Chapter One

1. Díaz de Arce, *Libro de la vida del próximo evangelico*; García, *Vida de el venerable Bernardino Alvarez*. García's biography was written for the purposes of advancing Alvarez's beatification. Both biographies are essentially hagiographies.
2. Díaz de Arce, *Libro de la vida del próximo evangelico*, 1-10. Díaz de Arce's biography of Alvarez was originally published in 1652. Throughout this text, I will be citing the eighteenth-century reprint.
3. Díaz de Arce, 15-16.
4. Díaz de Arce, 43-44.
5. Díaz de Arce, 43-44. On the spiritual gardening metaphor in narratives of Spanish colonization, see Cañizares-Esguerra, *Puritan Conquistadors*, chap. 5.
6. The property for the original hospital was donated by two *vecinos* of Mexico City, Miguel de Dueñas and his wife, Isabel de Ojeda. Díaz de Arce, *Libro de la vida del próximo evangelico*, 41-42; Muriel, *Hospitales de la Nueva España*, 1:188.
7. Muriel, *Hospitales de la Nueva España*, 1:187-88.
8. García, *Vida de el venerable Bernardino Alvarez*, 37-38.
9. Arrom has identified and discussed this trope and its uses in connection to the foundational story of Mexico City's Poor House. See Arrom, *Containing the Poor*, 32. European examples include the story establishment of the Hospital de los Inocentes in Valencia. See Tropé, *Locura y sociedad en la Valencia*, 28-30.
10. My discussion of San Hipólito's role in the broader evangelizing project is indebted to Guenter Risse's two seminal articles on hospital development in New Spain and Robert Ricard's classic study of the "spiritual conquest" of Mexico, all of which emphasize the hospital's deployment in the Americas for the purposes of religious conversion. See Risse, "Shelter and Care for Natives and Colonists" and "Medicine in New Spain," 12-63; Ricard, *Spiritual Conquest of Mexico*, 155-61.
11. See, for instance, Vaughn, *Curing Their Ills*; Sadowsky, *Imperial Bedlam*.
12. The phrase "tool of empire" comes from Headrick, *Tools of Empire*.
13. Borah, "Social Welfare and Social Obligation in New Spain," 45.
14. Leon-Portilla, "Las Comunidades Mesoamericanas ante la institución de los hospitales para Indios," 196-97; Venegas Ramirez, *Regimen hospitalario*, 9.
15. Quoted in Guijarro Oliveras, "Política Sanitaria en las Leyes de Indias," 66-67.
16. Risse, "Medicine in New Spain," 41-42.
17. On poor relief in Spain, see Arrizabalaga, "Poor Relief in Counter-Reformation Castile"; Lopez Terrada, "Health Care and Poor Relief in the Crown of Aragon"; Martz, *Poverty and Welfare in Habsburg Spain*; Brodman, *Charity and Welfare*; Flynn, *Sacred Charity*.

18. Borah, "Social Welfare and Social Obligation in New Spain," 45.

19. Arrom, *Containing the Poor*, 32. On the ideology of charity, see Brodman, *Poverty and Religion*, esp. chap. 1.

20. On hospitals for Indians in New Spain, see Venegas Ramirez, *Regimen hospitalario*; Howard, *Royal Indian Hospital*.

21. Risse, "Shelter and Care for Natives and Colonists," 67.

22. Gante, "Carta de Fray Pedro de Gante," 52.

23. Risse, "Medicine in New Spain," 20–21.

24. On the role of nurses as spiritual models, see Ricard, *Spiritual Conquest of Mexico*, 155–61.

25. *Recopilación de Leyes de los Reynos de las Indias*, Lib. I, Tit. IV, Ley I; quoted in Borah, "Social Welfare and Social Obligation in New Spain," 47.

26. Borah, "Social Welfare and Social Obligation in New Spain," 47.

27. Gabriela Ramos has noted that the "position of the king as protector of the poor was always unstable," and that the Church too vied for this role. Ramos, "Indian Hospitals and Government in the Colonial Andes," 189.

28. Milton, *Many Meanings of Poverty*, 6–11.

29. On the miserable status of the Indian, see Ramos, "Indian Hospitals and Government," 189; Castañeda Delgado, "La condición miserable del Indio." On the Valladolid debate and the notion that natives were natural children, see Pagden, *Fall of Natural Man*, chap. 4.

30. Risse, "Medicine in New Spain," 33–41. On the activities of the Protomedicato in New Spain, see Lanning, *The Royal Protomedicato*.

31. Huguet-Termes and Arrizabalaga, "Hospital Care for the Insane in Barcelona," 84; see also Park, "Healing the Poor," 26–45.

32. Huguet-Termes and Arrizabalaga, "Hospital Care for the Insane in Barcelona," 86–88.

33. On this institution, see Tropé, *Locura y sociedad en la Valencia*. In the sixteenth century, the hospital was subsumed into the Hospital General as part of a broader hospital consolidation project initiated by state reformers.

34. Nalle, *Mad for God*, 158–59; Tropé, *Locura y sociedad en la Valencia*, 30–32.

35. Porter, "Madness and Its Institutions," 179–80; Scull, "The Asylum, Hospital, and Clinic," 101–2. Ahmed Ragab offers a detailed description of the activities that took place within Islamic mad wards. See Ragab, *Medieval Islamic Hospital*, 193–99. Michael W. Dols has observed that these wards developed in tandem with the introduction of Galenism into the Arab world. See *Manjun*, 112–16.

36. González Duro, *Historia de la Locura en España*, vol. 1. See also López Alonso, *Locura y sociedad en Sevilla*; Viquera, "Los hospitales para locos e 'inocentes' en Hispanoamerica."

37. Nalle, *Mad for God*, 158.

38. Huguet-Termes and Arrizabalaga, "Hospital Care for the Insane in Barcelona," 101.

39. Nalle, *Mad for God*, 158–60.

40. Cheryl English Martin has conducted the most extensive research on the Order of San Hipólito's formation, activities, and internal organization, as well as the

various hospitals they administered. See Martin, "San Hipólito Hospitals of Colonial Mexico." Petitions to create a formal order began in the late sixteenth century, and Alvarez insisted that alongside the traditional monastic vows of poverty, chastity, and obedience, the order's members follow a fourth vow to *hospitalidad* (hospitality). It was not until 1700, however, that Pope Innocent XII officially recognized the brothers, who were known throughout New Spain as the *hipólitos*, as an autonomous religious order. Prior to that point, they operated first as a brotherhood and then as a congregation. See Muriel, *Hospitales de la Nueva España*, 1: 203-204.

41. AGN, Hospitales, vol. 73, exp. 2, fol. 74r.

42. Seed, *Ceremonies of Possession*, 3. Seed argues that the Spanish, unlike the French or English, were far more willing to establish claim through warfare, thus making battle sites all the more significant. See Seed, *Ceremonies of Possession*, chap. 3.

43. This holiday has been analyzed and reconstructed by Barbara Mundy. See Mundy, *Death of Aztec Tenochtitlan*, 95-96.

44. In both Spain and Mexico, the feast of the Holy Innocents developed into a quasi-April Fool's day, involving jokes and pranks. See Foster, *Culture and Conquest*, 104-5.

45. AGN, Clero Regular y Secular, vol. 65, exp. 1, fol. 27v.

46. The most detailed analysis of the Zaragoza hospital in the sixteenth century is Baquero, *Bosquejo Histórico*, chap. 3.

47. The Order of San Hipólito's 1616 statutes contain detailed specifications for how these relief convoys were to be conducted. See AGN, Tierras, vol. 3082, exp. 1, fols. 7v-8v.

48. AGN, Clero Regular y Secular, vol. 65, exp. 1, fol. 27v; Díaz de Arce, *Libro de la vida del próximo evangelico*, 55-60; Muriel, *Hospitales de la Nueva España*, 1:207-8; Martin, "San Hipólito Hospitals," 75-76.

49. García, *Vida de el venerable Bernardino Alvarez*, 37.

50. García, 37, 110.

51. AGN, Hospitales, vol. 73, exp. 3, fols. 228v, 234v.

52. AGN, Hospitales, vol. 45, exp. 9, fols. 382r-v.

53. Risse, "Medicine in New Spain," 39. A similar practice occurred in colonial Peru. See Ramos, "Indian Hospitals and Government in the Colonial Andes," 192-93.

54. AGN, Obras Pías, vol. 3, fols. 132r-v; AGN, Indiferente Virreinal, caja 4122, exp. 6, fols. 1r-2r; *La administración de Fray Antonio María de Bucareli y Ursúa*, 170.

55. AGN, Hospitales, vol. 45, exp. 9, fols. 366v-367r.

56. AGN, Indiferente Virreinal, caja 0930, exp. 2, fol. 12r.

57. Van Deusen, "'Alienated' Body," 13.

58. AGN, Tierras, vol. 3082, exp. 1, fol. 18r.

59. Marroqui, *La Ciudad de México*, 583-84; Muriel, *Hospitales de la Nueva España*, 1:196.

60. AGN, Hospitales, vol. 73, exp. 2, fol. 70r.

61. On the Order of San Hipólito's sugar plantations, see Martin, "San Hipólito Hospitals," chap. 5. See also Martin, "Crucible of Zapatismo."

62. Marroqui, *La Ciudad de México*, 583-84; Muriel, *Hospitales de la Nueva España*, 1:210-211.

63. I have not been able to locate the original decree. Instead, I cite a copy included in the hospital's records dated to 1764, when the decree appears to have been reinforced with greater urgency. AGN, Indiferente Virreinal, caja 0974, exp. 18, fol. 14r.

64. AGN, Inquisición, vol. 218, exp. 3, fols. 80r-v. See also Jaffary, *False Mystics*, 149–50.

65. AGN, Inquisición, vol. 329, exp. 5. Quoted in Sacristán, *Locura e Inquisición*, 122.

66. Ramos, "Indian Hospitals and Government."

67. Arrom, *Containing the Poor*, 89–92, 100–102; Chase, "Medical Care for the Poor in Mexico City," 159. See also Milton, *Many Meanings of Poverty*.

68. Although Cheryl D. Martin observes that the brothers of San Hipólito became more worldly following Alvarez's death and slackened in spiritual zeal, she nonetheless concludes that the statutes give a rough approximation of the hospital's administration in the seventeenth century. Martin, "San Hipólito Hospitals," 81.

69. This plan can be found in AGN, Tierras, vol. 3802, exp. 8. Its precise date is unclear. Although it is located alongside documents dating to 1701–2, the plan appears to have no relation to these documents. Moreover, it is also not clear if the ground plan belongs to the Hospital de San Hipólito or one of the other eight institutions administered by the brotherhood. The archival description identifies the illustration as the Convent of San Hipólito in Mexico City, but the document itself makes no clear reference to its status as such. If the layout indeed represents San Hipólito, then the illustration predates 1700, as the hospital seems to have stopped admitting women by the late seventeenth century, if not much earlier.

70. For a discussion of the cruciform plan and other architectural hospital arrangements, see Henderson, *Renaissance Hospital*, 81–88, 151–61.

71. The earliest set of surviving records of patient admissions dates from 1697–1706; it makes no reference to female patients. Thus, if San Hipólito did admit women, it ceased to do so some time before the 1690s.

72. Tropé, *Locura y sociedad*, 47–50.

73. For a sustained discussion of how early modern hospitals incorporated the dual project to heal the body and soul, see Henderson, *Renaissance Hospital*.

74. Specifically, the hospital's kitchen staff is referred to as being either Indian, Black, or "some other" (*qualquiera*). AGN, Tierras, vol. 3082, exp. 1, fol. 19v.

75. AGN, Indiferente Virreinal, caja 0930, exp. 2.

76. AHSS, Fondo Hospitales y Hospicios, Sección Hospital de San Hipólito, exp. 8. There is evidence that the other hospitals administered by the brotherhood owned slaves as well. See Martin, "San Hipólito Hospitals," 89–90.

77. AGN, Tierras, vol. 3082, exp. 1, fols. 16v–17r; Van Deusen, "'Alienated' Body," 10.

78. It is unclear whether San Hipólito enjoyed the regular services of a physician. Although the statutes make reference to the presence of a physician on the hospital grounds, the other hospital records do not. In Spain, physicians were morally and legally obligated to minister to the poor free of charge, but as Lanning has discussed in his study of the Protomedicato, these rules were not easily enforced in the colonies, which faced a dearth of medical practitioners and pervasive corruption. Given these issues, it is likely that much of the medical work at the hospital was undertaken by the brothers themselves. See Lanning, *Royal Protomedicato*, chap. 8.

79. For the Hospital de los Innocentes in Seville, Carmen López Alonso observes that by the end of the sixteenth century, the physician had become a key presence, playing an important role in determining who was admitted to the hospital as well as in curative treatments. The same observation cannot be extended to San Hipólito. Even when, in the late eighteenth century, the hospital became more medical in orientation, physicians remained a peripheral presence, with the brothers of San Hipólito undertaking the majority of medical activities. On medical activities at the Hospital de los Inocentes in Seville, see López Alonso, *Locura y sociedad en Sevilla*, 264–96. Although John S. Leiby documents medical treatments performed by physicians at San Hipólito, I have examined his sources and cannot corroborate his evidence. Leiby, "San Hipólito's Treatment of the Mentally Ill."

80. AGN, Tierras, vol. 3087, exp. 1, fol. 15v.

81. AGN, Tierras, vol. 3087, exp. 1, fols. 17v, 18r.

82. AGN, Tierras, vol. 3087, fol. 18; Henderson, *Renaissance Hospital*, 163.

83. AGN, Tierras, vol. 3082, exp, 1, fol. 8v.

84. AGN, Hospitales, vol. 45, exp. 9, fols. 569r–v.

85. AGN, Tierras, vol. 3082, exp. 1, fols. 8v–9r.

86. AGN, Tierras, vol. 3082, exp. 1, fols. 8v–9r.

87. On this hospital, see Muriel, *Hospitales de la Nueva Espana*, 2:108–13; Berkstein Kanarek, "El Hospital del Divino Salvador"; Jiménez Olivares, "Hospital el Divino Salvador para mujeres dementes."

88. Elena Carrera, "Understanding Mental Disturbance in Sixteenth- and Seventeenth-Century Spain," 128–29.

89. The statutes indicated that the apothecary would be a member of the brotherhood; however, the earliest surviving book of medical receipts (dating to 1698) indicates that medicines were purchased from the apothecary shop of Urbano Martínez. The annotations are difficult to decipher. AGN, Indiferente Virreinal, caja 1627, exp. 7. On New World materia medica, see Estes, "Reception of American Drugs in Europe" and López Piñero and Pardo Tomás, "Contribution of Hernández to European Botany and Materia Medica," both in *Searching for the Secrets of Nature*; Huguet-Termes, "New World Materia Medica in Spanish Renaissance Medicine."

90. AGN, Hospitales, vol. 73, exp. 3, fol. 234v; Viesca Treviño and de la Peña, "Las enfermedades mentales en el Códice Badiano," 81.

91. For a discussion of the centrality of regimen to the careful management of the non-naturals in hospital care, see Horden, "Non-natural Environment."

92. I have consulted the following account books: AGN, Indiferente Virreinal, caja 1030, exp. 3–5; AGN, Indiferente Virreinal, caja 1004, exp. 3–6; AGN, Indiferente Virreinal, caja 0930, exp. 2–6.

93. The statutes instructed the cook to take orders from the head nurse concerning dietary modifications for specific patients. AGN, Tierras, vol. 3082, exp. 1, fol. 19v.

94. AGN, Indiferente Virreinal, caja 1004, exp. 4, fol. 44.

95. See, for instance, Midelfort, *History of Madness in Sixteenth-Century Germany*; Porter, *Mind-Forg'd Manacles*; Mellyn, *Mad Tuscans and Their Families*.

Chapter Two

1. AGN, Correspondencia de Virreyes, 1a series, vol. 96, exp. 1, fol. 1r.
2. *La administración de Fray Antonio María de Bucareli y Ursúa*, 419.
3. Viera, *Breve y compendiosa narración de la ciudad de Mexico*, 250.
4. AGN, Indiferente Virreinal, caja 0974, exp. 18, fol. 3r.
5. Minor repairs to the roof and other parts of the building were reported throughout the account books, esp. AGN, Indiferente Virreinal, caja 3785, exp. 22, fol. 56r. References to flooding and humidity can be found in the following: AGN, Indiferente Virreinal, caja 4749, exp. 37, fol. 1r; AHDF, vol. 2303, exp. 1, fol. 28r.
6. Muriel, "El modelo arquitectrónico," 116; AHDF, vol. 2303, exp. 1, fols. 28r–31r.
7. AGN, Obras Pías, vol. 3, exp. 10, fols. 125r–26r.
8. Writing about children and the legal category of minority in colonial Lima, Premo has noted that the Bourbon reforms "amplified royal paternalism as a political philosophy." See Premo, *Children of the Father King*, 14.
9. On these reforms see, Stein and Stein, *Apogee of Empire*; Paquette, *Enlightenment, Governance, and Reform*.
10. On the crown's use of the discourse of public happiness, see Paquette, *Enlightenment, Governance, and Reform*, chap. 2.
11. See Arrom, *Containing the Poor*; Ramirez, *Enlightened Immunity*; Few, *For All of Humanity*; A. Warren, *Medicine and Politics in Colonial Peru*; De Vos, "Research, Development, and Empire."
12. Important studies of church-state relations during this period include Taylor, *Magistrates of the Sacred*; Brading, *Church and State in Bourbon Mexico*; Farriss, *Crown and Clergy in Colonial Mexico*; Zahino Peñafort, *Iglesia y sociedad en México*.
13. Arrom, *Containing the Poor*, 72–73. See also Aceves Pastrana, *El Hospital General de San Andrés*; Milton, *Many Meanings of Poverty*.
14. A. Warren, *Medicine and Politics in Colonial Peru*, 119–20.
15. A. Warren, 48.
16. A. Warren, 17. See also Ramirez, *Enlightened Immunity*; Premo, *Children of the Father King*; Twinam, *Public Lives, Private Secrets*; Milton, *Many Meanings of Poverty*.
17. For a discussion of New Spain's mendicant orders and their varied corporate identities, see Melvin, *Building Colonial Cities of God*, chap. 2.
18. AGI, México, vol. 2744, s/f.
19. Martin, "San Hipólito Hospitals," 251.
20. AGI, México, vol. 2744, s/f.
21. AGI, México, vol. 2744, s/f; Martin, "San Hipólito Hospitals," 253–54; Canterla and Tovar, "La orden hospitalaria de San Hipólito," 136–37. Although the Pope issued his decrees in 1700, the bulls were not promulgated until 1702.
22. In 1640, New Spain's population was estimated to have been 1.5 million; a century later, it was between 1.5 and 3 million. The increase in the number of people of mixed ancestry and the demographic "recovery" of the Indigenous population were largely responsible for this population growth. Martínez, *Genealogical Fictions*, 228.
23. Sharon Bailey Glascow discusses the impact of urbanization on disease and public health. See Glascow, *Constructing Mexico City*, chap. 3.

24. AGN, Indiferente Virreinal, caja 4749, exp. 37, fol. 1r.

25. Cabrera y Quintero, *Escudo de Armas*, 423–24. On the cult of Our Lady of Guadalupe and the role of popular devotion during the epidemic, see Brading, *Mexican Phoenix*, esp. 119–45; Ramirez, *Enlightened Immunity*, chap.1.

26. These numbers appear to be exaggerated, given that San Hipólito accommodated somewhere between twenty and eighty patients during this period.

27. Cabrera y Quintero approximated that the hospital received 2,240 pesos for its daily food expenses, in addition to double this amount for medicines and other medical expenses. Cabrera y Quintero, *Escudo de Armas*, 424.

28. Cabrera y Quintero, *Escudo de Armas*, 424.

29. AGI, Mexico, vol. 2744, s/f.

30. AGI, Mexico, vol. 2745, s/f.

31. In 1741, Balbuena pleaded with the Council of Indies to pursue a reform of the order instead of its dissolution. He submitted a detailed report to the council describing the order's fallen condition (reiterating most of Vizzarón's complaints) as well as a plan for reform. AGI, Mexico, vol. 2745, s/f.

32. On Catholic reformism as opposed to state-sponsored campaigns, see Chowning, "Convent Reform, Catholic Reform, and Bourbon Reform in Eighteenth-Century New Spain."

33. Lehner, *Catholic Enlightenment*, 7.

34. AGI, Mexico, vol. 2745, s/f.

35. Lehner, *Catholic Enlightenment*, 4, 36–37.

36. AGN, Indiferente Virreinal, caja 2512, exp. 26, fol. 20r.

37. See Arrom, *Containing the Poor*, esp. chaps. 1–2.

38. AGI, Mexico, vol. 2744, s/f.

39. AGI, Mexico, vol. 2744, s/f.

40. A 1755 report indicated that the order had dwindled to nearly half its former size of 120 members. It further specified that 40 members had died while 13 or 14 had fled the convent. A fraction of the remaining 56 to 57 brothers were carrying out their sentences and could therefore only perform certain menial or internal tasks.

41. Zahino Peñafort, *Iglesia y sociedad en México*, 136–37.

42. A. Warren, *Medicine and Politics in Colonial Peru*.

43. AGN, Indiferente Virreinal, caja 0974, exp. 18, fol. 2v.

44. AGN, Indiferente Virreinal, caja 0974, exp. 18, fol. 3v.

45. AGN, Indiferente Virreinal, caja 0974, exp. 18, fol. 3v.

46. AGN, Indiferente Virreinal, caja 0974, exp. 18, fol. 3r. My emphasis.

47. AGN, Indiferente Virreinal, caja 0974, exp. 18, fol. 3r.

48. AGN, Indiferente Virreinal, caja 0974, exp. 18, fol. 3r.

49. AGN, Indiferente Virreinal, caja 0974, exp. 18, fol. 4v.

50. AGN, Indiferente Virreinal, caja 0974, exp. 18, fol. 3v.

51. Martha Few documents shifting meanings of "cure" with respect to smallpox inoculation. Few, *For All of Humanity*, 50–51.

52. AGN, Indiferente Virreinal, caja 0974, exp. 18, fol. 4v.

53. AGN, Indiferente Virreinal, caja 0974, exp. 18, fols. 13r–14v.

54. One member of the syndicate, Don José Martín Chavez, was reported to have contributed 18,000 pesos of his personal wealth, while other members of the board donated more than 4,000 pesos annually. Rivera Cambas, *Mexico pintoresco, artistico y monumental*, 385; AGN, Obras Pías, vol. 3, exp. 10, fols. 125r-v.

55. Marroqui, *La Ciudad de Mexico*, 585.

56. Arrom, *Containing the Poor*.

57. AHDF, Fondo Ayuntamiento Gobierno del Distrito Federal, Sección Hospitales e Iglesia de San Hipólito, vol. 2303, exp. 1, fols. 28r-31r.

58. *La administración de D. Frey Antonio María de Bucareli y Ursúa*, 167.

59. In her study of Mexico City's Poor House, Arrom emphasizes that while the crown enlarged its role in matters of public welfare, it was only capable of providing limited financial support; institutions like the Poor House instead relied on mixed sources of funding. See Arrom, *Containing the Poor*, chap. 2.

60. AHDF, Fondo Ayuntamiento Gobierno del Distrito Federal, Hospitales e Iglesia de San Hipólito, vol. 2303, exp. 1ff., fol. 18v; Marroqui, *La Ciudad de Mexico*, 585-86.

61. AGN, Indiferente Virreinal, caja 4122, exp. 6, fols. 1r-2r. On the complexity of hospital finances during the colonial period, see Cahill, "Financing Health Care in the Viceroyalty of Peru," 23-154; Arrom, *Containing the Poor*, 50-59.

62. *La administración de D. Frey Antonio María de Bucareli y Ursúa*, 169; Marraquoi, *La Ciudad de Mexico*, 586.

63. AGN, Indiferente Virreinal, caja 5380, exp. 3.

64. The quote references Silva Arrom's characterization of the financial organization of Mexico City's Poor House. See Arrom, *Containing the Poor*, 45.

65. These records are located at INAH, Fondo Hospital de los Naturales. See table A.1 in the appendix.

66. Muriel, "El modelo arquitectrónico," 19.

67. AGN, Correspondecia de Virreyes, vol. 96, exp. 1, fol. 1r.

68. AHDF, Fondo Ayuntamiento Gobierno del Distrito Federal, Sección Hospitales e Iglesia de San Hipólito, vol. 2303, exp. 1, fols. 28r-30r.

69. Although the architects Idelfonso de Iniesta Bejarano and Lorenzo Rodriguez were hired to survey the initial building, it is not clear what part they played in the hospital's redesign. The floor plan submitted by the viceroy to the king of Spain does not contain a signature to identify its creator. Given that Rodriguez was the main architect of the Royal Indian Hospital, it is possible he also redesigned San Hipólito, but there is no way to corroborate this hypothesis. Certainly, the design of the Royal Indian Hospital differs substantially from that of San Hipólito, as Muriel has pointed out. See Muriel, "El modelo arquitectrónico," 117.

70. Muriel, "El modelo arquitectrónico," 118.

71. Viera, *Breve y compendiosa narración de la ciudad de Mexico*, 250.

72. On this cross-shaped model and on hospital design more generally, see Henderson, *Renaissance Hospital*; Goldin, *Work of Mercy*, chap. 5. See also Park and Henderson, "'The First Hospital among Christians.'"

73. Muriel, "El modelo arquitectrónico," 119; Ballenger, "Modernizing Madness," 45.

74. Muriel, "El modelo arquitectrónico," 118.

75. Viera, *Breve y compendiosa narración de la ciudad de Mexico*, 250.
76. Viera, 251.
77. AGN, Indiferente Virreinal, caja 2187, exp. 2, fols. 45r–v.
78. AGN, Indiferente Virreinal, caja 2187, exp. 2, fol. 48v.
79. AGN, Indiferente Virreinal, caja 2187, exp. 2, fol. 50r.
80. I would like to credit my colleague, Corinna Treitel, for this observation.
81. AGN, Indiferente Virreinal, caja 4951, exp. 47, fol. 3v.
82. AGN, Indiferente Virreinal, caja 4951, exp. 47, fols. 10v–11r.
83. AGN, Indiferente Virreinal, caja 4951, exp. 47, fol. 51v.
84. AGN, Indiferente Virreinal, caja 4951, exp. 47, fol. 16r.
85. AGN, Indiferente Virreinal, caja 4951, exp. 47, fol. 119v.
86. AGN, Indiferente Virreinal, caja 4951, exp. 47, fol. 29v.
87. AGN, Indiferente Virreinal, caja 4951, exp. 47, fol. 61r. For a more detailed study of suicide in New Spain, see Tortorici, "Reading the (Dead) Body."
88. AGN, Indiferente Virreinal, caja 4951, exp. 47, fol. 27r.
89. AGN, Indiferente Virreinal, caja 4951, exp. 47, fol. 16r.
90. AGN, Indiferente Virreinal, caja 4951, exp. 47, fol. 67r.
91. AGN, Indiferente Virreinal, caja 4951, exp. 47, fol. 101r.
92. AGN, Indiferente Virreinal, caja 4951, exp. 47, fol. 36r.
93. Lindemann, *Medicine and Society in Early Modern Europe*, 44; see also Lederer, *Madness, Religion and the State*.
94. See Martínez, *Genealogical Fictions*, chap. 9.
95. To be sure, the racial background of a considerable portion of the patient population went unrecorded.
96. Twinam, *Public Lives, Private Secrets*, 26.
97. Arrom documents a similar trend for the capital's Poor House. See Arrom, *Containing the Poor*, 90.
98. AGN, Indiferente Virreinal, caja 4951, exp. 47, fol. 67r.
99. AGN, Indiferente Virreinal, caja 4951, exp. 47, fols. 78v–79r.
100. AGN, Indiferente Virreinal, caja 4951, exp. 47, fol. 28.
101. AGN, Indiferente Virreinal, caja 4951, exp. 47, fol. 51v.

Chapter Three

1. AGN, Inquisición, vol. 1076, exp. 2, fols. 240r–42v.
2. AGN, Inquisición, vol. 1076, exp. 2, fol. 143.
3. AGN, Inquisición, vol. 1076, exp. 2, fols. 345r–56r.
4. Ginzburg, "Inquisitor as Anthropologist"; see also Ginzburg, *Cheese and the Worms*.
5. Sellers-García, *Distance and Documents at the Spanish Empire's Periphery*, 17.
6. Sacristán, *Locura e Inquisición*, 23. For a refutation of the argument that mental illness was viewed as a consequence of sin, see Kroll and Bachrach, "Sin and Mental Illness in the Middle Ages."
7. Working with Inquisition cases from sixteenth- and seventeenth-century Spain, Dale Shuger has argued that the "emergence of 'mental disorder' . . . destabilized an

institution only equipped to deal with heretical souls and punishable bodies." See Shuger, "Madness on Trial," 277.

8. García-Ballester, "Galenism and Medical Teaching at the University of Salamanca"; García-Ballester, "Circulation and Use of Medical Manuscripts in Arabic"; Carrera, "Understanding Mental Disturbance in Sixteenth- and Seventeenth-Century Spain"; Foster, *Hippocrates' Latin American Legacy*. On the rise of psychiatry in Mexico, see Ballenger, "Modernizing Madness"; Rivera-Garza, "Dangerous Minds"; Somolinos d'Ardois, *Historia de la Psiquiatría en México*.

9. This view dates back to the Enlightenment itself, as prominent philosophers targeted the Inquisition as "the chief symbol of religious intolerance." See Peters, *The Inquisition*. On the Inquisition's role in policing Enlightenment thought, see Greenleaf, "Mexican Inquisition and the Enlightenment."

10. McMahon, *Enemies of the Enlightenment*.

11. For a discussion of trends in the historiography of the Spanish and Mexican Inquisitions, see De Bujanda, "Recent Historiography of the Spanish Inquisition"; Greenleaf, "Historiography of the Mexican Inquisition." More recent revisionist histories include, Silverblatt, *Modern Inquisitions*; Nesvig, *Ideology and Inquisition*; Nesvig, *Promiscuous Power*; Schaposchnik, *The Lima Inquisition*.

12. Boyer, *Lives of the Bigamists*, 16.

13. On the history of the Inquisition in sixteenth-century Mexico and its various phases, see Greenleaf, *Mexican Inquisition of the Sixteenth Century*.

14. Although Indians were excluded from the Inquisition's jurisdiction, the activities and beliefs of Indigenous communities were nevertheless monitored by local priests and the regular clergy, and by the episcopal courts of the Provisorato de Indios y Chinos. Moreover, as Laura Lewis has shown, Indians were often implicated in trials involving witchcraft through the selling of "powders, herbs, instructions, and cures" to non-Indians. Although they were not punished, Indians—and Indigenous culture and beliefs more broadly—were central to these witchcraft cases. See Lewis, *Hall of Mirrors*, 38–39.

15. Although only surveying the period up to 1700, Solange Alberro provides the following estimates: 34.4%, minor religious crimes; 18.8%, magic and witchcraft; 13.2%, sexual transgressions; 6.6.%, solicitation; 14.8%, heresy; 1%, idolatry and heterodoxy; 8.9%, civil crimes. See Alberro, *Inquisición y sociedad en Mexico*, 205.

16. Silverblatt, *Modern Inquisitions*, 57.

17. Kamen, *Spanish Inquisition*, 183, 196.

18. On the indeterminacy of Inquisition verdicts, see Silverblatt, *Modern Inquisitions*, 7, 65–70.

19. The indeterminacy of Inquisition cases has largely been discussed in the context of trials dealing with mystics and the discernment of spirits. Recent studies of mysticism have emphasized the hermeneutic challenges involved in determining sanctity from fraud, and divine from demonic possession. See, for instance, Keitt, *Inventing the Sacred*; Schutte, *Aspiring Saints*; Sluhovsky, *Believe Not Every Spirit*; Jaffary, *False Mystics*. Recently, Dale Shuger has extended this scholarship into the domain of madness. See Shuger, "Madness on Trial."

20. Lewis, *Hall of Mirrors*, 43. See also Shuger, *Don Quixote in the Archives*, 31–32.

21. Nalle, "Insanity and the Insanity Defense in the Spanish Inquisition."

22. Mellyn, *Mad Tuscans and Their Families*, 61–62; Nalle, "Insanity and the Insanity Defense in the Spanish Inquisition."

23. *Las Siete Partidas*, vol. 5, 8.

24. Shuger, *Don Quixote in the Archives*, 31; Tropé, *Locura y sociedad*, 186.

25. On medieval canonists and their interpretation of Roman law with respect to insanity, see Midelfort, *History of Madness*, 190–91.

26. Shuger, "Madness on Trial," 278. For a list of cases assembled chronologically from 1573 to 1738, see Sacristán, *Locura y disidencia*, 141–51 (index).

27. Shuger, "Madness on Trial," 277–78.

28. Shuger, 278.

29. Sluhovsky, *Believe Not Every Spirit*, 7. On the discernment of spirits in the Middle Ages and the construction of possession as a physiological phenomenon, see Caciola, *Discerning Spirits*.

30. Beecher, "Witches, the Possessed, and the Diseases of the Imagination," 105; Strocchia, "Women on the Edge," 63.

31. Sluhovsky, *Believe Not Every Spirit*, 191. The condition of melancholy, for instance, a disease of the imagination and emotions, offered only a narrow interpretation of possession, failing to furnish inquisitors with a humoral etiology for symptoms such as seizures and convulsions; at best, it provided a plausible answer only when considered in conjunction with the devil's influence. See Levack, *Devil Within*, 118–23.

32. Keitt, *Inventing the Sacred*, 168. See also Keitt, "Religious Enthusiasm, the Spanish Inquisition, and the Disenchantment of the World."

33. Keitt, *Inventing the Sacred*, 151; Sluhovsky, *Believe Not Every Spirit*, 191.

34. Cervantes, *Devil in the New World*, 136.

35. Behar, "Sex and Sin"; see also Few, *Women Who Lead Evil Lives*; Lewis, *Hall of Mirrors*.

36. See Jaffary, *False Mystics*, esp. chap. 5; Araya Espinoza, "De espirtuales a hystericas."

37. As Brian Levack as emphasized, the "notion that all possessions had natural, medical causes did not gain widespread support until the nineteenth century." Levack, *Devil Within*, 113.

38. For the sixteenth and seventeenth centuries, María Cristina Sacristán has documented nineteen instances in which the Inquisition deemed the suspect to be mad. For the eighteenth century, her appendixes record forty-two cases. See appendixes in *Locura e Inquisición en Nueva España* and *Locura y disidencia en el México ilustrado*.

39. Eimeric, *Manual de inquisidores*, 17–19; 44. This is a facsimile of the 1821 edition based on the sixteenth-century Spanish jurist Francisco Peña's annotated version.

40. Both Dale Shuger and Sara Nalle have noted the absence of torture in trials involving madness. See Nalle, "Insanity and the Insanity Defense in the Spanish Inquisition"; Shuger, "Madness on Trial"; Shuger, *Don Quixote in the Archives*. For Mexico, María Cristina Sacristán's two studies have also noted the absence of torture. See *Locura y Inquisición en Nueva España* and *Locura y Disidencia en el México Ilustrado*.

41. AGN, Inquisición, vol. 1117, exp. 4, fol. 89r.

42. AGN, Inquisición, vol. 1117, exp. 4, fols. 2r–v.

43. AGN, Inquisición, vol. 1117, exp. 4, fol. 84r.
44. AGN, Inquisición, vol. 1117, exp. 4, fols. 34r–v.
45. Schwartz, *All Can Be Saved*, 18.
46. Schwartz, 18.
47. This problem was not unique to insanity cases, as Maureen Flynn has shown in her study of blasphemy in sixteenth-century Spain. See Flynn, "Blasphemy and the Play of Anger," 29–56.
48. Flynn, "Blasphemy and the Play of Anger," 34.
49. Flynn, 40.
50. Flynn, 40. See also Villa-Flores, *Dangerous Speech*.
51. Shuger, "Madness on Trial," 28.
52. AGN, Inquisición, vol. 1058, fols. 152r–53r. In colonial Mexico, *cambujo* was a caste category that could signify several mixtures of different backgrounds, including Indigenous with African, *chino*, and *lobo* castes. As an adjective, *cambujo* also denoted swarthy skin tone.
53. AGN, Inquisición, vol. 1058, fol. 154r.
54. AGN, Inquisición, vol. 1058, fols. 165r–66r.
55. AGN, Inquisición, vol. 1058, fol. 171r.
56. AGN, Inquisición, vol. 1119, exp. 9, fol. 180rr.
57. AGN, Inquisición, vol. 1119, exp. 9, fol. 206v.
58. AGN, Inquisición, vol. 1119, exp. 9, fol. 173r.
59. AGN, Inquisición, vol. 1119, exp. 9, fol. 183r.
60. AGN, Inquisición, vol. 1119, exp. 9, fol. 199.
61. AGN, Inquisición, vol. 1119, exp. 9, fol. 205v.
62. AGN, Inquisición, vol. 1119, exp. 9, fol. 208v.
63. AGN, Inquisición, vol. 1119, exp. 9, fols. 206v–7r.
64. Shuger, "Madness on Trial," 281.
65. In this respect, the colonial population of New Spain differed markedly from that of Europe, or at least Italy, where as Elizabeth Mellyn has shown, early modern Tuscans skillfully employed medical terms and medical concepts regarding madness to craft arguments in Tuscan courts. See Mellyn, *Mad Tuscans and Their Families*, chap. 4
66. Gonzalez's case and the contents of his surviving writings and drawings have received some scholarly attention. See Albert, "Nuevas líneas de investigación"; Flores, "Tebanillo González, heteróclito." For a reproduction of some of Gonzalez's writings, see Flores, "Papeles de Tebanillo González."
67. I borrow this insight from Shuger, *Don Quixote in the Archives*, 31.
68. AGN, Inquisición, vol. 1505, exp. 3, fol. 109r.
69. AGN, Inquisición, vol. 1505, exp. 3, fols. 115v–16v.
70. AGN, Inquisición, vol. 1505, exp. 3, fol. 118r.
71. AGN, Inquisición, vol. 1505, exp. 3, fol. 131r.
72. AGN, Inquisición, vol. 1505, exp. 3, fols. 137r–v.
73. Albert, "Nuevas líneas de investigación," 707. See also Greenleaf, "Mexican Inquisition and the Enlightenment."
74. AGN, Inquisición, vol. 1505, exp. 3, fols. 139r–v.

75. Few, *Women Who Lead Evil Lives*, 52–53.
76. Tortorici, *Sins against Nature*, 89.
77. Monica Calabritto, "Medical and Moral Dimensions of Feminine Madness," 26. To be sure, Calabritto's comments refer to Renaissance Italy.
78. Jaffary, *False Mystics*, esp. chap. 5.
79. Bynum, "The Female Body and Religious Practice in the Later Middle Ages." On the relationship between female sexuality and popular devotion in New Spain, see Tortorici, "Masturbation, Salvation, and Desire."
80. Ruth Behar has documented a similar pattern for women guilty of practicing witchcraft. See Behar, "Sex and Sin," 34–54.
81. AGN, Inquisición, vol. 1162, exp. 34, fols. 385r–v.
82. AGN, Inquisición, vol. 1162, exp. 34, fol. 386v.
83. AGN, Inquisición, vol. 1162, exp. 34, fol. 387r.
84. AGN, Inquisición, vol. 1162, exp. 34, fols. 388r–389v.
85. AGN, Inquisición, vol. 1162, exp. 34, fol. 389v.
86. AGN, Inquisición, vol. 1009, exp. 15, fols. 311r–v.
87. AGN, Inquisición, vol. 1009, exp. 15, fols. 312r–v.
88. Sousa, "Devil and Deviance in Native Criminal Narratives from Early Mexico," 162.
89. AGN, Inquisición, vol. 1009, exp. 15, fol. 315r.
90. AGN, Inquisición, vol. 1009, exp. 15, fol. 323r.
91. AGN, Inquisición, vol. 1009, exp. 15, fol. 325r.
92. AGN, Inquisición, vol. 1009, exp. 15, fols. 327r–29r.
93. AGN, Inquisición, vol. 1009, exp. 15, fol. 331r.
94. AGN, Inquisición, vol. 1009, exp. 15, fol. 332r.
95. AGN, Inquisición, vol. 1009, exp. 15, fol. 335r.
96. Lederer, *Madness, Religion and the State in Early Modern Europe*, 1. Lederer suggests that psychiatry emerged from the practice of "spiritual physic."
97. Haliczer, *Sexuality in the Confessional*, 22.
98. AGN, Inquisición, vol. 1009, exp. 15, fol. 338r.
99. AGN, Inquisición, vol. 1009, exp. 15, fols. 342r–v.
100. AGN, Inquisición, vol. 1009, exp. 15, fols. 344r–v.
101. AGN, Inquisición, vol. 1009, exp. 15, fol. 347r.
102. AGN, Inquisición, vol. 1009, exp. 15, fol. 374v.
103. AGN, Inquisición, vol. 1009, exp. 15, fol. 348r.
104. AGN, Inquisición, vol. 1009, exp. 15, fol. 346v.
105. AGN, Inquisición, vol. 1009, exp. 15, fol. 349r.
106. Strocchia has made this observation in connection to forced monarchization and patterns of attempted suicide in early modern Italian convents. See Strocchia, "Women on the Edge."
107. Van Deusen, *Between the Sacred and the Worldly*, 59. Van Deusen's study deals with the case of colonial Peru. On the development of *recogimientos* in colonial Mexico, see Muriel, *Los recogimientos de mujeres*.
108. *Gaceta de Mexico*, vol. 1, no. 5, 998.

109. Greenleaf, "Mexican Inquisition and the Enlightenment," 183–84.
110. Greenleaf, 184–85.

Chapter Four

1. AGN, Inquisición, vol. 1086, exp. 1. The auto-da-fé appears on fols. 98r–99v.
2. In the inquisitorial courts, punishments often combined spiritual penance with corporal penalties. Penitents had their sins abjured either *de levi* (for minor crimes) or *de vehementi* (for graver ones). In cases involving serious heresy, the convicted were "relaxed"—that is, released to state authorities for execution—although this was quite rare. See Kamen, *Spanish Inquisition*, 200–204.
3. AGN, Inquisición, vol. 1086, exp. 1, fol. 103r.
4. AGN, Inquisición, vol. 1086, exp. 1, fols. 105r–v.
5. AGN, Inquisición, vol. 1086, exp. 1, fol. 105v. Specifically, Peña y Brizuela cited the work of the natural philosopher Olivia Sabuco (1562–1622), who explored connections between the body and emotions.
6. AGN, Inquisición, vol. 1086, exp. 1, fols. 106r–7v.
7. See Sacristán, *Locura e Inquisición en Nueva España*.
8. Green, *Inquisition: Reign of Fear*. On the pedagogical and performative function of the auto-da-fé, see Cañeque, "Theater of Power."
9. For a summary of the Enlightenment construction of the Inquisition, see Peters, *The Inquisition*, 155–88.
10. See Mott, "Rule of Faith over Reason."
11. AGN, Inquisición, vol. 1117, exp. 4, fols. 177v–18r.
12. Although some have described Zacchia as the father of forensic medicine, this is an anachronistic characterization. For a discussion that situates Zacchia's work within a long history of medicalization, see Mellyn, *Mad Tuscans and Their Families*, 161–92.
13. Quoted in Mellyn, *Mad Tuscans and Their Families*, 161, 177.
14. AGN, Inquisición, vol. 1117, exp. 4, fol. 118v.
15. AGN, Inquisición, vol. 1117, exp. 4, fol. 124v.
16. AGN, Inquisición, vol. 1117, exp. 4, fol. 126r.
17. Bouley, *Pious Postmortems*; Vidal, "Miracles, Science, and Testimony in Post-Tridentine Saint-Making"; Pomata, "Malpighi and the Holy Body."
18. De Renzi, "Witnesses of the Body."
19. I borrow the term "medical turn" from Mellyn, *Mad Tuscans and Their Families*, 130.
20. Tortorici, "Sexual Violence, Predatory Masculinity, and Medical Testimony"; *Sins against Nature*, 96–100.
21. Jaffary, *False Mystics*, 139–44.
22. Hernández Sáenz, *Learning to Heal*, 5.
23. Jaffary, *False Mystics*, 155; Hernández Sáenz, 27.
24. Venegas, *Compendio de la Medicina Practica*, 209–10.
25. Venegas, 210.
26. Venegas, 212.

27. Pardo-Tomás and Martinez-Vidal, "Victims and Experts," 15–16. See also Jiménez Olivares, *Los Medicos en el Santo Oficio*.
28. Pardo-Tomás and Martinez-Vidal, "Victims and Experts," 14; Hernández Sáenz, 21–23.
29. This argument has been most powerfully made by Timothy D. Walker, who focuses on eighteenth-century Portugal. See Walker, *Doctors, Folk Medicine, and the Inquisition*. For New Spain, see Martha Few, *Women Who Lead Evil Lives*, esp. chap. 4.
30. AGN, Inquisición, vol. 1206, exp. 2, fols. 64r–v.
31. AGN, Inquisición, vol. 1206, exp. 2, fols. 69v–70r.
32. AGN, Inquisición, vol. 1206, exp. 2, fol. 77r.
33. AGN, Inquisición, vol. 1206, exp. 2, fol. 76r.
34. Venegas, *Compendio de la Medicina Practica*, 109.
35. Sousa, "Devil and Deviance," 162.
36. I borrow this term from Shuger, "Madness on Trial," 290.
37. AGN, Inquisición, vol. 1206, exp. 2, fol. 104v.
38. AGN, Inquisición, vol. 1206, exp. 2, fols. 108v–9r.
39. AGN, Inquisición, vol. 1206, exp. 2, fol. 115r.
40. Esteyneffer, *Florilegio medicinal*, 154–55.
41. For an examination of representations of melancholy in Baroque Spain, see Barta, *Melancolía y cultura*. In another text, Barta offers a more philosophical musing of melancholy as distinctive to Mexican national identity. See Barta, *Jaula de la melancolía*. I take a cue here from Elizabeth Mellyn, who positions her social history of madness in early modern Italy against studies that have privileged melancholy as a representation rather than a lived experience. See Mellyn, *Mad Tuscans and their Families*.
42. AGN, Inquisición, vol. 865, exp. 1, fol. 507v.
43. AGN, Inquisición, vol. 865, exp. 1, fols. 467r–v.
44. AGN, Inquisición, vol. 865, exp. 1, fols. 468r–69v.
45. AGN, Inquisición, vol. 865, exp. 1, fols. 480r–85r.
46. AGN, Inquisición, vol. 865, exp. 1, fol. 478v.
47. AGN, Inquisición, vol. 865, exp. 1, fol. 499r.
48. AGN, Inquisición, vol. 865, exp. 1, fol. 500r.
49. AGN, Inquisición, vol. 865, exp. 1, fols. 505r–v.
50. AGN, Inquisición, vol. 865, exp. 1, fols. 526r–27r.
51. On the rise of the moral treatment and its indebtedness to religious forms of consolation, see Goldstein, *Console and Classify*, 200–210.
52. AGN, Inquisición, vol. 865, exp. 1, fols. 521r–22r.
53. AGN, Inquisición, vol. 865, exp. 1, fol. 532r.
54. AGN, Inquisición, vol. 865, exp. 1, fol. 538r.
55. AGN, Inquisición, vol. 1354, exp. 1, fols. 5v–7r.
56. AGN, Inquisición, vol. 1354, exp. 1, fol. 11v.
57. AGN, Inquisición, vol. 1354, exp. 1, fols. 49v–50r, 53v.
58. AGN, Inquisición, vol. 1354, exp. 1, fol. 118r. On mechanical explanations of melancholy, see S. W. Jackson, "Melancholia and Mechanical Explanation" and "Melancholia and the Waning of Humoral Theory."

59. AGN, Inquisición, vol. 1354, exp. 1, fols. 18v–19v.
60. AGN, Inquisición, vol. 1354, exp. 1, fol. 120r.
61. AGN, Inquisición, vol. 1354, exp. 1, fol. 121r.
62. AGN, Inquisición, vol. 1354, exp. 1, fols. 198r–v.
63. AGN, Inquisición, vol. 1354, exp. 1, fol. 203r.
64. Sacristán, *Locura e Inquisición en Nueva España*, 119–20. On the centrality of the family to the management of madness in the early modern period, see Mellyn, *Mad Tuscans and Their Families*.
65. AGN, Inquisición, vol. 218, exp. 3, fols. 80r–v. See also Jaffary, *False Mystics*, 149–50.
66. Quoted in Cohen, *Martyr*, 181.
67. On penal servitude in Spain, see Pike, *Penal Servitude in Early Modern Spain*.
68. I base this estimate on the work of María Cristina Sacristán, who has combed the inquisitorial archives for cases involving madness. For the period between 1571 and 1760, she has identified twenty-five cases dealing with madness; for the period between 1760 and 1810, she has identified fifty-eight cases (including secular criminal trials). Of the latter group, she states that a third of them resulted in the suspect's transfer to a mental hospital of some sort. Most of these suspects were male and were sent to San Hipólito, although one suspect was sent to the Hospital de Santissima Trinidad (also known as the Hospital de San Pedro), which was reserved for clerics suffering from age-related dementia. This estimate holds if we expand the timetable to encompass the period 1700–1821 and only include Inquisition cases, as I have done. Many of the cases cited by Sacristán—that is, those dealing explicitly with the Hospital de San Hipólito—are also analyzed in this chapter. See Sacristán, *Locura e Inquisición en Nueva España* and *Locura y disidencia en el México ilustrado*. In Spain, the Inquisition also used hospitals for similar purposes. See Tropé, "Locura y Inquisición en la España del siglo XVII" and "Inquisición y locura en la España del siglo XVI y XVII"; Nalle, *Mad for God*.
69. Bennassar, "Patterns of the Inquisitorial Mind."
70. AGN, Inquisición, vol. 1117, exp. 3, fol. 125v.
71. AGN, Inquisición, vol. 1013, exp., 1, fol. 249r.
72. See AGN, Inquisición, vol. 1086, exp. 1, fol. 105v; AGN, Inquisición, vol. 1117, exp. 3, fol. 249r. In the case of Felipe Alvarez, the *calificadores* cited Zacchia to defend this point.
73. AGN, Indiferente Virreinal, caja 5536, exp. 25, fols. 1v–2r.
74. María Cristina Sacristán makes a similiar argument, in labeling San Hipólito as a "laboratory for diagnostics." See *Locura y disidencia en al México ilustrado*, 82.
75. See Smith, "Laboratories."
76. AGN, Inquisición, vol. 1013, exp. 1, fols. 229r–33v. On freemasonry and its connection to the "radical Enlightenment," see Jacob, *Radical Enlightenment*.
77. AGN, Inquisición, vol. 1013, exp. 1, fol. 236.
78. AGN, Inquisición, vol. 1013, exp. 1, fols. 246r–v.
79. AGN, Inquisición, vol. 1013, exp. 1, fol. 249r.
80. AGN, Inquisición, vol. 1013, exp. 1, fol. 248v.
81. AGN, Inquisición, vol. 1013, exp. 1, fols. 249r–v.

82. AGN, Inquisición, vol. 1086, exp. 1, fols. 110r–v.
83. AGN, Inquisición, vol. 1086, exp. 1, fols. 112v–113r.
84. AGN, Inquisición, vol. 1086, exp. 1, fols. 113r–v. This passage is very confusing, and it appears that one of the reasons for Silva's outbursts was that, as a prisoner of the Inquisition, he was denied some of the sacraments. Apparently, he was still allowed to confess, which he refused.
85. AGN, Inquisición, vol. 1086, exp. 1, fols. 113v–14r.
86. AGN, Inquisición, vol. 1086, exp. 1, fol. 115r.
87. AGN, Inquisición, vol. 1086, exp. 1, fol. 116r.
88. AGN, Inquisición, vol. 1086, exp. 1, fols. 116v–17r.
89. AGN, Inquisición, vol. 1086, exp. 1, fols. 119r–20v.
90. AGN, Inquisición, vol. 1086, exp. 1 fols. 118r–v.
91. AGN, Inquisición, vol. 1352, exp. 2, fols. 1v, 12v.
92. AGN, Inquisición, vol. 1352, exp. 2, fol. 12v.
93. AGN, Inquisición, vol. 1352, exp. 2, fol. 21v.
94. AGN, Inquisición, vol. 1352, exp. 2, fol. 34r.
95. AGN, Inquisición, vol. 1352, exp. 2, fols. 74r–75r.
96. AGN, Inquisición, vol. 1352, exp. 2, fols. 78r–82v.

Chapter Five

1. AGN, Indiferente Virreinal, caja 3472, exp. 4, fols. 1r–8r.
2. Here, I build on the observations of Elizabeth Mellyn, who documents similar concerns and dynamics for criminal cases involving madness in early modern Italy. See Mellyn *Mad Tuscans*, esp. chap. 2.
3. The notion of a "great confinement" comes from Foucault's *Madness and Civilization*.
4. Scardaville, "(Hapsburg) Law and (Bourbon) Order," 508. For a more detailed discussion of the urban underclass, see Haslip-Viera, "The Underclass."
5. Villaroel, *Enfermedades politicas que padece la capital*, 16.
6. Haslip-Viera, *Crime and Punishment*, 45; Scardaville, "(Hapsburg) Law and (Bourbon) Order," 510. On the Acordada's activities see, MacLachlan, *Criminal Justice in Eighteenth Century Mexico*.
7. Haslip-Viera, *Crime and Punishment*, 47.
8. Haslip-Viera, 48; Scardaville, "(Hapsburg) Law and (Bourbon) Order," 511.
9. Scardaville, "(Hapsburg) Law and (Bourbon) Order," 512.
10. Voekel, "Peeing on the Palace," 183. Paquette also argues that the political concept of public happiness facilitated the state's ability to expand its function and influence in society. See Paquette, *Enlightenment, Governance, and Reform*, chap. 2.
11. Voekel, "Peeing on the Palace." Voekel is referring more generally to acts of impropriety committed by the popular classes. I extend this insight to the arena of the criminal courts, where similar language appears to have been employed.
12. Scardaville, "(Hapsburg) Law and (Bourbon) Order," 512.
13. Haslip-Viera, *Crime and Punishment*, 43. Haslip-Viera notes a "conservative opposition" to proposals for criminal justice reform, and that even Lardizábal y Uribe

"defended the continued imposition of the death penalty on those persons considered beyond redemption."

14. Buffington, *Criminal and Citizen in Modern Mexico*, 12–13.

15. Haslip-Viera, *Crime and Punishment*, 43. On Beccaria, see Bierne, *Inventing Criminology*, chap. 1.

16. Lardizábal y Uribe, *Discurso sobre las penas*, 101.

17. Lardizábal y Uribe, 102.

18. Scardaville, "(Hapsburg) Law and (Bourbon) Order," 513, 520.

19. Scardaville, 511.

20. Scardaville, 514–15.

21. Scardaville, 516. The ideas of penal reformers like Beccaria and Lardizábal were not implemented until the postcolonial period. See Buffington, *Criminal and Citizen in Modern Mexico*, chap. 1.

22. Premo, *Children of the Father King*, 21–22; Cutter, *Legal Culture of Northern New Spain*, 31–32.

23. Haslip-Viera, *Crime and Punishment*, 37.

24. Scardaville, "Justice by Paperwork," 989.

25. Scardaville, 989–90.

26. On the protections offered to legal minors (including Indians), see Premo, *Children of the Father King*, esp. chap. 1.

27. *Las Siete Partidas*, vol. 5, 1343.

28. *Las Siete Partidas*, vol. 5, 8.

29. Hevia Bolaños, *Curia Philipica*, 202.

30. Hevia Bolaños, 202.

31. Hevia Bolaños, 202.

32. Hevia Bolaños, 202.

33. Elizabeth Mellyn also emphasizes a culture of experimentation and negotiation in early modern Florence with respect to how criminal and civil justices, working both in conflict and in collaboration with families, devised ad hoc solutions for caring for the mentally disturbed, including the criminally insane. However, in her account, which focuses on the mid-fourteenth through mid-seventeenth centuries, hospitals figure only marginally, and it was the family that acted as the main custodial institution for the insane. See Mellyn, *Mad Tuscans and Their Families*.

34. This summary of arrest and trial procedure is based on my reading of the following: Haslip-Viera, *Crime and Punishment*; Cutter, *Legal Culture of Northern New Spain*, chap. 3; Spores, *Mixtecs in Ancient and Colonial Times*, chap. 8

35. Historians have long remarked on the at times arbitrary and political nature of committal, especially in the French institutions of the Old Regime, where enemies of the state and political rivals were often unjustly confined alongside the mad in general hospitals and *maisons de santé*. See Ackerknecht, "Political Prisoners in French Mental Institutions before 1789"; and, of course, Foucault, *Madness and Civilization*. On the "politics of committal" in England, see Andrews et al., *History of Bethlem*, chap. 19.

36. AGN, Criminal, vol. 667, exp. 2, fols. 73r–78r.

37. AGN, Criminal, vol. 667, exp. 2, fols. 84r–v.

38. For an interesting and in some ways parallel case involving an Indian "mad messiah," whose deranged ideas resonated with those of Indian peasants engaged in the struggle for independence, see Van Young, "Millennium on the Northern Marches."

39. Martínez, *Genealogical Fictions*, 92; see also Villella, "'Pure and Noble Indians.'"

40. Martínez, *Genealogical Fictions*, 92.

41. AGN, Criminal, vol. 667, exp. 2, fols. 84r–v.

42. AGN, Criminal, vol. 667, exp. 2, fol. 84v.

43. Haslip-Viera, *Crime and Punishment*, 38–39; Premo, *Children of the Father King*, 32–34.

44. Solórzano Pereira, *Politica Indiana*, 2:623.

45. Owensby, *Empire of Law and Indian Justice*, 56.

46. The source of Chimalpopoca's "immunity" is unclear. Although the Indians were granted protection from persecution by the Inquisition, they could be tried by the criminal courts. It is possible that the immunity was granted by the Spanish king to whom Chimalpopoca beseeched for mercy, as noted in the main text, although the records are ambiguous.

47. AGN, Criminal, vol. 667, exp. 2, fols. 73r–78r.

48. See Zeitlin, *Cultural Politics in Colonial Tehuantepec*, chaps. 5 and 6.

49. On rebellions in the Andean highlands, see C. Walker, *Tupac Amaru Rebellion*; C. Walker, *Smoldering Ashes*; Serulnikov, *Subverting Colonial Authority*; Thomson, *We Alone Will Rule*.

50. AGN, Criminal, vol. 667, exp. 2, fol. 85v.

51. AGN, Criminal, vol. 667, exp. 2, fol. 87v.

52. AGN, Criminal, vol. 667, exp. 2, fols. 91v–92r.

53. AGN, Criminal, vol. 667, exp. 2, fol. 99r.

54. AGN, Criminal, vol. 667, exp. 2, fol. 117v.

55. On the varieties of punishment in the Spanish Empire and its connection to state-building, see Czeblakow, "Prison by Any Other Name."

56. AGN, Criminal, vol. 9, exp. 5, fols. 62r–v. The surgeon's report describing Cruz's injuries appears on fols. 56r–57r.

57. AGN, Criminal, vol. 9, exp. 5, fols. 138r–39r.

58. AGN, Criminal, vol. 9, exp. 5, fol. 140.

59. AGN, Criminal, vol. 9, exp. 5, fol. 141.

60. AGN, Criminal, vol. 28, exp. 5, fols. 145r–47v.

61. Scardaville, "Alcohol Abuse and Tavern Reform," 644–47. On drinking patterns in the countryside, see Taylor, *Drinking, Homicide, and Rebellion*.

62. Taylor, *Drinking, Homicide, and Rebellion*, 64–66, 91.

63. Johnson and Lipsett-Rivera, *Faces of Honor*, 12; Johnson, "Dangerous Words, Provocative Gestures, and Violent Acts," 132.

64. AGN, Criminal, vol. 28, exp. 5, fol. 147r.

65. AGN, Criminal, vol. 28, exp. 5, fol. 148r.

66. AGN, Criminal, vol. 28, exp. 5, fol. 149r.

67. AGN, Criminal, vol. 28, exp. 5, fol. 149r.

68. AGN, Criminal, vol. 28, exp. 5, fols. 150r–v.

69. AGN, Criminal, vol. 28, exp. 5, fol. 154r.

70. AGN, Criminal, vol. 28, exp. 5, fol. 154v. My emphasis.
71. AGN, Criminal, vol. 28, exp. 5, fols. 154v–55r.
72. Hevia Bolaños, *Curia Philipica*, 202.
73. AGN, Criminal, vol. 28, exp. 5, fols. 155v–56r.
74. AGN, Criminal, vol. 28, exp. 5, fol. 160r.
75. Herzog, *Upholding Justice*, 9.
76. AGN, Criminal, vol. 712, exp. 3, fols. 197r, 199r.
77. AGN, Criminal, vol. 712, exp. 3, fol. 198r.
78. AGN, Criminal, vol. 712, exp. 3, fols. 208v–9r.
79. AGN, Criminal, vol. 712, exp. 3, fols. 199r–206r.
80. AGN, Criminal, vol. 712, exp. 3, fol. 206r.
81. Although women in nineteenth-century Mexico City generally married later in life, the mean age, according to an 1811 census, was 22.7 years, placing María Getrudis well past her prime to marry. Arrom, *Women of Mexico City*, 116–17.
82. AGN, Criminal, vol. 712, exp. 3, fols. 209v–12r.
83. AGN, Criminal, vol. 712, exp. 3, fols. 228r–29v.
84. In the 1811 census, 22 percent of the women residing in Mexico City were enumerated as single; most of these were between the ages of forty-five and fifty-four, an indication that they never married. Arrom, *Women of Mexico City*, 111.
85. Socolow, *Women of Colonial Latin America*, 66–67. In the colonial Spanish America, the other major socio-group likely to engage in legal marital unions were Indians, particularly those residing in rural Indigenous communities or living on missions. The *castas* and poor Spaniards were more likely to engage in both short- and long-term informal unions. Socolow, 70.
86. Socolow, 68.
87. Lipsett-Rivera, "Slap in the Face of Honor."
88. AGN, Criminal, vol. 712, exp. 3, fol. 200r.
89. AGN, Criminal, vol. 712, exp. 3, fols. 238v–39r.
90. AGN, Criminal, vol. 712, exp. 3, fols. 339v–40r.
91. AGN, Criminal, vol. 712, exp. 3, fols. 339v–340r.
92. AGN, Criminal, vol. 712, exp. 3, fols. 340r–v.
93. The initial medical report is located in AGN, Criminal, vol. 712, exp. 3, fols. 228v–29v.
94. AGN, Criminal, vol. 712, exp. 3, fols. 246r–47r.
95. AGN, Criminal, vol. 712, exp. 3, fols. 249r–v.
96. AGN, Criminal, vol. 712, exp. 3, fols. 251r–52v.
97. AGN, Criminal, vol. 712, exp. 3, fols. 252r–v.
98. AGN, Criminal, vol. 712, exp. 3, fols. 255r–v.
99. AGN, Criminal, vol. 712, exp. 3, fols. 257r–v.
100. AGN, Criminal, vol. 712, exp. 3, fols. 259r–v.
101. AGN, Criminal, vol. 712, exp. 3, fols. 265r–66v.
102. AGN, Criminal, vol. 712, exp. 3, fol. 268r.
103. AGN, Hospitales, vol. 62, exp. 5, fol. 134r.
104. AGN, Hospitales, vol. 62, exp. 5, fols. 129–130.
105. AGN, Hospitales, vol. 62, exp. 5, fol. 134.

106. AGN, Hospitales, vol. 62, exp. 5, fols. 117–118.
107. AGN, Hospitales, vol. 62, exp. 5, fols. 158r–59r.
108. AGN, Hospitales, vol. 62, exp. 5, fol. 152.
109. AGN, Hospitales, vol. 62, exp. 5, fol. 140.
110. AGN, Hospitales, vol. 62, exp. 5, fols. 167r–68r.
111. AGN, Hospitales, vol. 62, exp. 5, fols. 172r–v. San Andres was a general hospital in Lima that had a ward for mad patients.
112. AGN, Hospitales, vol. 62, exp. 5, fol. 177r.
113. AGN, Hospitales, vol. 62, exp. 5, fol. 190r.
114. AGN, Hospitales, vol. 62, exp. 5, fol. 216r.
115. AGN, Hospitales, vol. 62, exp. 5, fol. 214r.
116. On elite views toward poverty, mendacity, and vagrancy, see Sacristán, "Filantropismo, improductividad, y delincuencia"; Arrom, *Containing the Poor*, chap. 1.
117. See Spierenburg, *Prison Experience*, chap. 2; Finzsch and Jütte, *Institutions of Confinement*.
118. Elizabeth Mellyn has emphasized the centrality of the family in providing long-term custodial solutions in cases involving the criminally insane prior to the establishment of mental hospitals. See Mellyn, *Mad Tuscans and Their Families*, esp. chap. 2.
119. AGN, Criminal, vol. 360, exp. 1, fols. 1r–2r.
120. AGN, Criminal, vol. 360, exp. 1, fols. 2v, 167r.
121. AGN, Criminal, vol. 360, exp. 1, fols. 57r–60r.
122. AGN, Criminal, vol. 360, exp. 1, fols. 50r–v; 74r–v.
123. AGN, Criminal, vol. 360, exp. 1, fol. 155r.
124. Haslip-Viera, *Crime and Punishment*, 88–92.
125. AGN, Criminal, vol. 360, exp.1, fols. 149r–v.
126. AGN, Criminal, vol. 360, exp. 1, fols. 149v–50r.
127. AGN, Criminal, vol. 360, exp. 1, fol. 202v.

Conclusion

1. Lynch, *Spanish American Revolutions*, 304–6.
2. Schwaller, *History of the Catholic Church in Latin America*, 121.
3. Silvia Arrom has also noted the scarity of records for the Poor House in the early decades of the nineteenth century, a pattern, she observes, that recurred whenever the institution "weathered trying times." Arrom, *Containing the Poor*, 159.
4. Sacristán, *Locura y disidencia en el México ilustrado*, 64. On the intersection of madness and revolutionary rhetoric, see Van Young, "Millennium on the Northern Marches."
5. Arrom, *Containing the Poor*, 158; Sánchez Uriarte, *Entre la misericordia y el desprecio*, 45; Howard, *Royal Indian Hospital*, 71. On local rebellions on the eve of independence, see Van Young, *Other Rebellion*.
6. Quoted in Arrom, *Containing the Poor*, 160; see AGN, Policía, vol. 30, fol. 1r.

7. On this decree and its implementation in the Americas, see Chowning, "The Consolidación de Vales Reales in the Bishopric of Michoacán"; Hamnett, "Appropriation of Mexican Church Wealth."

8. AGN, Indiferente Virreinal, caja 0974, exp. 17, fols. 1rr-2. The Royal Indian Hospital also appears to have discontinued making payments to the Hospital de San Lázaro for the treatment of Indigenous patients suffering from leprosy. See Sánchez Uriarte, *Entre la misericordia y el desprecio*, 45.

9. Ballenger, "Modernizing Madness," 63.

10. AGN, Hospitales, vol. 24, exp. 18, fols. 413r-v.

11. AGN, Hospitales, vol. 24, exp. 18, fols. 415v, 414v-15r.

12. AGN, Hospitales, vol. 24, exp. 18, fols. 418r-v.

13. AGN, Hospitales, vol. 24, exp. 18, fol. 420.

14. Muriel, *Hospitales de la Nueva España*, 2:283-85. See also Mendoza García, "La secularización de los hospitales y el ayuntamiento en la ciudad de México."

15. Domínguez, "A State Within a State."

16. AHDF, Hospitales e Iglesia de San Hipólito, vol. 2300, exp. 16, fol. 1r.

17. AHDF, Hospitales e Iglesia de San Hipólito, vol. 2300, exp. 13, fol. 1r

18. Rivera Cambas, *México pintoresco, artistico y monumental*, 1:388; AGN, Indiferente Virreinal, caja 5746, exp. 18.

19. Ballenger, "Modernizing Madness," 65.

20. Ballenger, 67-68.

21. Calderon de la Barca, *Life in Mexico*, quoted in Ballenger, "Modernizing Madness," 65.

22. Rivera-Garza, "Dangerous Minds."

23. Arrom, *Containing the Poor*, 207. Arrom borrows the quote from the historian Armida de Gonzalez.

24. Ballenger, "Modernizing Madness," 73-74.

25. Ballenger, 78-79.

26. Rivera-Garza, "Dangerous Minds," 42.

27. Rivera-Garza, 43.

28. Goldstein, *Console and Classify*, 197-210.

29. Ballenger, "Modernizing Madness," 177-88, 117-18, and chap. 3 more generally.

Bibliography

Archival Sources

Archivo General de la Indias, Seville, Spain
  México
Archivo General de la Nación, Mexico City, Mexico
  Bienes Nacionales
  Carceles y Presidios
  Clero Regular y Secular
  Correspondencia de Virreyes
  Criminal
  Gobierno Virreinal
  Hospitales
  Indiferente Virreinal
  Inquisición
  Obras Pías
  Templos y Conventos
  Tierras
Archivo Histórico de la Secretaria de Salud, Mexico City, Mexico
  Fondo Beneficiencia Pública, Sección Establecimientos Hospitalarios, Serie Hospital de San Hipólito
  Fondo Hospitales y Hospicios, Sección Hospital de San Hipólito
  Fondo Hospitales y Hospicios, Sección Hospital del Divino Salvador
Archivo Histórico del Distrito Federal, Mexico City, Mexico
  Fondo Ayuntamiento Gobierno del Districto Federal, Sección Hospital del Divino Salvador
  Fondo Ayuntamiento Gobierno del Districto Federal, Sección Hospitales e Iglesia de San Hipólito
  Fondo Ayuntamiento Gobierno del Districto Federal, Sección Temporalidades, Jesuitas
Instituto Nacional de Antropología e Historia, Mexico City, Mexico
  Fondo Hospital Real de los Naturales

Published Primary Sources

Cabrera y Quintero, Cayetano de. *Escudo de Armas de México*. Mexico, 1746.
Calderón de la Barca, Francis. *Life in Mexico*. Berkeley: University of California Press, 1983.
Covarrubias Orozco, Sebastián de. *Tesoro de la lengua castellana, o española*. Madrid, 1611.

Díaz de Arce, Juan. *Libro de la vida del próximo evangelico, el venerable Padre Bernardino Alvarez*. Mexico, 1762.

Dorantes de Carranza, Baltasar. *Sumaria relación de las cosas de la Nueva España*. Edited by José Maria de Agreda y Sánchez. Mexico City: Museo Nacional, 1902. Manuscript first written in 1604.

Eimerich, Nicolau. *Manual de inquisidores para uso de Las inquisiciones de España y Portugal*. Nabu Press, 2010.

Esteyneffer, Juan. *Florilegio medicinal*. Mexico, 1712.

Fernández de Lizardi, José Joaquín. *The Mangy Parrot: The Life and Times of Periquillo Sarniento, Written by Himself for His Children*. Translated by David L. Frye. Indianapolis: Hackett, 2004. Originally published in Spanish as *El periquillo sarniento* in 1816.

Gaceta de México. Vol. 1, no. 5. Mexico, 1722.

Gante, Pedro de. "Carta de Fray Pedro de Gante al Emperador D. Carlos." *Cartas de Indias*. No. 8. Madrid, 1877.

García, Francisco. *Vida de el venerable Bernardino Alvarez, fundador de el Orden de la Caridad*. Madrid, 1678.

Hevia Bolaños, Juan de. *Curia Philipica*. Madri, 1790. Originally published in 1603.

La administración de D. Frey Antonio María de Bucareli y Ursúa. Mexico: Talleres Gráficos de la Nación, 1936.

Lardizábal y Uribe, Manuel de. *Discurso sobre las penas*. Mexico, 1776.

Las Siete Partidas. Vol. 1, *The Medieval Church: The World of Clerics and Laymen*. Translated by Samuel Parsons Scott. Edited by Robert I. Burns. Philadelphia: University of Pennsylvania Press, 2001.

Las Siete Partidas. Vol. 5, *Underworlds: The Dead, the Criminal, and the Marginalized*. Translated by Samuel Parsons Scott. Edited by Robert I. Burns. Philadelphia: University of Pennsylvania Press, 2001.

Recopilación de Leyes de los Reynos de las Indias. Tomo 1. Consejo de la Hispanidad, 1943.

Rivera Cambas, Manuel. *México pintoresco, artístico y monumental*. 3 vols. Mexico, DF: Imprenta de la Reforma, 1800-83.

Solórzano Pereira, Juan de. *Politica Indiana*. Vol. 2. Madrid, 1739.

Venegas, Juan Manuel. *Compendio de la medicina practica*. Mexico, 1788.

Viera, Juan de. *Breve y compendiosa narracion de la ciudad de Mexico, corte y cabeza de toda la America septentrional*. *La ciudad de Mexico en el siglo XVIII (1690-1780)*. Edited by Gonzalo Obregón. Mexico, D.F.: Consejo Nacional Para la Cultura y las Artes, 1990.

Villaroel, Hipólito. *Enfermedades politicas que padece la capital de esta Nueva España*. Mexico, D.F.: Editorial Joaquin Mortiz, 2002.

Secondary Sources

Aceves Pastrana, Patricia. *El Hospital General de San Andrés: la modernización de la medicina novohispana 1770-1883*. Mexico, D.F.: Universidad Autónoma Metropolitana, 2002.

Ackerknecht, Erwin H. "Political Prisoners in French Mental Institutions before 1789, during the Revolution, and under Napoleon I." *Medical History* 19 (1975): 250–55.

Aguirre, Carlos A., and Robert Buffington, eds. *Reconstructing Criminality in Latin America*. Wilmington, DE: Scholarly Resources, 2000.

Alberro, Solange. *Inquisición y sociedad en Mexico 1571–1700*. Mexico, D.F.: Fondo de Cultral Económica, 1988.

Albert, Salvador Bernabéu. "Nuevas líneas de investigación: Tebanillo González, un loco ante la inquisición mexicana (1789–1790)." *Anuario de Estudios Americanos* 75, no. 2 (2018): 699–729.

Alexander, Franz G., and Sheldon T. Selesnick. *The History of Psychiatry: An Evaluation of Psychiatric Thought from Prehistoric Times to the Present*. New York: Harper & Row, 1967.

Allderidge, Patricia. "Bedlam: Fact or Fantasy?" *The Anatomy of Madness: Essays in the History of Psychiatry*. Vol. 2, *Institutions and Society*, edited by W. F. Bynum, Roy Porter, and Michael Sheperd, 17–33. London: Routledge, 1985.

Anderson, Warwick. *Colonial Pathologies: American Tropical Medicine, Race, and Hygiene in the Philippines*. Durham, NC: Duke University Press, 2006.

Andrews, Jonathan, Asa Briggs, Roy Porter, Penny Tucker, and Keir Waddington. *The History of Bethlem*. London: Routledge, 1997.

Araya Espinoza, Alejandra. "De espirituales a histéricas: Las beatas del siglo XVIII en la Nueva España." *Historia* 37, no. 1 (2004): 5–32.

Arrizabalaga, Jon. "Poor Relief in Counter-Reformation Castile: An Overview." In *Health Care and Poor Relief in Counter-Reformation Europe*, edited by Ole Peter Grell, Andrew Cunningham, and Jon Arrizabalaga, 151–76. London: Routledge, 1999.

Arrom, Silvia Marina. *Containing the Poor: The Mexico City Poor House, 1774–1871*. Durham, NC: Duke University Press, 2000

———. *The Women of Mexico City, 1790–1857*. Stanford, CA: Stanford University Press, 1985.

Ballenger, Stephanie. "Modernizing Madness: Doctors, Patients and Asylums in Nineteenth-Century Mexico." PhD diss., University of California, Berkeley, 2009.

Barry, Jonathan, and Colin Jones. *Medicine and Charity Before the Welfare State*. London: Routledge, 1991.

Barta, Roger. *Melancolía y Cultura: Las enfermedades del alma en el Siglo de Oro*. Barcelona: Editorial Anagrama S.A., 2001.

———. *La jaula de la melancolía: identidad y metamorphosis del Mexicano*. Mexico, DF: Delbolsillo, 2005.

Baquero, Aurelia. *Bosquejo histórico del Hospital Real y General de Nuestra Señora de la Gracía de Zaragoza*. Zaragoza: Seccíon de Estudios Médicos Aragoneses, Institución "Fernando el Católico," 1952.

Beecher, Donald. "Witches, the Possessed, and the Diseases of the Imagination." In *Diseases of the Imagination and Imaginary Disease in the Early Modern Period*, edited by Yasmin Haskell, 103–38. Turnhout: Brepols, 2011.

Behar, Ruth. "Sex and Sin: Witchcraft and the Devil in Late-Colonial Mexico." *American Ethnologist* 14, no. 1 (1987): 34–54.

———. "Sexual Witchcraft: Colonialism and Women's Powers: Views from the Inquisition." In *Sexuality and Marriage in Colonial Latin America*, edited by Asunción Lavrin. Lincoln: University of Nebraska Press, 1992.

Bennassar, Bartolomé. "Patterns of the Inquisitorial Mind as the Basis for a Pedagogy of Fear." In *The Spanish Inquisition and the Inquisitorial Mind*, edited by Angel Alcalá, 177–84. New York: Columbia University Press, 1987.

Berkstein Kanarek, Celia. "El Hospital del Divino Salvador." Tésis de Licenciatura. Universidad Nacional Autónoma de México, 1981.

Bertucci, Paola. *Artisanal Enlightenment: Science and the Mechanical Arts in Old Regime France*. New Haven, CT: Yale University Press, 2017.

Bierne, Piers. *Inventing Criminology: Essays on the Rise of "Homo Criminalis."* Albany: State University of New York Press, 1993.

Bleichmar, Daniela. *Visible Empire: Botanical Expeditions and Visual Culture in the Hispanic Enlightenment*. Chicago: The University of Chicago Press, 2012.

Bobb, Bernard E. *The Viceregency of Antonio Maria Bucareli in New Spain, 1771–1779*. Austin: University of Texas Press, 1962.

Borah, Woodrow. "Social Welfare and Social Obligation in New Spain: A Tentative Assessment." *Congreso internacional de Americanista, España 1964: Actas y Memorias* 36, no. 4 (1966): 45–57.

Bouley, Bradford. *Pious Postmortems: Anatomy, Sanctity, and the Catholic Church in Early Modern Europe*. Philadelphia: University of Pennsylvania Press, 2017.

Boyer, Richard. *The Lives of the Bigamists: Marriage, Family, and Community in Colonial Mexico*. Abridged ed. Albuquerque: University of New Mexico Press, 1995.

Brading, D. A. *Church and State in Bourbon Mexico: The Diocese of Michoacán, 1749–1810*. Cambridge: Cambridge University Press 1994.

———. *The First America: The Spanish Monarchy, Creole Patriots, and the Liberal State, 1492–1867*. Cambridge: Cambridge University Press, 1991.

———. *Mexican Phoenix, Our Lady of Guadalupe: Image and Tradition across Five Centuries*. Cambridge: Cambridge University Press, 2001.

———. "Tridentine Catholicism and Enlightened Despotism in Bourbon Mexico." *Journal of Latin American Studies* 15, no. 1 (1983): 1–22.

Brodman, James William. *Charity and Welfare: Hospitals and the Poor in Medieval Catalonia*. Philadelphia: University of Pennsylvania Press, 1998.

Buffington, Robert M. *Criminal and Citizen in Modern Mexico*. Lincoln: University of Nebraska Press, 2000.

Burns, Kathryn. *Colonial Habits: Convents and the Spiritual Economy of Cuzco, Peru*. Durham, NC: Duke University Press, 1999.

Burton, Jeffrey D., and Ulrich L. Lehner. *Enlightenment and Catholicism in Europe: A Transnational History*. Notre Dame: University of Notre Dame Press, 2014.

Butterwick, Richard. "Peripheries of the Enlightenment: An Introduction." In *Peripheries of Enlightenment: Studies in Voltaire and the Eighteenth Century*, edited by Richard Butterwick, Simon Davies, and Gabriel Sánchez-Espinosa, 1–16. Oxford: Oxford University Press, 2008.

Bynum, Caroline Walker. "The Female Body and Religious Practice in the Later Middle Ages." In *Fragmentation and Redemption: Essays on Gender and the Human Body in Medieval Religion*, 181–238. New York: Zone Books, 1992.

Caciola, Nancy. *Discerning Spirits: Divine and Demonic Possession in the Middle Ages*. Ithaca, NY: Cornell University Press, 2003.

Cahill, David. "Financing Health Care in the Viceroyalty of Peru: The Hospitals of Lima in the Late Colonial Period." *Americas* 52, no. 2 (1995): 123–54.

Calabritto, Monica. "A Case of the Melancholic Humor and *Dilucida Intervalla*." *Intellectual History Review* 18, no. 1 (2008): 139–54.

———. "Medical and Moral Dimensions of Feminine Madness: Representing Madwomen in the Renaissance." *Forum Italicum* 36, no. 1 (2002): 26–52.

Calderón Narváez, Guillermo. "Hospitales psiquiátricos de México: desde la colonia hasta la acutalidad." *Revista mexicana de neurología y psiquiatria* 7, no. 3 (1966): 111–26.

Callahan, William J. "The Problem of Confinement: An Aspect of Poor Relief in Eighteenth-Century Spain." *Hispanic American Historical Review* 51, no. 1 (1971): 1–24.

Cañeque, Alejandro. "Theater of Power: Writing and Representing the Auto de Fe in Colonial Mexico." *Americas* 52, no. 3 (1996): 321–43.

Cañizares-Esguerra, Jorge. *How to Write the History of the New World: Histories, Epistemologies, and Identities in the Eighteenth-Century Atlantic World*. Stanford, CA: Stanford University Press, 2001.

———. *Nature, Empire, and Nation: Exploration of the History of Science in the Iberian World*. Stanford, CA: Stanford University Press, 2006.

———. "New World, New Stars: Patriotic Astrology and the Invention of Indian and Creole Bodies in Colonial Spanish America, 1600–1650." *American Historical Review* 104, no. 1 (1999): 33–68.

———. *Puritan Conquistadors: Iberianizing the Atlantic, 1550–1700*. Stanford, CA: Stanford University Press, 2006.

Canterla, Francisco, and Martín de Tovar. "La orden hospitalaria de San Hipólito Mártir hasta la fecha de su reforma." *Anuario de Estudios Americanos* 37 (1980): 127–55.

Carbajal López, David. "Exclaustración o continuidad: conventos hosptiales y frailes en Veracruz, 1820–1834." *Ulúa* 11 (2008): 45–70.

Carrera, Elena. "Anger and the Mind-Body Connection in Medieval and Early Modern Medicine." In *Emotions and Health, 1200–1700*, edited by Elena Carrera, 95–146. Leiden: Brill, 2013.

———. "Understanding Mental Disturbance in Sixteenth- and Seventeenth-Century Spain: Medical Approaches." *Bulletin of Spanish Studies* 87, no. 8 (2010): 105–36.

Castañeda Delgado, Paulino. "La condición miserable del Indio y sus privilegios." *Anuario de Estudios Americanos* 28 (1971): 245–335.

Cervantes, Fernando. *The Devil in the New World: The Impact of Diabolism in New Spain*. New Haven, CT: Yale University Press, 1994.

Chase, Bradley Lewis. "Medical Care for the Poor in Mexico City, 1770–1810: An Aspect of Spanish Colonial *Beneficencia*." PhD diss., University of Maryland, 1975.

Chowning, Margaret. "The Consolidación de Vales Reales in the Bishopric of Michoacán." *Hispanic American Historical Review* 69, no. 3 (1989): 451–78.

———. "Convent Reform, Catholic Reform, and Bourbon Reform in Eighteenth-Century New Spain: The View from the Nunnery." *Hispanic American Historical Review* 85, no. 1 (2005): 1–37.

Cohen, Martin A. *The Martyr: Luis de Caravajal, a Secret Jew in Sixteenth-Century Mexico*. Albuquerque: University of New Mexico Press, 1973.

Cope, Douglas. *The Limits of Racial Domination: Plebian Society in Colonial Mexico City, 1660–1720*. Madison: University of Wisconsin Press, 1994.

Cueto, Marcos, and Steven Palmer. *Medicine and Public Health in Latin America: A History*. Cambridge: Cambridge University, 2015.

Cunningham, Andrew. *The Medical Enlightenment in the Eighteenth Century*. Cambridge: Cambridge University Press, 1997.

Cutter, Charles R. *The Legal Culture of Northern New Spain, 1700–1810*. Albuquerque: University of New Mexico Press, 1995.

Czeblakow, Agnieszka. "A Prison by Any Other Name: Incarceration in Seventeenth and Eighteenth-Century Audiencia de Quito." PhD diss., Emory University, 2011.

Daston, Lorraine. "Afterword: The Ethos of Enlightenment." In *The Sciences of Enlightened Europe*, edited by William Clark, Jan Golinski, and Simon Schaffer. Chicago: University of Chicago Press, 1999.

De Bujanda, Jesús M. "Recent Historiography of the Spanish Inquisition (1977–1988): Balance and Perspective." In *Cultural Encounters: The Impact of the Inquisition in Spain and the New World*, edited by Mary Elizabeth Perry and Anne J. Cruz, 221–47. Berkeley: University of California Press, 1991.

De Renzi, Silvia. "Medical Expertise, Bodies, and the Law in Early Modern Courts." *Isis* 98 (2007): 315–22.

———. "Witnesses of the Body: Medico-legal Cases in Seventeenth-Century Rome." *Studies in the History and Philosophy of Science* 33 (2002): 219–42.

De Vos, Paula. "The Art of Pharmacy in Seventeenth and Eighteenth Century Mexico." PhD diss., University of California, Berkeley, 2001.

———. "Research, Development, and Empire: State Support of Science in the Later Spanish Empire." *Colonial Latin American Review* 15, no. 1 (2006): 55–79.

Digby, Anne. *Madness, Morality, and Medicine: A Study of the York Retreat 1796-1914*. Cambridge: Cambridge University Press, 1985.

Dols, Michael W. *Manjun: The Madman in Medieval Islamic Society*. Oxford: Clarendon Press, 1992.

Domínguez, Juan Pablo. "A State Within a State: The Inquisition in Enlightenment Thought." *History of European Ideas* 43, no. 4 (2017): 376–388.

Edington, Claire. *Beyond the Asylum: Mental Illness in French Colonial Vietnam*. Ithaca, NY: Cornell University Press, 2019.

———. "Going in and Getting out of the Colonial Asylum: Families and Psychiatric Care in French Indochina." *Comparative Studies in Society and History* 55, no. 3 (2013): 725–55.

Eghigian, Greg, ed. *The Routledge History of Madness and Mental Health*. New York: Routledge, 2017.
Ernst, Waltraud. *Mad Tales from the Raj: Colonial Psychiatry in South Asia, 1800-58*. London: Anthem Press, 2010.
Estes, J. Worth. "The Reception of American Drugs in Europe, 1500-1650." In *Searching for the Secrets of Nature: The Life and Works of Dr. Francisco Hernandez*, edited by Simon Varey, Rafael Chabrán, and Dora B. Weiner, 111-21. Stanford, CA: Stanford University Press, 2000.
Ewalt, Margaret R. *Peripheral Wonders: Nature, Knowledge, and Enlightenment in Eighteenth-Century Orinoco*. Lewisburg, NJ: Bucknell University Press, 2008.
Fanon, Frantz. *The Wretched of the Earth*. Translated by Richard Philcox. New York: Grove Press, 2005. First published 1963 by Grove Press.
Farriss, Nancy. *Crown and Clergy in Colonial Mexico, 1759-1821: The Crisis of Ecclesiastical Privilege*. London: Athlone Press, 1968.
Few, Martha. *For All of Humanity: Mesoamerican and Colonial Medicine in Enlightenment Guatemala*. Tucson: University of Arizona Press, 2015.
———. *Women Who Lead Evil Lives: Gender, Religion, and the Politics of Power in Colonial Guatemala*. Austin: University of Texas Press, 2002.
Few, Martha, Zeb Tortorici, and Adam Warren. *Baptism Through Incision: The Postmortem Cesarean Operation in the Spanish Empire*. University Park: The Pennsylvania State University Press, 2020.
Fields, Sherry. *Pestilence and Headcolds: Encountering Illness in Colonial Mexico*. New York: Columbia University Press, 2008.
Finzsch, Norbert, and Robert Jütte, eds. *Institutions of Confinement: Hospitals, Asylums, and Prisons in Western Europe and North America, 1500-1950*. Cambridge: Cambridge University Press, 1996.
Flores, Enrique. "Papeles de Tebanillo González." *Revista de Literaturas Populares* 12, no. 1 (2012): 5-44.
———. "Tebanillo González, heteróclito," *Litoral* 43 (2011): 62-80.
Flynn, Maureen. "Blasphemy and the Play of Anger in Sixteenth-Century Spain." *Past and Present* 149 (1995): 29-56.
———. *Sacred Charity: Confraternities and Social Welfare in Spain, 1400-1700*. London: Macmillan Press, 1989.
Foster, George M. *Culture and Conquest: America's Spanish Heritage*. New York: Wenner-Gren Foundation for Anthropological Research, 1960.
———. *Hippocrates' Latin American Legacy: Humoral Medicine in the New World*. Langhorne, PA: Gordon and Breach. 1994.
Foucault, Michel. *Discipline and Punish: The Birth of the Prison*. Translated by Alan Sheridan. New York: Vintage Books, 1995. First American edition published 1978 by Pantheon.
———. *Madness and Civilization: A History of Insanity in the Age of Reason*. Translated by Richard Howard. New York: Vintage Books, 1988. First American edition published 1965 by Pantheon.
García-Ballester, Luis. "The Circulation and Use of Medical Manuscripts in Arabic in 16th Century Spain." *Journal for the History of Arabic Science* 3, no. 2 (1979): 183-99.

———. "Galenism and Medical Teaching at the University of Salamanca in the Fifteenth Century." *Dynamis* 20 (2000): 209-47.
Gay, Peter. *The Enlightenment: An Interpretation*. Vol. 2, *The Science of Freedom*. New York: W. W. Norton, 1969.
Gerbi, Antonello. *The Dispute of the New World: The History of a Polemic, 1750-1900*. Pittsburgh: University of Pittsburgh Press, 1973.
Giles, Mary E. *Women and the Inquisition: Spain and the New World*. Baltimore: Johns Hopkins University Press, 1999.
Ginzburg, Carlo. *The Cheese and the Worms: The Cosmos of a Sixteenth-Century Miller*. Baltimore: Johns Hopkins University Press, 1980.
———. "The Inquisitor as Anthropologist." In *Clues, Myth, and the Historical Method*, translated by John Tedeschi and Anne C. Tedeschi. Baltimore: Johns Hopkins University Press, 1989.
Glascow, Sharon Bailey. *Constructing Mexico City: Colonial Conflicts over Culture, Space and Authority*. London: Palgrave Macmillan, 2010.
Goldberg, Ann. *Sex, Religion, and the Making of Modern Madness: The Eberbach Asylum and German Society, 1815-1849*. Oxford: Oxford University Press, 1999.
Goldin, Grace. *Work of Mercy: A Picture History of Hospitals*. Boston: Boston Mills Press, 1994.
Goldstein, Jan. *Console and Classify: The French Psychiatric Profession in the Nineteenth Century*. Cambridge: Cambridge University Press, 1987. Reprinted with a new afterword by the author. Chicago: University of Chicago Press, 2001. Page references are to the 2001 edition.
Gómez,, Pablo F. *The Experiential Caribbean: Creating Knowledge and Healing in the Early Modern Atlantic*. Chapel Hill: University of North Carolina Press, 2017.
Gonzalbo Aizpuru, Pilar. "Violencia y discordia en las relaciones personales en la ciudad de Mexico a fines del siglo XVIII." *Historia Mexicana* 51, no. 2 (2001): 233-59.
González Duro, Enrique. *Historia de la Locura en España*. 3 vols. Madrid, 1994.
Goodheart, Lawrence B. *Mad Yankees: The Hartford Retreat for the Insane and Nineteenth-Century Psychiatry*. Amherst: University of Massachusetts Press, 2003.
Green, Toby. *Inquisition: Reign of Fear*. New York: St. Martin's Press, 2007.
Greenleaf, Richard E. "Historiography of the Mexican Inquisition: Evolution of Interpretations and Methodologies." In *Cultural Encounters: The Impact of the Inquisition in Spain and the New World*, edited by Mary Elizabeth Perry and Anne J. Cruz, 248-76. Berkeley: University of California Press, 1991.
———. "The Inquisition in Eighteenth-Century New Mexico." *New Mexico Historical Review* 60, no. 1 (1985): 29-60.
———. "The Mexican Inquisition and the Enlightenment, 1763-1805." *New Mexico Historical Review* 41, no. 3 (1966): 181-96.
———. *The Mexican Inquisition of the Sixteenth Century*. Albuquerque: University of New Mexico Press, 1969.
Grell, Ole Peter, and Andrew Cunningham, eds. *Medicine and Religion in Enlightenment Europe*. New York: Routledge, 2017.
Grell, Ole Peter, Andrew Cunningham, and Jon Arrizabalaga, eds. *Health Care and Poor Relief in Counter-Reformation Europe*. London: Routledge, 1999.

Gruzinski, Serge. *The Conquest of Mexico: The Incorporation of Indian Societies into the Western World, 16th–18th Centuries*. Translated by Eileen Corrigan. Cambridge: Polity Press, 1993.

Guerra, Francisco. *El hospital en Hispanoamerica y Filipinas, 1492–1898*. Madrid: Ministerio de Sanidad y Consumo, 1994.

Guijarro Oliveras, J. "Politica Sanitaria en las Leyes de Indias," *Archivo Iberoamericano de Historia de la Medicina y antropología médica* 9 (1957): 255–62.

Gutting, Gary. "Foucault and the History of Madness." In *The Cambridge Companion to Foucault*, edited by Gary Gutting, 49–73. Cambridge: Cambridge University Press, 2005.

Haliczer, Stephen. *Sexuality in the Confessional: A Sacrament Profaned*. New York: Oxford University Press, 1996.

Hamnett, Brian R. "The Appropriation of Mexican Church Wealth by the Spanish Bourbon Government: The 'Consolidación de Vales Reales,' 1805–1809." *Journal of Latin American Studies* 1, no. 2 (1969): 85–113.

Haslip-Viera, Gabriel. *Crime and Punishment in Late Colonial Mexico City, 1692–1810*. Albuquerque: University of New Mexico Press, 1999.

———. "The Underclass." In *Cities and Society in Colonial Latin America*, edited by Louisa Schell Hoberman and Susan Midgen Socolow, 285–312. Albuquerque: University of New Mexico Press, 1986.

Headrick, Daniel. *Tools of Empire: Technology and European Imperialism in the Nineteenth Century*. Oxford: Oxford University Press, 1991.

Henderson, John. *The Renaissance Hospital: Healing the Body and Healing the Soul*. New Haven, CT: Yale University Press, 2006.

Hernández Sáenz, Luz María. *Learning to Heal: The Medical Profession in Colonial Mexico, 1767–1831*. New York: Peter Lang, 1997.

Herzog, Tamar. *Defining Nations: Immigrants and Citizens in Early Modern Spain and Spanish America*. New Haven, CT: Yale University Press, 2003.

———. *Upholding Justice: Society, State, and the Penal System in Quito, 1650–1750*. Ann Arbor: University of Michigan Press, 2004.

Hesse, Carla. "Towards a New Topography of Enlightenment." *European Review of History* 13, no. 3 (2006): 499–508.

Horden, Peregrine. "A Non-natural Environment: Medicine without Doctors and the Medieval European Hospital." In *The Medieval Hospital and Medical Practice*, edited by Barbara S. Bowers, 133–46. Aldershot: Ashgate, 2007.

Houston, R.A. *Madness and Society in Eighteenth-Century Scotland*. Oxford: Oxford University Press, 2000.

———. "Clergy and Care of the Insane in Eighteenth-Century Britain." *Church History* 73.1 (2004): 114–138.

Howard, David A. *The Royal Indian Hospital of Mexico City*. Tempe: Arizona State University, 1980.

Huguet-Termes, Teresa. "New World Materia Medica in Spanish Renaissance Medicine: From Scholarly Reception to Practical Impact." *Medical History* 45, no. 3 (2001): 359–76.

Huguet-Termes, Teresa, and Jon Arrizabalaga. "Hospital Care for the Insane in Barcelona, 1400–1700." *Bulletin of Spanish Studies: Hispanic Studies and Researches on Spain, Portugal and Latin America* 87, no. 8 (2010): 81–104.

Jackson, Lynette. *Surfacing Up: Psychiatry and Social Order in Colonial Zimbabwe, 1908–1968*. Ithaca, NY: Cornell University Press, 2005.

Jackson, Stanley W. *Melancholia and Depression from Hippocratic Times to Modern Times*. New Haven, CT: Yale University Press, 1986.

―――. "Melancholia and Mechanical Explanation in Eighteenth-Century Medicine." *Journal of the History of Medicine and the Allied Sciences* 38 (1983): 298–319.

―――. "Melancholia and the Waning of Humoral Theory." *Journal of the History of Medicine* 33 (1978): 367–76.

Jacob, Margaret C. *The Secular Enlightenment*. Princeton: Princeton University Press, 2019.

―――. *The Radical Enlightenment: Pantheists, Freemasons, and Republicans*. London: Allen and Unwin, 1981.

Jaffary, Nora E. *False Mystics: Deviant Orthodoxy in Colonial in Mexico*. Lincoln: University of Nebraska Press, 2004.

―――. *Reproduction and Its Discontents: Childbirth and Contraception from 1750 to 1905*. Chapel Hill: University of North Carolina Press, 2017.

Jiménez Olivares, Ernestina. "Hospital el Divino Salvador para mujeres dementes." *Cirujia y cirujanos* 64, no. 6 (1996): 175–78.

―――. "La atención de los enfermos mentales." In *Historia general de la medicina en México*, vol. 4, *Medicina novohispana, Siglo XVIII*, edited by Carlos Viesca Treviño, Martha Eugenia Rodríguez Pérez, and Xóchitl Martínez Barbosa, 227–32. Mexico, D.F.: UNAM, Facultad de Medicina, 2001.

―――. *Los Medicos en el Santo Oficio*. Mexico, D.F.: U.N.A.M., 2000.

―――. *Psiquiatria e Inquisición: Procesos A Enfermos Mentales*. Mexico, D.F.: U.N.A.M., 1992.

Johnson, Lyman L. "Dangerous Words, Provocative Gestures, and Violent Acts." In *The Faces of Honor in Colonial Latin America: Sex, Shame and Violence*, edited by Lyman L. Johnson and Sonya Lipsett-Rivera, 127–51. Albuquerque: University of New Mexico Press, 1998.

Johnson, Lyman L., and Sonya Lipsett-Rivera, eds. *The Faces of Honor in Colonial Latin America: Sex, Shame and Violence*. Albuquerque: University of New Mexico Press, 1998.

Jones, Colin. *The Charitable Imperative: Hospitals and Nursing in Ancien Régime and Revolutionary France*. London: Routledge, 1989.

Kamen, Henry. *The Spanish Inquisition: A Historical Revision*. New Haven, CT: Yale University Press, 1998.

Keitt, Andrew W. *Inventing the Sacred: Imposture, Inquisition, and the Boundaries of the Supernatural in Golden Age Spain*. Leiden: Brill, 2005.

―――. "Religious Enthusiasm, the Spanish Inquisition, and the Disenchantment of the World." *Journal of the History of Ideas* 65, no. 2 (2004): 231–50.

Keller, Richard C. *Colonial Madness: Psychiatry in French North Africa*. Chicago: University of Chicago Press, 2007.

Kroll, Jerome, and Bernard Bachrach. "Sin and Mental Illness in the Middle Ages." *Psychological Medicine* 14, no. 3 (1984): 507–14.

Kromm, J. E. "Archives and Sources: Goya and the Asylum at Saragossa." *Society for the Social History of Medicine* 1, no. 1 (1988): 79–89.

Lanning, John Tate. *The Royal Protomedicato: The Regulation of the Medical Profession in the Spanish Empire*. Durham, NC: Duke University Press, 1985.

Larkin, Brian. *The Very Nature of God: Baroque Catholicism and Religious Reform in Bourbon Mexico City*. Albuquerque: University of New Mexico Press, 2010.

Lavrin, Asunción. Ed. *Sexuality and Marriage in Colonial Latin America*. Lincoln: University of Nebraska Press, 1989.

———. "Sexuality in Colonial Mexico: A Church Dilemma." In *Sexuality and Marriage in Colonial Latin America*, edited by Asunción Lavrin, 47–95. Lincoln: University of Nebraska Press, 1989.

Lederer, David. *Madness, Religion and the State in Early Modern Europe: A Bavarian Beacon*. Cambridge: Cambridge University Press, 2009.

Lehner, Ulrich. *The Catholic Enlightenment: The Forgotten History of a Global Movement*. Oxford: Oxford University Press, 2016.

Leiby, John S. "San Hipolito's Treatment of the Mental Ill in Mexico City, 1589–1650." *Historian* 54, no. 3 (1992): 491–98.

Leon-Portilla, Miguel. "Las Comunidades Mesoamericanas ante la institución de los hospitales para Indios." *Boletín de la Sociedad Mexicana de Historia y Filosofía de la Medicina* 44 (1983): 195–216.

Levack, Brian. *The Devil Within: Possession and Exorcism in the Christian West*. New Haven, CT: Yale University Press, 2013.

Lewis, Elizabeth Franklin, Mónica Bolufer Peruga, and Catherine M. Jaffe, eds. *The Routledge Companion to the Hispanic Enlightenment*. New York: Routledge, 2020.

Lewis, Laura E. *Hall of Mirrors: Power, Witchcraft, and Caste in Colonial Mexico*. Durham, NC: Duke University Press, 2003.

Lindemann, Mary. "Murder, Melancholy and the Insanity Defence in Eighteenth-Century Hamburg." In *Medicine, Madness and Social History: Essays in Honour of Roy Porter*, edited by Roberta Bivins and John V. Pickstone, 161–72. London: Palgrave Macmillan, 2007.

Lippy, Charles. H., Robert Choquette, and Stafford Poole. *Christianity Comes to the Americas, 1492–1776*. New York: Paragon House, 1992.

Lipsett-Rivera, Sonya. "A Slap in the Face of Honor." In *The Faces of Honor in Colonial Latin America: Sex, Shame and Violence*, edited by Lyman L. Johnson and Sonya Lipsett-Rivera, 179–200. Albuquerque: University of New Mexico Press, 1998.

———. *Gender and the Negotiation of Daily Life in Mexico, 1750–1856*. Lincoln: University of Nebraska Press, 2012.

López Alonso, Carmen. *Locura y sociedad en Sevilla: Historia del hospital de los inocentes (1436?–1840)*. Sevilla: Diputación Provincial, 1988.

López Piñero, José M., and José Pardo Tomás. "The Contribution of Hernández to European Botany and Materia Medica." In *Searching for the Secrets of Nature: The Life and Works of Dr. Francisco Hernández*, edited by Simon Varey, Rafael Chabrán, and Dora B. Weiner, 122–37. Stanford, CA: Stanford University Press, 2000.

López Terrada, María Luz. "Health Care and Poor Relief in the Crown of Aragon." In *Health Care and Poor Relief in Counter-Reformation Europe*, edited by Ole Peter Greel, Andrew Cunningham, and Jon Arrizabalaga, 177–200. London: Routledge, 1999.

Lozano Armendares, Teresa. *La criminalidad en la Ciudad de México, 1800–1821*. Mexico, D.F.: Universidad Nacional Autónoma de México, 1987.

Lynch, John. *Bourbon Spain, 1700–1808*. Oxford: Blackwell, 1989.

———. *The Spanish American Revolutions, 1808–1826*. New York: Norton, 1973.

MacDonald, Michael. *Mystical Bedlam: Madness, Anxiety and Healing in Seventeenth-Century England*. Cambridge: Cambridge University Press, 1983.

MacLachlan, Colin M. *Criminal Justice in Eighteenth Century Mexico: A Study of the Tribunal of the Acordada*. Berkeley: University of California Press, 1974.

Mahone, Sloan, and Megan Vaughn. *Psychiatry and Empire*. New York: Palgrave Macmillan, 2007.

Marroqui, José María. *La Ciudad de Mexico*. 2nd ed. Mexico: J. Medina, 1969.

Martin, Cheryl English. "The San Hipólito Hospitals of Colonial Mexico, 1566–1702." PhD diss., Tulane University, 1976.

———. "Crucible of Zapatismo: Hacienda *Hospital* in the Seventeenth Century." *The Americas* 38, no. 1 (1981): 31–43.

Martínez, María Elena. *Genealogical Fictions: Limpieza de Sangre, Religion, and Gender in Colonial Mexico*. Stanford, CA: Stanford University Press, 2008.

Martz, Linda. *Poverty and Welfare in Habsburg Spain: The Example of Toledo*. Cambridge: Cambridge University Press, 1983.

Mazzotti, Massimo. *The World of Maria Gaetana Agnesi, Mathematician of God*. Baltimore: Johns Hopkins University Press, 2007.

McKendrick, Geraldine, and Angus MacKay. "Visionaries and Affective Spirituality during the First Half of the Sixteenth Century." In *Cultural Encounters: The Impact of the Inquisition in Spain and the New World*, edited by Mary Elizabeth Perry and Anne J. Cruz, 93–104. Los Angeles: University of California Press, 1991.

McMahon, Darrin M. *Enemies of the Enlightenment: The French-Counter Enlightenment and the Making of Modernity*. Oxford: Oxford University Press, 2001.

Meléndez, Mariselle. *Deviant and Useful Citizens: The Cultural Production of the Female Body in Eighteenth-Century Peru*. Nashville: Vanderbilt University Press, 2011.

Meléndez, Mariselle, and Karen Stolley. "Enlightenments in Ibero-America." *Colonial Latin American Review* 24, no. 1 (2015): 1–16.

Mellyn, Elizabeth W. *Mad Tuscans and Their Families: A History of Mental Disorder*. Philadelphia: University of Pennsylvania Press, 2014.

Melvin, Karen. *Building Colonial Cities of God: Mendicant Orders and Urban Culture in New Spain*. Stanford, CA: Stanford University Press, 2012.

Mendoza García, J. Edgar. "La secularización de los hospitales y el ayuntamiento en la ciudad de México ante el decreto de supresión de órdenes monacales, 1820–1822." *Andamios* 15, no. 38 (2018): 339–364.

Messbarger, Rebecca, Christopher M. S. Johns, and Philip Gavitt, eds. *Benedict XIV and the Enlightenment: Art, Science, and Spirituality*. Toronto: University of Toronto Press, 2016.

Midelfort, H. C. Erik. *A History of Madness in Sixteenth-Century Germany*. Stanford, CA: Stanford University Press, 1999.

———. "Madness and Civilization in Early Modern Europe: A Reappraisal of Michel Foucault." In *After the Reformation: Essays in Honor of J. H. Hexter*, edited by Barbara C. Malament. Philadelphia: University of Pennsylvania Press, 1980.

———. *Mad Princes of Renaissance Germany*. Charlottesville, VA: University Press of Virginia, 1994.

Milton, Cynthia E. *The Many Meanings of Poverty: Colonialism, Social Compacts, and Assistance in Eighteenth-Century Ecuador*. Stanford, CA: Stanford University Press, 2007.

Mott, Margaret. "The Rule of Faith over Reason: The Role of the Inquisition in Iberia and New Spain." *Journal of Church and State* 40, no. 1 (1998): 57–81.

Mundy, Barbara. *The Death of Aztec Tenochtitlan, the Life of Mexico City*. Austin: University of Texas Press, 2018.

Muriel, Josefina. "El modelo arquitectrónico de los hospitales para dementes en la Nueva España." *Retabolo barroco á la memoria de Francisco de la Maza*. Mexico, D.F.: U.N.A.M., 1974.

———. *Hospitales de la Nueva España*. 2 vols. Mexico, D.F.: Editorial Jus, 1956–1960.

———. *Los recogimientos de mujeres: Respuesta a una problemática social novohispana*. Mexico, D.F.: U.N.A.M., 1974.

Nalle, Sara Tighman. "Insanity and the Insanity Defense in the Spanish Inquisition." Paper presented at the Society for Spanish and Portuguese Studies, San Juan, Puerto Rico, April 1992.

———. *Mad for God: Bartolomé Sanchez, the Secret Messiah of Cardenete*. Charlottesville: University of Virginia Press, 2001.

Nesvig, Martin Austin. *Ideology and Inquisition: The World of the Censors in Early Mexico*. New Haven, CT: Yale University Press, 2009.

———. *Promiscuous Power: An Unorthodox History of New Spain*. Austin: University of Texas Press, 2018.

Nye, David. "The Evolution of the Concept of Medicalization in the Late Twentieth Century." *Journal of the History of the Behavioral Sciences* 39, no. 2 (2003): 115–29.

Ordorika Sacristán, Teresa. "¿Herejes o Locos?" *Cuicuilco* 45 (2009): 139–62.

Owensby, Brian P. *Empire of Law and Indian Justice in Colonial Mexico*. Stanford, CA: Stanford University Press, 2008.

Pagden, Anthony. *The Fall of Natural Man: The American Indian and the Origins of Comparative Ethnology*. Cambridge: Cambridge University Press, 1982.

Paquette, Gabriel, ed. *Enlightened Reform in Southern Europe and Its Atlantic Colonies, c. 1750–1830*. London: Ashgate, 2009.

———. *Enlightenment, Governance, and Reform in Spain and Its Empire, 1759–1808*. New York: Palgrave Macmillan, 2008.

Pardo-Tomás, José, and Àlvar Martínez-Vidal. "Victims and Experts: Medical Practitioners and the Spanish Inquisition." In *Coping with Sickness: Medicine, Law, and Human Rights: Historical Perspectives*, edited by John Woodward and Robert Jütte, 11–27. Sheffield: European Association for the History of Medicine and Health Publications, 2000.

Park, Katharine. "Healing the Poor: Hospitals and Medical Assistance in Renaissance Florence." In *Medicine and Charity before the Welfare State*, edited by Jonathan Barry and Colin Jones, 26–45. London: Routledge, 1991.

Perez, Joseph. *The Spanish Inquisition: A History*. New Haven, CT: Yale University Press, 2006.

Peters, Edwards. *The Inquisition*. Berkeley: University California Press, 1989.

Philo, Chris. "Edinburgh, Enlightenment, and the Geographies of Unreason." In *Geography and Enlightenment*, edited by David N. Livingstone and Charles W. J. Withers, 372–98. Chicago: University of Chicago Press, 1999.

Pike, Ruth. *Penal Servitude in Early Modern Spain*. Madison: University of Wisconsin Press, 1983.

Pomata, Gianna. "Malpighi and the Holy Body: Medical Experts and Miraculous Evidence in Seventeenth-Century Italy." *Renaissance Studies* 21, no. 4 (2007): 568–85.

Porter, Roy. "Foucault's Great Confinement." In *Rewriting the History of Madness: Studies in Foucault's "Histoire de la folie*,*"* edited by Arthur Still and Irving Velody, 119–25. London: Routledge, 1992.

———. *Madness: A Brief History*. Oxford: Oxford University Press, 2002.

———. "Madness and Its Institutions." In *Medicine in Society: Historical Essays*, edited by Andrew Wear, 277–301. Cambridge: Cambridge University Press, 1992.

———. "Mental Illness." In *The Cambridge Illustrated History of Medicine*, edited by Roy Porter, 278–303. Cambridge: Cambridge University Press, 1996.

———. *Mind-Forg'd Manacles: A History of Madness in England from the Restoration to the Regency*. London: Athlone Press, 1987.

———. "The Patient's View: Doing Medical History from Below." *Theory and Society* 14, no. 2 (1985): 175–98.

Porter, Roy, W. F. Bynum, and Michael Shepard, eds. *The Anatomy of Madness: Essays in the History of Psychiatry*. 3 vols. London: Tavistock, 1985–88.

Premo, Bianca. *Children of the Father King: Youth, Authority, and Legal Minority in Colonial Lima*. Chapel Hill: University of North Carolina Press, 2005.

———. *The Enlightenment on Trial: Ordinary Litigants and Colonialism in the Spanish Empire*. Oxford: Oxford University Press, 2017.

Ragab, Ahmed. *The Medieval Islamic Hospital: Medieval, Religion, and Charity*. New York: Cambridge University Press, 2015.

Ramirez, Paul. *Enlightened Immunity: Mexico's Experiments with Disease Prevention in the Age of Reason*. Stanford, CA: Stanford University Press, 2018.

Ramirez Moreno, Samuel. "History of the First Psychopathic Institution on the American Continent." *American Journal of Psychiatry* 99, no. 2 (1942): 194–95.

Ramos, Christina. "Beyond the Columbian Exchange: Medicine and Public Health in Colonial Latin America." *History Compass*, 19, no. 8 (August 2021): 1–13.

Ramos, Gabriela. "Indian Hospitals and Government in the Colonial Andes." *Medical History* 57, no. 2 (2013): 186–205.

Rawlings, Helen. *The Spanish Inquisition*. Malden, MA: Blackwell, 2006.

Ricard, Robert. *The Spiritual Conquest of Mexico: An Essay on the Apostolate and the Evangelizing Methods of the Mendicant Orders in New Spain*. Translated by Lesley Byrd Simpson. Berkeley: University of California Press, 1966.

Risse, Guenter B. *Hospital Life in Enlightenment Scotland: Care and Teaching at the Royal Infirmary of Edinburgh*. New York: Cambridge University Press, 1986.

———. "Medicine in New Spain." *Medicine in the New World: New Spain, New France, and New England*, edited by Ronald L. Numbers, 12-63. Knoxville: University of Tennessee Press, 1987.

———. "Medicine in the Age of Enlightenment." In *Medicine in Society: Historical Essays*, edited by Andrew Wear, 149-95. Cambridge: Cambridge University Press, 1992.

———. *Mending Bodies, Saving Souls: A History of Hospitals*. New York: Oxford University Press, 1999.

———. "Shelter and Care for Natives and Colonists: Hospitals in Sixteenth-Century New Spain." In *Searching for the Secrets of Nature: The Life and Works of Dr. Francisco Hernandez*, edited by Simon Varey, Rafael Chabrán, and Dora B. Weiner, 65-81. Stanford, CA: Stanford University Press, 2000.

Rivera-Garza, Cristina. "Dangerous Minds: Changing Psychiatric Views of the Mentally Ill in Porfirian Mexico, 1876-1911." *Journal of the History of Medicine* 56 (2001): 36-67.

Rosenberg, Charles E. "Framing Disease: Illness, Society, and History." In *Framing Disease: Studies in Cultural History*, edited by Charles Rosenberg and Janet Golden. New Brunswick: Rutgers University Press, 1992.

Rothman, David. *The Discovery of the Asylum: Social Order and Disorder in the New Republic*. Rev. ed. New Brunswick: Aldine Transaction, 2011. First published 1971 by Little Brown (Boston).

Rumbaut, Ruben D. "Bernardino Alvarez: New World Psychiatric Pioneer." *American Journal of Psychiatry* 127, no. 9 (1971): 1217-21.

Sacristán, María Cristina. "Filantropismo, improductividad, y delincuencia en algunos textos novohispanos sobre pobres, vagos, y mendico (1782-1794)." *Relaciones* 36 (1988): 21-32.

———. "El pensamiento ilustrado ante los grupos marginados de la ciudad de México, 1767-1824." In *La ciudad de México en la primera mitad del siglo XIX*, vol. 1, *Economía y estructura urbana*, edited by Regina Hernández Franyuti, 187-249. Mexico, D.F.: Instituto de Investigaciones Dr. José María Luis Mora, 1994.

———. *Locura e Inquisición en Nueva España, 1571-1760*. Mexico: El Colegio de Michoacan 1992.

———. *Locura y disidencia en el México ilustrado, 1760-1810*. Mexico: El Colegio de Michoacan, 1994.

———. "Sexualidad feminina y condicion genérica en el México ilustrado." *Tramas. Subjetividad y procesos sociales* 5 (1993): 251-66.

Sadowsky, Jonathan. *Imperial Bedlam: Institutions of Madness in Colonial Southwest Nigeria*. Berkeley: University of California Press, 1999.

Safier, Neil. *Measuring the New World. Enlightenment Science in South America*. Chicago: University of Chicago Press, 2008.

Scardaville, Michael C. "Alcohol Abuse and Tavern Reform in Late Colonial Mexico." *Hispanic American Historical Review* 60, no. 4 (1980): 643-71.

———. "Crime and the Urban Poor: Mexico City in the Late Colonial Period." PhD diss., University of Florida, 1977.

———. "(Hapsburg) Law and (Bourbon) Order: State Authority, Popular Unrest, and the Criminal Justice System in Bourbon Mexico City." *Americas* 50, no. 4 (1994): 501–25.

———. "Justice by Paperwork: A Day in the Life of a Court Scribe in Bourbon Mexico City." *Journal of Social History* 36, no. 4 (2003): 979–1007.

Schaposchnik, Ana E. *The Lima Inquisition: The Plight of Crypto-Jews in Seventeenth-Century Peru*. Madison: University of Wisconsin Press, 2017.

Schmidt, Jeremy. *Melancholy and the Care of the Soul: Religion, Moral Philosophy, and Madness in Early Modern England*. Aldershot: Ashgate, 2007.

Schutte, Anne Jacobson. *Aspiring Saints: Pretense to Holiness, Inquisition, and Gender in the Republic of Venice 1618–1715*. Baltimore: Johns Hopkins University Press, 2001.

Schwaller, John Frederick. *The History of the Catholic Church in Latin America: From Conquest to Revolution and Beyond*. New York: New York University Press, 2011.

Schwartz, Stuart. *All Can Be Saved: Religious Tolerance and Salvation in the Iberian Atlantic World*. New Haven, CT: Yale University Press, 2008.

Scull, Andrew. "The Asylum, Hospital, and Clinic." In *The Routledge History of Madness and Mental Health*, edited by Greg Eghigian, 101–14. New York: Routledge, 2017.

———. *The Most Solitary of Afflictions: Madness and Society in Britain, 1700–1900*. New Haven, CT: Yale University Press, 1993.

Seed, Patricia. *Ceremonies of Possession in Europe's Conquest of the New World, 1492–1640*. Cambridge: Cambridge University Press, 1995.

———. "Social Dimensions of Race: Mexico City, 1753." *Hispanic American Review* 62, no. 4 (1982): 559–606.

Sellers-García, Sylvia. *Distance and Documents at the Spanish Empire's Periphery*. Stanford, CA: Stanford University Press, 2013.

Serulnikov, Sergio. *Subverting Colonial Authority: Challenges to Spanish Rule in the Eighteenth-Century Southern Andes*. Durham, NC: Duke University Press.

Shuger, Dale. *Don Quixote in the Archives: Madness and Literature in Early Modern Spain*. Edinburgh: Edinburgh University Press, 2012.

———. "Madness on Trial." *Journal of Spanish Cultural Studies* 10, no. 3 (2009): 277–97.

Silverblatt, Irene. *Modern Inquisitions: Peru and the Colonial Origins of the Civilized World*. Durham, NC: Duke University Press, 2004.

Sluhovsky, Moshe. *Believe Not Every Spirit: Possession, Mysticism, and Discernment in Early Modern Catholicism*. Chicago: University of Chicago Press, 2007.

Smith, Pamela. "Laboratories." In *The Cambridge History of Science*, vol. 3, *Early Modern Science*, edited by Katharine Park and Lorraine Daston, 290–305. Cambridge: Cambridge University Press, 2006.

Socolow, Susan Midgen. *The Women of Colonial Latin America*. Cambridge: Cambridge University Press, 2000.

Somolinos d'Ardois, Germán. *Historia de la psiquiatría en México*. Mexico, D.F.: Secretaría de Educación Pública, 1976.

Sorkin, David. *The Religious Enlightenment: Protestant, Jews, and Catholics from London to Vienna*. Princeton: Princeton University Press, 2008.

Sousa, Lisa. "The Devil and Deviance in Native Criminal Narratives from Early Mexico." *Americas* 59, no. 2 (2002): 161–79.
Spary, E.C. *Eating the Enlightenment: Food and the Sciences in Paris, 1670–1760*. Chicago: University of Chicago Press, 2012.
Spierenburg, Pieter. *The Prison Experience: Disciplinary Institutions and Their Inmates in Early Modern Europe*. New Brunswick: Rutgers University Press, 1991.
Spores, Ronald. *The Mixtecs in Ancient and Colonial Times*. Norman: University of Oklahoma Press, 1986.
Stein, Stanley J., and Barbara H. Stein. *Apogee of Empire: Spain and New Spain in the Age of Charles III, 1759–1789*. Baltimore: Johns Hopkins University Press, 2003.
Stoler, Ann, and Frederick Cooper. "Between Metropole and Colony: Rethinking a Research Agenda." *Tensions of Empire: Colonial Cultures in a Bourgeois World*. Berkeley: University of California Press, 1997.
Stolley, Karen. *Domesticating Empire. Enlightenment in Spanish America*. Nashville: Vanderbilt University Press, 2013.
Strocchia, Sharon. "Women on the Edge: Madness, Possession, and Suicide in Early Modern Convents." *Journal of Medieval and Early Modern Studies* 45, no. 1 (2015): 53–77.
Suarez, Marcela. *Hospitales y sociedad en la ciudad de Mexico del siglo XVI*. Mexico, D.F.: Universidad Autónoma Metropolitana, División de Ciencias Sociales y Humanidades, 1988.
Takats, Sean. *The Expert Cook in Enlightenment France*. Baltimore: Johns Hopkins University Press, 2011.
Taylor, William B. *Drinking, Homicide, and Rebellion in Colonial Mexican Villages*. Stanford, CA: Stanford University Press, 1979.
———. *Magistrates of the Sacred: Priests and Parishioners in Eighteenth-Century Mexico*. Stanford, CA: Stanford University Press, 1996.
Thompson, John D., and Grace Goldin, *The Hospital: A Social and Architectural History*. New Haven, CT: Yale University Press, 1975.
Thomson, Sinclair. *We Alone Will Rule: Native Andean Politics in the Age of Insurgency*. Madison: University of Wisconsin Press, 2003.
Tilly, Helen. *Africa as a Living Laboratory: Empire, Development, and the Problem of Scientific Knowledge, 1870–1950*. Chicago: University of Chicago Press, 2011.
Toribio Medina, José. *Historia del Tribunal del Santo Oficio de la Inquisición de México*. Mexico, D.F.: Conaculta, 2010.
Tortorici, Zeb. "Masturbation, Salvation, and Desire: Connecting Sexuality and Religiosity in Colonial Mexico." *Journal of the History of Sexuality* 16, no. 3 (2007): 355–72.
———. "Reading the (Dead) Body: Histories of Suicide in New Spain." In *Death and Dying in Colonial Spanish America*, edited by Martina Will de Chaparro and Miruna Achim, 53–77. Tucson: University of Arizona Press, 2011.
———. "Sexual Violence, Predatory Masculinity, and Medical Testimony in New Spain." *Osiris* 30, no. 1 (2015): 272–94.
———. *Sins against Nature: Sex and Archives in Colonial New Spain*. Durham, NC: Duke University Press, 2018.

Tropé, Hélène. "Inquisición y locura en la España del siglo XVI y XVII." *Bulletin of Spanish Studies* 87, no. 8 (2010): 57–79.

———. "Locura y Inquisición en la España del siglo XVII." *Norte de Salud Mental* 8, no. 36 (2010): 90–101.

———. *Locura y sociedad en la Valencia de los siglos XV al XVII*. Valencia: Diputació de Valencia, 1994.

Twinam, Ann. *Public Lives, Private Secrets: Gender, Honor, Sexuality and Illegitimacy in Colonial Spanish America*. Stanford, CA: Stanford University Press, 1999.

Van Deusen, Nancy E. "The 'Alienated' Body: Slaves and Castas in the Hospital de San Bartolomé in Lima, 1680–1700." *Americas* 56, no. 1 (1999): 1–30.

———. *Between the Sacred and the Worldly: The Institutional and Cultural Practice of Recogimiento in Colonial Lima*. Stanford, CA: Stanford University Press, 2001.

Van Young, Eric. "Millennium on the Northern Marches: The Mad Messiah of Durango and Popular Rebellion in Mexico, 1800–1815." *Comparative Studies in Society and History* 28, no. 3 (1986): 385–413.

———. *The Other Rebellion: Popular, Violence, Ideology, and the Struggle for Independence, 1810–1821*. Stanford, CA: Stanford University Press, 2001.

Vaughn, Megan. *Curing Their Ills: Colonial Power and African Illness*. Stanford, CA: Stanford University Press, 1991.

Venegas Ramirez, Carmen. *Regimen hospitalario para los indios en la Nueva Espana*. Mexico City: Instituto Nacional de Antropologia y Hisoria, 1973.

Vidal, Fernando. "Miracles, Science, and Testimony in Post-Tridentine Saint-Making." *Science in Context* 20, no. 3 (2007): 481–508.

Viesca Treviño, Carlos, and Igancio de la Peña. "Las enfermedades mentales en el Códice Badiano." *Estudios de Cultura Nahautl* 12 (1976): 79–84.

Villa-Flores, Javier. *Dangerous Speech: A Social History of Blasphemy in Colonial Mexico*. Tucson: University of Arizona Press, 2006.

Villella, Peter B. "'Pure and Noble Indians, Untainted by Inferior Idolatrous Races': Native Elites and the Discourse of Blood Purity in Late Colonial Mexico." *Hispanic American Review* 91, no. 4 (2011): 633–63.

Viquera, Carmen. "Los hospitales para locos e 'inocentes' en Hispanoamerica y sus antecedentes Españoles." *Revista Española de Antropología Americana* 5 (1970): 341–84.

Voekel, Pamela. *Alone before God: The Religious Origins of Modernity in Mexico*. Durham, NC: Duke University Press, 2002.

———. "Peeing on the Palace: Bodily Resistance to Bourbon Reforms in Mexico City." *Journal of Historical Sociology* 5, no. 2 (1992): 183–208.

Walker, Charles. *Smoldering Ashes: Cuzco and the Creation of Republican Peru, 1780–1840*. Durham, NC: Duke University Press, 1999.

———. *The Tupac Amaru Rebellion*. Boston: Belknap Press, 2016.

Walker, Timothy. *Doctors, Folk Medicine, and the Inquisition: The Repression of Magical Healing in Portugal during the Enlightenment*. Leiden: Brill, 2005.

Warren, Adam. *Medicine and Politics in Colonial Peru: Population Growth and the Bourbon Reforms*. Pittsburgh: University of Pittsburgh Press, 2010.

Warren, Fintan B. *Vasco de Quiroga and His Pueblo-Hospitals of Santa Fe*. Washington, DC: Academy of American Franciscan History, 1963.

Weber, David J. *Bárbaros: Spaniards and their Savages in the Age of Enlightenment*. Oxford: Oxford University Press, 2005.

Weiner, Dora B. "The Brothers of Charity and the Mentally Ill in Pre-revolutionary France." *Social History of Medicine* 2, no. 3 (1989): 321–37.

———. "The Madman in the Light of Reason: Enlightenment Psychiatry: Part I. Custody, Therapy, Theory and the Need for Reform." *History of Psychiatry and Medical Psychology*, edited by Edwin R. Wallace IV and John Each, 255–77. New York: Springer, 2008.

———. "The Madman in the Light of Reason: Enlightenment Psychiatry: Part II. Alienists, Treatises, and the Psychologic Approach in the Era of Pinel." *History of Psychiatry and Medical Psychology*, edited by Edwin R. Wallace IV and John Each, 281–303. New York: Springer, 2008.

Zahino Peñafort, Luisa. *Iglesia y sociedad en México, 1765–1800: Tradición, reforma y reacciones*. Mexico, D.F.: U.N.A.M., 1996.

Zeitlin, Judith Francis. *Cultural Politics in Colonial Tehuantepec: Community and State among the Isthmus Zapotec, 1500–1750*. Stanford, CA: Stanford University Press, 2005.

Zilboorg, Gregory. *A History of Medical Psychology*. In collaboration with George W. Henry. New York: Norton, 1941.

Index

Age of Enlightenment, 7, 167
"Age of Revolutions," 175
alcohol use, 124, 156–58
Algeria, 14
alumbradismo (illuminism), 119, 133
Alvarez, Bernardino (founder of San Hipólito), 17, 23–25, 26, 30, 32, 35, 57, 198n40
Alvarez, Felipe Antonio (friar, defendant), 91–94, 117–18, 134
Alvarez, Rafaela Ignacia (defendant), 106–7, 111
Amor de Dios (hospital for syphilitics), 29
Anderson, Warwick, 12
Apelo, Mauricia Josefa de (defendant, patient), 107–11, 125
Apodaca, Juan Ruíz de (viceroy), 176
Arangado y Chavez, Diego, 128
arbitrio judicial (judicial discretion), 148–49
architecture, 15–16, 40–42, 62, 65, 67; monastic model, 41, 41
Armarero, Mariano (Inquisition staff physician), 142
Arpide, Manuel de (priest), 124
Arrieta, Pedro de (inquisitor), 108–9
Aspe y Aguirre, Teodoro Francisco de (accuser), 80–84
asylum, as term, 22
auto-da-fé (act of faith), 114, 117
auto-denunciation, 105–11
avería (tax on merchant convoys), 64

Balbotín, Manuel (governing counselor), 177–78
Balbuena, José (official), 56–57, 202n31
Barberá, Felipe (official), 56–57
Barrero, Gabriel (physician), 132–33
Beccaria, Cesare, 11, 19, 146–47

Benedict XIV, 56
Bermudez, Juan José (physician), 164, 165
Bestan, Juan de Dios Loreto (priest), 114
Bethlehem (Bedlam) hospital (London), 4
Bicêtre hospital (Paris, France), 4, 112
bigamy, 127–31
"birth of the prison," 170
blasphemy, 93–94, 106, 124–25
body, mechanical models of, 120, 132
Bonaparte, Joseph, 175
Borah, Woodrow, 27
Bourbon model, 7–8; Consolidación de Vales Reales, 176; dynasty, 52; enlightened absolutism, 13, 50, 52–53, 64, 145, 201n8; legal foundations of, 147; reforms under, 13, 16, 18–19, 47, 48–50, 56–58, 61–62, 69, 144–45, 170–71; and Royal Indian Hospital, 36
Bucareli y Ursúa, Antonio María de (viceroy), 48–50, 61–62, 177
Butterwick, Richard, 13

cabildo (municipal council), 33, 162
Cabrera, Juan de (friar), 53
Cabrera y Quintero, Cayetano de, 54–55, 202n27
Calabritto, Monica, 104
Calderón, José María (defendant, patient), 131–33, 135
Calderón de la Barca, Frances (wife of Spanish minister), 178
calificadores (evaluators or consultants), 85, 91–92, 118
Campos, Juan Gregorio (Inquisition staff physician), 90–91, 109
Candide (Voltaire), 11
Cañete, Joseph Ruíz (defendant, priest, patient), 135–36

Carvajal, Luis de (the Younger), 134
Casa de Recogidas, 163, 164
Casasola, Mariano José (*comisario*), 98–99
castes. *See* race-caste system (*sistema de castas*)
Castille, kingdom of, 147
Castillo, José (physician), 141
Castro, José de (prior general), 69
Catholic Church: "Catholic Enlightenment," 11, 56; Council of Trent, 56; evangelical agenda, 25; index of prohibited books, 112; legitimized by charitable institutions, 27, 47; nursing orders, 52–53; paternalism of, 25; Protestant threat to, 87–88; reform of, 51, 53, 56; reinforced by hospital services, 47. *See also* Inquisition (Holy Office)
"ceremonies of possession," 33
certificate of health, 164, 166
certificates of mental illness/letters of recommendation for admission, 75–76, 80–81, 96
Cervantes, Fernando, 89
Cevallos, Manuel (*alcalde*), 169
charity (*caridad*), 5, 33
Charles III, 58, 112; *instrucción* (instruction) of 1776, 63–64, 69
Charles IV, 58, 175
Charles V, 28–29
Chichimecas, 23
Chimalpopoca, Manuel Antonio (defendant, patient), 150–54, 214n46
clergy/priests: age-related dementia, 6, 211n68; as confessors, 109–10; as key agents of medicalization, 10; letters of recommendation from, 75–76; medical training, 43; as physicians of the soul, 109; primary responsibility for institutional care, 8; role in care of *pobres dementes*, 42–43; in Spanish American colonial setting, 6. *See also* Inquisition (Holy Office); Order of San Hipólito (*hipólitos*); San Hipólito, Hospital de

cocoxcalli, as Nahuatl term for hospital, 27
Codex Osuna, 27
Colegio de San Fernando, 178
Colima, José (physician), 164
colonialism, 1–10, 195n38; appropriation of former battlegrounds or religious sites, 32–33; colonial law (*derecho indiano*); 147; colonies as laboratories of modernity, 6, 13; destabilized authority of, 12, 147, 168; and *hospitalidad*, 27–30; Iberian models adapted to, 25–27, 46–47; improvisational nature of, 32, 46–47; intersection with madness and medicine, 14; legal codes, 147–50; San Hipólito as laboratory of, 8–10, 13, 136–42, 146; San Hipólito as limited tool of governance, 17, 27, 40, 46; spatial dimension of, 35; subjectivity of colonized as akin to madness, 14; violence of, 46. *See also* Bourbon model
Compendio de la medicina practica (Venegas), 120, 124
confinement, 3; as ad hoc arrangement, 12, 14, 18, 37, 135, 138, 171, 213n33; "great confinement" narrative, 6, 47, 144; narrative of mass internment as misleading, 47
Congregación de la Purísima, 63
conquistadores, 13–14, 17
consolation, religious, 180
Consolidación de Vales Reales (Consolidation of Royal Bonds), 176
convents, 22–23, 48, 111, 179; *convento-hospital* (convent-hospital), 22
Cooper, Frederick, 195n38
Cortés, Hernán (conquistador), 17, 23–24, 29, 33, 35
Cosio, Francisco (convict, patient), 168–70
Council of Indies, 34, 53, 55, 202n31
Council of Trent (1545–63), 88
Counter-Reformation, 56, 89–90
Count of Moctezuma. *See* Chimalpopoca, Manuel Antonio (defendant, patient)

courts. *See* criminal courts (*sala del crimen*); Inquisition (Holy Office)
Covarrubias Orozco, Sebastián de, 21
Creoles (*criollos*), 85, 175; culture, 33, 47; as patients, 5, 38–40, 75–76
criminal courts (*sala del crimen*), 8, 18–19, 79, 86, 144–45, 214n46; appointed physicians for, 21–22; and insanity defense, 152, 162–63; legal protections, 148; *locos furiosos* in, 143, 148–49, 155–58; no precedent for mental illness in Spanish law, 149; paternalistic leniency in sentencing, 19, 147, 152–54, 157–59; procedural norms of, 150; San Hipólito as prison of last resort, 155–59. *See also* jurisprudence
Cruz, Antonio de la (defendant, patient), 127–31, 135
Cruz, Ignacio (victim), 155
crypto-Judaism, 88, 134
Cubo, Rafael (defendant, patient), 171–73
cure, 31–32, 45, 133, 180; *curar* (to cure), 60; dual focus on mind and body, 42–43; "talking cure," 112
Curia Philipica (Bolaños), 148–49

Day of the Holy Innocents, 33
defense attorney (*defensor*), 150, 158
De la Borda, Joseph (employer), 80–81
Delgadillo, Atanasio Guadalupe (defendant, patient), 155–56
demencia, as term, 21
demencia parcial (partial madness), 90
demente, as term, 21, 29
demonological treatises, 108
denunciations, 93–94, 98, 124; auto-denunciation, 105–11
derecho de asilo eclesiastico (ecclesiastical asylum), 154
devil/Satan, 107–9, 125, 161, 206n31; diabolism, 89
dialogue, diagnostic power of, 129
Díaz, Porfirio, 2
Díaz de Arce, Juan, 23–25
Dirección de Beneficencia Pública, 179

discourse, 8, 14
diseases, 9, 28; categories of madness, 96; *matlazahuatl* (typus), 54–55; preternatural etiology of, 88
Dorantes, Francisco (surgeon), 128, 129–31
Dorantes de Carranza, Baltasar (official), 13–14

Echegoyen, Juan Pablo (defendant, patient), 134–35, 137–38
Edict of Faith, 93
Edington, Claire, 15
Eimeric, Nicolau (friar), 90
El Consejo Superior de Salubridad (Superior Health Council), 178
England, 2, 4
"enlightened piety" (*la piedad ilustrada*), 53
Enlightenment, 2; Age of Enlightenment, 7, 167; anti-clerical elements of, 53, 56; "Catholic," 11, 56; centrality of the periphery to, 13; geographies of, 8–9; utility, language of, 51, 59–60. *See also* Hispanic Enlightenment
entendimiento (reasoning), 148, 152, 158
escapes and escape attempts, 12, 19, 73–74, 136, 140, 142, 154–55, 167–73; state impotence exposed by, 147, 168
Escudo de Armas de México (Cabrera y Quintero), 54–55
españoles (Spaniards), 38, 76
Esteyneffer, Juan (physician), 126
Europe, 1–4, 6, 30, 195n38. *See also* Bourbon model; France; Habsburg model; Spain

Faculty of Medicine, 178
families of patients, 36, 74, 87, 133, 216n115; required to take custody, 170–71
Fanon, Frantz, 14
fatuidad (fatuity), 125, 135, 152
fear, pedagogy of, 134
feast days and holidays, 33, 36, 44, 46, 64, 69

Index 241

Feijoo, Benito (priest), 117
Ferdinand VII, 175, 176
Ferris, Francisco (defendant, patient), 140–42
fevers, thought to be cause of frenzy (*frenesi*), 41, 45, 120, 138
Few, Martha, 15, 99
Fierro (physician), 138
Figueroa, Eucebio (friar, surgeon), 141, 176–77
fiscal (prosecuting judge), 169–70; Inquisition courts, 126, 128, 131–32; secular criminal courts, 151–53
Florilegio medicinal (Esteyneffer), 126
Flynn, Maureen, 93
Folger, Cristobal de (priest), 110
Foucault, Michel, 8, 112, 194n17; "great confinement" narrative, 6, 47
France, 4, 213n35; French Revolution, 2, 11–12, 99, 112, 131
free will, doctrine of, 16, 91, 147
frenzy (*frenesi*), 45. *See also locos furiosos* (violently insane persons)
Fuente, Matheo de la, 139
furiosos. *See locos furiosos* (violently insane persons)

Gaceta de Mexico (periodical), 111–12
Galenism, 31–32, 45
Gálvez, José de (visitor-general), 48, 64
Gante, Pedro de (friar), 28–29
García, Francisco (priest), 24–25, 35
Garcia, José Mariano (defendant, patient), 156–59
García Jove, Don Pedro José (attorney), 163
Garza, Cristina Rivera, 179
Gay, Peter, 9–10
General Hospital for Dementes, 141
geographies of Enlightenment, 8–9
Ginzburg, Carlo, 16, 81
Goldstein, Jan, 180
Gómez de Cervantes, Francisco Javier (visitor-general), 56–57

González, José Ventura (Tebanillo). *See* Tebanillo (José Ventura González)
González Calderón, Don José (official), 63, 64
González de Andia, Julian Vicente (inquisitor), 91, 106, 115
Goya, Francisco de, 7, 11
Granada, 30–31
Granados, Pedro (friar), 139
Green, Toby, 117
Greenleaf, Richard, 112
gremio de panaderos (public granary), 63
Guanajuato (city), 176
Guerrero, Fernando (physician), 132–33
Guerrero, Vicente (surgeon), 177
Gutiérrez, Manuel Joseph (official), 156

Habsburg model, 7, 46–47, 50, 52, 179; paternal rule, 17, 27, 46, 147
Haliczer, Stephen, 109
Havana, transportation to, 114, 139, 171
head nurse (*enfermero mayor*), 42, 43, 60, 78–79
heresy, 209n2; *alumbradismo* (illuminism), 119, 133; *alumbrados* (false mystics), 38, 104–5; cases before the Inquisition, 91–95; Catholic doctrine challenged, 91; and feigned madness, 90–92, 95; interiority, focus on, 82, 84, 86–92; *locos* not capable of committing, 86; political, 99; requirements for, 86; revolutionary politics conflated with, 11–12
Herrera, Felipe (surgeon), 156
Hevia Bolaños, Juan de (jurist), 148–49
Hidalgo, Miguel (priest, insurgent), 175–76
hipólitos. *See* Order of San Hipólito
Hippolytus, Saint, 24, 33, 46, 64
Hispanic Enlightenment: compromise between tradition and innovation, 60, 69, 116–17; San Hipólito as colonial laboratory of, 6, 8–10, 12–13, 136–42, 146; San Hipólito as microcosm of, 8, 18–19, 51, 61, 79. *See also* Enlightenment; New Spain

historiographies, 6–7, 16–17
Holy Innocents, Feast of, 46
Holy Office. *See* Inquisition (Holy Office)
Holy Week, 33
Hospital de Colom (Barcelona), 30
Hospital de Convalecientes y Desamparados (Hospital of Convalescents and the Defenseless), 32. *See also* San Hipólito, Hospital de
Hospital de la Concepción de Nuestra Señora, 23–24, 29, 32, 33, 35
Hospital de la Santa Creu (Barcelona), 31
Hospital del Divino Salvador, 6, 10, 15, 109, 111–12, 164–65
Hospital de los Inocentes (Sevilla), 32, 200n79
Hospital de los Inocentes (Valencia), 30, 31, 42
Hospital de San Hipólito. *See* San Hipólito, Hospital de
Hospital de San Lázaro (hospital for lepers), 29, 39
Hospital de San Roque (Puebla), 52
hospitality (*hospitalidad*), 17, 24, 27–37, 49, 181; crisis in, 51–58
Hospital of Convalescents, 24. *See also* San Hipólito, Hospital de
Hospital Real y General de Nuestra Señora de Gracia (Zaragoza), 7, 32, 34, 42
hospitals: development of in New Spain, 24, 27–28; Islamic, 5, 30–31; proselytization function of, 28–29; as site of conflict between secular and sacred, 50. *See also specific hospitals*
humoral medicine, 31–32, 45, 68, 83, 88, 115, 119. *See also melancolia* (melancholy)
hygienic concerns, 43, 50, 68
hypochondria, 120–21, 170

Iberia: charity provision as tradition of, 5–6, 17; hospitals in, 3, 30–31, 33
Ilustración. See Hispanic Enlightenment
ilustrados (men of enlightened thinking), 11

immigrants, sheltered at San Hipólito, 34–35
Indies, 13–14; edicts for, 147
indigenous peoples: botany and pharmacy, 45; Chimalpopoca, trial of, 150–54; Christianization agenda for, 28–29; cost of care for, 36, 64; exempt from Inquisition, 205n14; and Inquisition, 85, 108; and insanity defense, 152; and insurgencies, 153, 175–76; *medio real de hospital* (tribute) paid by, 36; paternalism toward, 152–54; as patients, 38–39, 76, 77, *183–84*; pre-Hispanic lineages, 151; recent converts (*plantas nuevas*), 24; *república de indios* (Indian republic), 151. *See also* Royal Indian Hospital (Hospital Real de los Naturales)
indios (Indians), 38
Iniesta Bejarano, Idelfonso de (architect), 62, 203n69
Innocent XII, 53, 198n40
inocente, as term, 21
inocentes. See locos inocentes (feebleminded and harmless- persons)
Inquisition (Holy Office), 8, 10–11, 80–113, 211n68; archival materials, 15–16, 81; *audiencias* (formal hearings), 86; auto-da-fe (act of faith), 114, 117; *calificadores* (evaluators or consultants), 85, 91–92, 118; challenges of madness to, 84–92; changes in approach, 83–84; compromise verdicts, 96; crypto-Judaism persecuted by, 88; eighteenth-century worldview of, 142; as enemy of the Enlightenment, 84; *familiares* (functionaries), 122; familiarity with physicians, 121–22; feigned madness, concern about, 90–92, 95; fifteenth-century procedures adapted for eighteenth century, 12; heresy as fraction of cases, 85; Holy Office of 1571, 85; humane function of, 12, 112–13, 135; and indigenous peoples, 85, 105; interiority, focus on, 18–19,

Index 243

Inquisition (Holy Office) (*continued*)
82, 84, 86–93, 97, 112–13, 143; juxtaposition of tradition and innovation, 116–17; lenience shown by, 16, 82–83, 87, 89, 108, 111, 123; list of crimes prosecuted, 205n15; and medical expertise, 83, 87, 94, 116, 119, 123–24, 129, 133; medicalization, role in, 10–11, 16, 18–19, 83, 88–89, 112, 116, 142; offensive speech rendered nonsensical by, 92–97; pedagogy of fear, 134; physicians on staff, 90–91, 109, 121–22, 125, 133, 138, 142; and political heresy, 99; procedures of (*procesos*), 85–86; questioning of witnesses, 85, 87, 95–98; as rational conscious, 111; resurgence of after French Revolution, 112; San Hipólito as an outlet for confining and treating mad suspects, 89, 133–36; San Hipólito as colonial laboratory for, 136–42, 146; secret cells, 121, 132, 134, 138; sixteenth- and seventeenth-century, 88–89; state, connection with, 11–12, 84–85; stereotypes of, 11, 18, 82, 84–85, 86, 117, 205n9; *sumaria* (summary), 85, 150; and Tebanillo's sketches, 97–104; terminology used for madness, 21; and witchcraft accusations, 80–81; women's auto-denunciation, 105–11. *See also* Catholic Church

insania, 130

insanity defense, 10, 18–19, 84; appearance of in sixteenth century, 87–88; applied to formerly sane persons, 115; Catholic Church protected by, 92; medical models deployed by defendants, 129; and secular criminal courts, 152, 162–63; used by indigenous peoples, 152. *See also* madness (*locura*)

interiority, 18–19, 82, 84, 86–93, 112–13, 143; physicians' role in determining, 116–17; and speech acts, 93

Isabel of Castile, 27

Isla del Carmen, 143

Islamic hospitals, 5, 30–31
Iturbide, Agustín de, 177
Iturrigaray (Viceroy), 143

Jaffary, Nora, 104–5
Jesuits, 48, 52, 63
Jiménez, Don Miguel María (physician), 167
Jofré, Gilaberto, 30
judgment or reason (*juicio, razón*), 8, 10, 20–21, 38, 81, 83, 93–95, 108, 114; *entendimiento* (reasoning), 148, 152, 158; *juicio natural* (natural judgment), 128; *juicio trastornado* (disordered judgment), 132
jurisprudence: *arbitrio judicial*, 148–49; civil law codes, 87; colonial law (*derecho indiano*), 147; *derecho Castellano* (Castilian law), 148; *entendimiento* (reasoning), 148, 152; *Las Siete Partidas*, 87, 148; medieval laws, 19, 87, 147–48; Roman, 87, 147, 148; written doctrines (*derecho vulgar*), 147. *See also* criminal courts (*sala del crimen*)

Keitt, Andrew, 88
knowledge production, 6–10, 137. *See also* medicalization; medical knowledge and treatments
kuraka (local lord), 153

Labastida, Sebastián, 1–3
La Castañeda psychiatric facility, 2, 178, 180–81
Lardizábal y Uribe, 19, 145–47, 174, 212–13n13
Larrea, Francisco (inquisitor), 107–8
Las Siete Partidas, 87, 148
Lewis, Laura, 86
Libro de la vida del próximo evangelico (Díaz de Arce), 23–25
limpieza de sangre (purity of blood), 122, 151
Lipsett-Rivera, Sonya, 162
loco, as term, 20

locos furiosos (violently insane persons), 4–5, 21, 24, 35, 44–45, 68–69, 136; building damage by, 48; cages (*jaulas*) for, 44, 46, 65; criminals, 8, 18–19, 78–79; deaths at hands of, 59; indigenous people as, 150–54, 214n46; mania, 120, 139, 165–66; in secular criminal courts, 143, 148–49, 155–67

locos inocentes (feebleminded and harmless- persons), 21, 24, 34, 43–44, 46

locura, as term, 4. *See also* madness (*locura*)

Locura e Inquisición en Nueva España, 1571–1760 (Sacristán), 16

Locura y disidencia en el México ilustrado, 1760–1810 (Sacristán), 16

Lomarriba, Francisco (official), 157

Lope de Aguirre (El Loco), 13–14

López, Francisco (friar), 43

Los locos de Valencia (Lope de Vega), 4

lucid intervals (*intervals*), 21, 83, 123, 133, 139, 149

madness (*locura*): amorous passion (*locos de amores*), 163; categories, 30, 40, 76, 96, 122; as condition of poverty, 3, 31, 40, 75–76, 180; European treatment of, 1–2; feigned, 90–92, 95, 117–18, 123, 128, 135–36, 167–73; gendered forms of, 105–11, 161–62; as hereditary, 81–82, 120; inability to unspecify, 125–26; lucid intervals (intervals),21, 83, 123, 133, 139, 149; medicalization of, 10, 79–80, 83, 204–5n7; as part of life, 181; as physical condition, 3, 19; physicians' role in diagnosing, 122–26; and political subversion, 28, 30, 84, 99, 131, 150–52, 175, 213n35; sanity lost during confinement, 83, 114–15, 134–35, 137–38, 143, 156, 168; and social order, 3, 12, 18–19, 30, 38, 59–60, 95; terminology for, 20–22, 120. *See also* insanity defense; melancolia (melancholy)

Malleus Maleficarum, 108

mania, 120, 139, 165–66

marriage, 161–62, 215n85; bigamy, 127–31

Marroqui, José María, 37

Martínez, José (friar), 141–42

Martínez, Joseph (prior general), 168

Martínez, María Elena, 151

masculine culture, 129, 157

Maximilian and Charlotte, 179

Mayorga Martín de (viceroy), 144–45, 151

McMahon, Darrin, 84

Meave, Don Ambrosio (official), 63

medical discourse, 19, 207n65

medical expertise, 6, 16, 18–19, 87, 96–97, 180; and criminal courts, 167; and Inquisition, 83, 87, 94, 116, 119, 123–24, 129, 133; nurses, testimony of, 137–38. *See also* physicians; psychiatry

medicalization, 3, 114–42; and expansion of *pobre demente* category, 76; Inquisition's role in, 10–11, 16, 18–19, 83, 88–89, 112; in late eighteenth century, 15; limits to, 73, 125–26, 130, 132–33; physicians as witnesses of the mind and body, 117–21; and religious concerns, 19; San Hipólito as colonial laboratory, 6, 136–42

medical knowledge and treatments: cure of body and soul as dual function of, 42–43; cures sought for patients, 31–32, 60; Enlightenment advances in, 9–10; fevers thought to be cause of frenzy (*frenesi*), 41, 45, 120, 138; humoral medicine, 31–32, 45, 68, 83, 88, 115, 119; Iberian medical models, 45–47; indigenous botany and pharmacy, 45; lunar observations, 129; regimen (diet, rest, exercise), 45; "spiritual physic," 75; therapeutic capabilities, 73; traditional forms of healing, 54

medical turn, 119

medieval laws, 19, 87, 147–48

melancolía (melancholy), 45, 80, 84, 114–15, 126–33, 132, 206n31, 210n41; hypochondria, 120–21

Mellyn, Elizabeth, 20, 207n65, 210n41, 213n33
Mendoza, Diego (defendant), 95–96, 135
mental, as term, 20
mental disorder, 19–20; as inherited, 82
mental disorder/illness. *See* madness (*locura*)
mental hospital, as term, 22
merchants' guild (*consulado*), 50, 63, 64
metropole and periphery, 13, 50
Mexica Empire (Aztecs), 5, 17, 24
Mexican War of Independence, 2, 175–76
Mexico: erasure of from psychiatric origin story, 3–4; independence from Spain (1821), 1, 10, 20, 174; modernization campaign, 2. *See also* colonialism; New Spain; Spanish Empire
Mexico City: administrative and police districts (*cuartel* system), 144–45; *cabildo* (municipal council), 33, 162; disasters and epidemics, 17, 48, 54–55, 61, 62; financial crisis, 176; hospitals, 29–30; merchants' guild (*consulado*), 50, 63, 64; municipal government (*ayuntamiento*), 50, 58–63, 177; Poor House (Hospicio de Pobres), 62; regidor (governing counselor), 177; smaller hospitals in, 6; torrential rain, 48; urbanization, 54; welfare institutions, 2
Michoacan, 28
micro-history, 16
Midelfort, H. C. Erik, 20
miserables (wretched or unfortunate people), 29, 46, 76, 152
modernization: reforms under Bourbons, 13, 16, 18–19, 47, 48–50, 56–58, 61–62, 69, 144–45, 170–71; religious interest in, 60; remodeling and reopening of San Hipólito, 8, 17–18, 48–51, 79, 139, 144
monarchy, Spanish: as benevolent distributor of charity, 5, 29, 47; as divine and absolute authority, 11; French overthrow of, 19, 175, 179; power curbed by *córtes*, 19–20. *See also* Bourbon model; Habsburg model; state

monomania, 90
Montezuma, 24, 33
Montúfar, Alonso de, 24, 32
Moors, 29
moral hypervigilance, 106
moral treatment, 4, 112, 179–80
Morelos, José María (priest, insurgent), 175–76
Moreno y Jove, Maria Manuela (victim), 159–60
Muriel, Josefina, 65
mysticism, 88–90, 104–5; *alumbradismo* (illuminism), 119, 133; *alumbrados* (false mystics), 38, 104–5

nahualism, 108
Nalle, Sara T., 31
Napoleon, 19, 175
Navarro de Isla, Pedro (inquisitor), 127
negros (Blacks), 38, 76
New Christians, 88
New Spain, 1–6; decline of, 46–47, 170–74, 175–77; hospital development in, 24, 27–28; modern policing in, 144; population, 201n22; re-creation of Spanish societies in, 5; rural areas, 144, 153; Spanish institutional models adapted to, 25–27, 30–40, 46–47; two-tiered model of sociopolitical organization, 36, 38–39. *See also* Mexico
North Africa, hospitals in, 30
nurses, 8, 137; head nurse (*enfermero mayor*), 42, 43, 70, 78–79. *See also* Order of San Hipólito (*hipólitos*)

On Crime and Punishment (Beccaria), 146
Ordenanzas de pobladores (1753), 29
Order of San Hipólito (*hipólitos*), 8, 32, 198n40; abolishment of, 177; abolishment of, call for, 55–56; alms seeker (*hermano demandante*), 42, 44, 57; apothecary (*boticario*), 42, 45, 200n89; ascension in status, 1700, 53; brother in charge of congregations (*hermano general*), 43; chief brother (*hermano*

mayor), 42; complaints about lack of spiritual rigor and discipline, 17, 47, 52–56; decline in membership, 57, 202n40; disingenuous members, 53; dissolution of, 20; financial abuses alleged, 55; healing skills of brothers, 22; medical training, 58; novices, prohibition against admitting, 57, 59; nurses, 137; official bookkeeper (*procurador conventual*), 56–57; Peña as prior general of, 57–61; *recua* (system of transport), 34–35; reform efforts, 17, 48, 51; statutes, 40, 43, 199n68. *See also* San Hipólito, Hospital de

origin stories, 3–4, 17, 23–27, 26, 32
orphans (*huérfanos*), 78
Our Lady of Guadalupe, cult of, 54
Ovando, Nicolas de, 27

Palacio of the Inquisition, 178
passiones de animo (emotions), 118, 128–30
paternalism, 25; Habsburg model, 17, 27, 46, 147; leniency in sentencing, 19, 147, 152–54, 157–59
patients: admissions lists, 69–79, 71, 72, *183–91*; certificates of mental illness and letters of recommendation, 75–76, 80–81, 96; Communion required of, 43; criminally insane, 19, 60, 87, 149, 213n33; *criollos* as, 5, 38–40, 75–76; discharge notes, 73; of economic means, 37–38, 59; escapes and escape attempts, 12, 19, 73–74, 136, 140, 147, 154–55, 167–73; *estos infelices* (these unhappy ones), 49; families of, 36, 74, 87, 133, 216n115; foot washing of, 43; funding of own hospitalization, 37, 140; honorific titles, 40; indigenous people as, 38–39, 76, 77, *183–84*; mortality rate, 74; prisoners as, 78–79; slaves as, 36–38, 74; treatment measures, 43–44; turnover, 73–75; "unknown parentage," 78. *See also* women
Peña, José de la (friar, prior general), 57–61, 140

Peña y Brizuela, Juan Joseph de la (physician), 114–15
Peña y Brizuelas, Vicente de la (physician), 139
Peters, Edward, 12
Philo, Chris, 8
philosophes, 9–10, 112
physical coercion and restraints (*prisiones*), 1–2, 21, 30–31, 42–44; cages (*jaulas*), 35, 44, 46, 64–65; shackles (*grillos*), 156; special chamber (*aposento*), 44
physicians, 199n78, 200n79; certificates of mental illness written by, 75; decentered in Spanish American colonial setting, 6; as *familiares* (functionaries), 122; Inquisition's familiarity with, 121–22; as key witnesses, 116; legitimacy of, 119, 122; limits on medical expertise of, 125–26, 130, 132–33; medical training, 119–20; as peripheral, 6, 10, 14–15, 21–22, 116, 200n79; and professionalization, 2, 15, 50, 58, 120; role in diagnosing *locura*, 122–26; technical terminology used by, 120; tensions with *hipólitos*, 140, 142; university-trained, 6, 10, 43, 79, 116, 119, 122; as witnesses of the mind and body, 117–21. *See also* medical expertise
Pichardo, Antonio (priest), 109–11
piedad ilustrada (enlightened piety), 9
Pinel, Philippe, 2, 4, 7, 112, 179
pobres dementes (poor mad people), 4; as flexible category, 40, 76, 96; *locos inocentes*, 21, 24, 34, 43–44, 46; *locos inocentes* (feebleminded and harmless-persons), 21, 24, 34, 43–44, 46; at San Hipólito, 5, 33. *See also locos furiosos* (violently insane persons); madness (*locura*)
pobres inocentes y faltos de juico (feebleminded poor and those without judgment), 43
policía (rational order), 9, 145
policing: administrative and police districts (*cuartel* system), 144–45; reformers, 145–47

political subversion, 28, 30, 84, 99, 131–33, 150–54, 175, 213n35; revolutionary activity and thought, policing of, 11–12, 99, 112, 131–32, 141, 144
Poor House (Hospicio de Pobres), 62, 110, 203n59
Porfiriato, 2, 83, 178, 180
possession, spiritual, 21, 37], 82, 88–90, [206nn31
poverty, 3, 31, 40, 62, 75–76, 180
prisons, public, 172–73
professionalization, 2, 15, 50, 58, 120
Protestantism, 87, 112
Protomedicato, tribunal of, 30
psychiatry, 3–4, 112, 178, 179–80. See also medicalization
psychosomatic forms of spirituality, 88
public good (*beneficio común*), 59
public happiness (*felicidad pública*), 9, 50
public health (*salud pública*), 9, 48–49
Puebla de los Ángeles (city), 6
punishments, 209n2, 212–13n13; auto-da-fé (act of faith), 114, 117; confession and penance, 102; Havana, transportation to, 139, 171; shame, 114; torture, 90, 93, 121

Quaestiones medico-legales (Zacchia), 117–18

race-caste system (*sistema de castas*), 5, 38–40; and architecture, 65; *cambujo*, 207n52; *castas* (mixed-blood *mestizos, mulatos,* and *moriscos*), 38–39, 76; *castizas*, 162; *gente baja* (underclass), 145; in hospital work designations, 42; and Inquisition, 108; *ladino* (Hispanicized Indian), 169; *limpieza de sangre* (purity of blood), 122, 151; and marriage, 161–62, 215n85; and patient treatment, 59; women's role in upholding, 159, 165
Rada, Francisco (physician for Inquisition), 125–26, 139, 142, 153–54
Ramos, Gabriela, 38

rationalism, 18–19, 58, 61, 70, 84, 117, 125, 146–47; models of madness, 10, 116, 120, 123
Real Audiencia, 176
real cédula (1596), 37
Real Sala del Crimen, 169
reason. *See* judgment or reason (*juicio, razón*)
recogimiento/casas de recogimiento, 111–12
reconquista (reconquest), 29
Recopilación de leyes de los reinos de las Indias, 148
recua (system of transport), 34–35
Reformation, 11, 87
rehabilitation, 145
Renzi, Silvia de, 119
republic of Indians (*república de indios*), 36, 151
republic of Spaniards (*república de españoles*), 36, 151
Revillagigedo, Viceroy, 69, 145
revolutionary activity and thought, policing of, 11–12, 99, 112, 131–32, 141, 144
riña (superficial fight), 157
Robles, José Antonio, 157
Rodriguez, Lorenzo (architect), 62, 203n69
Rodriguez Moreno, Nicolas (royal secretary), 54
Roman jurisprudence, 87, 147, 148
Royal and Pontifical University of Mexico, 30
Royal Indian Hospital (Hospital Real de los Naturales), 30, 35, 36, 54, 64, 176, 203n69, 216–17n8; records of patients at San Hipólito, 76, 183–84
Ruiz, Felipe (friar, head nurse), 70, 95, 138

Sabuco, Olivia, 209n5
Sacristán, María Cristina, 15–16
Salpêtrière hospital (Paris, France), 4, 112
San Hipólito, Church of, 5–6, 32, 33, 67
San Hipólito, Hospital de: 1601 viceregal mandate, 37, 61; account books, 15, 36, 40, 45–46; adaptation of Old World

antecedents by, 12, 17, 27, 30, 32, 46–47; as alternative to prisons, 60; as an outlet for confining and treating mad suspects, 89, 133–36; archival record, 15–16, 34–36, 40–42, 45–46; *asesorías* (offices), 67–68; charitable and practical services provided by, 33–34; as colonial laboratory of Hispanic Enlightenment, 6, 8–10, 12–13, 136–42, 146; as convalescent hospital, 5, 17, 30, 32, 37, 46; *criollos* as patients in, 5, 38–40, 75–76; crisis in hospitality, 51–58; cure of body and soul as dual function of, 42–43; as custodial space, 143–74; damage to, 48–49, 61, 62; decline of, 1, 17, 47, 48–49, 51–56, 59, 173–74, 176–79; as eclectic mix, 146–47; economic syndicate, 58, 61, 203n54; and evasion of law by patients, 167–68; finances, 17, 33, 35–36, 49–65, 69, 176–78; funding strategies for, 57–61, 63–64; governing board, 61; ground plan, 40–42, 41, 65–68, 66, 67, 199n69, 203n69; heterogeneity of occupants, 34–35, 38–40, 39, 47; hospital life, 27, 40–47; immigrants sheltered at, 34–35; Labastida's comments on, 1–3; as limited tool of colonial governance, 17, 27, 40, 46; list of criminal inmates, 185–91; location of, 32–33, 180–81; as microcosm of Hispanic Enlightenment, 8, 18–19, 51, 61, 79; modeled on Spanish antecedents, 26–27; origin story, 3–4, 17, 23–27, 26, 32; physical coercion and restraints, 21, 31, 43, 44, 46, 65, 156; physicians as peripheral at, 6, 10, 21–22, 200n79; as prison of last resort, 155–59; private cells, 48, 65, 66, 67; remodeling and reopening of, 8, 17–18, 48–51, 61–69, 66, 67, 79, 139, 144; slaves at, 36–37, 38; social history of, 6–7, 14; social order preserved by confinements, 19, 30, 38; Spanish Crown, role in, 37–38; state, dependence on, 173; statutes, 36, 40–44, 198n47; sugar plantations owned by, 37; transition from to psychiatry, 178–79; treatment measures at, 43–45; utilitarian mission of, 17–18, 47, 51, 74, 144–45. *See also* hospitality (*hospitalidad*); Order of San Hipólito (*hipólitos*)

sanity: lost while detained, 83, 114–15, 134–35, 137–38, 143, 156, 168; restored in confinement, 60, 164, 171–72; as slippery spectrum, 83

San Juan de Ulua, port of, 34

San Pedro, Hospital de, 6

San Roque hospital, 6

Scardaville, Michael, 145, 147

secularism, rise of, 51–53. *See also* criminal courts (*sala del crimen*); modernization

Seed, Patricia, 33

Shuger, Dale, 87, 96

Sierra, Felipe (convict, patient), 168–69

Silva, José de (defendant, patient), 114–17, 134, 138–39, 212n84

Silverblatt, Irene, 11, 85

sin, 86–87, 93; conscious will as precondition for, 87; as illness, 121; as voluntary, 83, 102, 107; women's requests for pardon, 105–7

slaves, 36–38, 42, 74

Sluhovsky, Moshe, 88

social Darwinism, 180

social engineering, 13, 145

social order, 3, 12, 18–19, 59–60, 95; preserved by confinements, 19, 30, 38

Solórzano Pereira, Juan de, 152

Spain: "black legend" (*leyenda negra*), 11, 84–85; cordon sanitaire, 99; *córtes* parliament), 19–20, 177; medieval, 83; *reconquista* (reconquest), 29; revolutionary era, 7; universities, 14

Spanish Empire, 5, 9, 17, 50, 56, 89, 155; collapse of, 19–20; institutional models adapted to New World, 12, 17, 27, 30, 32, 46–47; reorganization of under Charles III and IV, 58

speech acts: blasphemy, 93–94, 106; offensive, 92–97; personal confession, 93

spiritual counseling, 6
state: centralization, 3, 7–8, 13, 18, 52, 58, 170; expansion, logic of, 58; impotence exposed by escapes and escape attempts, 147, 168; and Inquisition, 11–12, 85; intersection of church, state, and society, 51. *See also* Bourbon model; colonialism; Habsburg model; monarchy, Spanish
St. Luke's Hospital (London), 2
Stoler, Ann, 195n38
sugar plantations, 37

tabla de carniceria (a tax on the butchering of cattle), 61, 63
Tebanillo (José Ventura Gonzalez), 97–104, 100–105
Tehuantepec, isthmus of, 153
Tello de Meneses, Francisco Xavier (physician), 165–67
templos de piedad (temples of piety and compassion), 28
temporalidades (Jesuit assets), 63
teniente provincial (provincial deputy), 171
Tenochtitlán (city), 5, 17, 24, 33
Teotihuacan (village), 155
Tesoro de la lengua castellana, o española (Covarrubias Orozco), 21
Toribio, Jose (physician), 106–7
Torres, María Getrudis (defendant, patient), 159–67, 160, 168
Tortorici, Zeb, 16, 101
torture, 90, 93, 121, 134
Triano, José Ruiz (physician), 132–33
Tribunal of the Acordada, 79, 144, 171
Tupac Amaru II, 153

universities, New Spain, 30
utility, language of, 51, 59–60, 144–47, 153, 166, 173

Valley of Mexico, 28
van Deusen, Nancy, 111

Vasquez, José (physician), 164
Vega, Juan de la (defendant, patient), 94–96, 137
Venegas, Juan Manuel, 120, 124
Viera, Juan de (priest), 48, 65, 68–69
Villaroel, Hipólito (lawyer), 144
Vizarrón y Eguiarreta, Juan Antonio, 52–53, 55–57
Voekel, Pamela, 145
Voltaire ("Wolter"), 9, 11, 131, 141

Warren, Adam, 50, 58
watchmen (guardafaroles),145
witchcraft (*hechicería*), 80–81, 85, 89
witnesses: and Inquisition, 85, 87, 94–98, 101, 117–21; *lo vido ocularmente* ("I saw it ocularly"), 101; unreliable, 121, 124, 141. *See also* medical expertise; physicians
"Wolter" (Voltaire), 9, 141
women, 44, 215n84; auto-denunciation and pathology, 105–11; confined in *casas de recogimiento*, 111–12; madness of as arising from body, 104; and magic rituals, 99; and marriage, 161–62; poor mad women (*pobres mujeres dementes*), 6, 10, 15, 41–42; religious, madness attributed to, 89; and secular criminal courts, 159–67; "uterine fury" attributed to, 21, 109

Yard with Lunatics (Goya), 7
York Retreat (London), 2

Zacchia, Paolo (physician and jurist), 117–18, 209n12
Zaragoza hospital (Spain), 7, 32, 34, 42
Zarate, Felipe (defendant, patient), 124–26, 132, 135
Zetina, Pedro José (defendant, patient), 143
Zuniga, Juan Jose de (physician), 128–31

www.ingramcontent.com/pod-product-compliance
Lightning Source LLC
Chambersburg PA
CBHW020602251125
35938CB00022B/473